Student Workbook for

Modern Dental Assisting

Student Workbook for

Modern Dental Assisting

Eleventh Edition

Doni L. Bird, CDA, RDA, RDH, MA
Director of Allied Dental Education
Santa Rosa Junior College
Santa Rosa, California

Debbie S. Robinson, CDA, MS
Research Assistant Professor and Research Study Coordinator
University of North Carolina
Chapel Hill, North Carolina

SAUNDERS

3251 Riverport Lane
St. Louis, Missouri 63043

STUDENT WORKBOOK FOR MODERN DENTAL ASSISTING   ISBN: 978-1-4557-7454-8

Notices

ISBN: 978-1-4557-7454-8

Vice President and Publisher: Linda Duncan
Content Strategist: Kristin Wilhelm
Senior Content Development Specialist: Courtney L. Sprehe
Manuscript Development: Sarah Vora
Publishing Services Manager: Hemamalini Rajendrababu
Project Manager: Anitha Sivaraj
Cover Designer: Gopalakrishnan Venkatram

Printed in the United States of America

Last digit is the print number: 9 8 7 6 5 4 3 2 1

Contents

Introduction

This student workbook is designed to help you prepare for and master the preclinical, clinical, and administrative procedures presented in *Modern Dental Assisting,* Eleventh Edition. It is designed so that the pages can be easily removed, submitted if required, and placed in your notebook with the corresponding lecture notes. Workbook chapters correspond directly to chapters in the textbook, and each contains questions and exercises designed to help you practice, comprehend, and master the chapter content.

CHAPTER EXERCISES

Chapters include a variety of exercises, such as short-answer questions, which are taken from the chapter's learning outcomes; fill-in-the-blank statements that stem from the key terms of the chapter; multiple-choice questions that parallel the recall questions in the chapter; and case studies and activities that tie in the chapter topics and use knowledge from other chapters and the *Interactive Dental Office,* which is hosted on the companion Evolve website. You will also find recommended video clips listed at the end of applicable chapters to watch on the accompanying Evolve site.

The chapter exercises are intended to help you study and better understand the information presented in the corresponding chapter of the textbook. Please take the time to work through them carefully. Answers to the workbook exercises are available through your instructor.

In addition, we are thrilled to introduce Dentrix software to the MDA Workbook for this edition. The importance of a student's comprehension of a dental software system is imperative. The student will be introduced to both the business and clinical areas of dentistry. A DVD is included with this workbook, and the instructions on how to download the software can be found on the Evolve website. Chapters 26, 28, 62, and 63 provide practice exercises on how to use the system, along with additional exercises that incorporate the patients from the Interactive Dental Office.

COMPETENCY SHEETS

A competency is a system that is used to evaluate mastery of preclinical, clinical, administrative, and advanced skills. The competency sheets included within this workbook are designed to give you the opportunity to practice a skill until mastering it. A space on the form allows for three different evaluations: self, peer, and instructor and/or dentist. The evaluation system has been enhanced to provide an objective grading scale. This truly reflects a step-by-step competency of each procedure at all levels. A space for reviewer comments is available, along with an area for documentation of evaluation, date, and grade.

For each procedure in the textbook, a competency sheet is included at the end of the corresponding workbook chapter. Each competency sheet appears individually so that you can submit each one as it is completed to your instructor or supervisor if necessary.

FLASHCARDS

Flashcards are made up of key information from the textbook and include information on the sciences, medical emergencies, infection control, radiography, dental materials, instruments, and dental procedures and specialties. The flashcards in the back of this workbook are easily removed from the workbook to become a bonus study tool.

We wish you much success in your studies and your chosen profession of dental assisting!

Doni L. Bird
Debbie S. Robinson

1 History of Dentistry

SHORT-ANSWER QUESTIONS

1. Describe the role of Hippocrates in history.

2. State the basic premise of the Hippocratic Oath.

3. Name the first woman to graduate from a college of dentistry.

4. Name the first woman to practice dentistry in the United States.

5. Name the first African American woman to receive a dental degree in the United States.

6. Name the first African American to receive the DMD degree from Harvard University.

7. Discuss the contributions of Horace H. Hayden and Chapin A. Harris.

8. Describe two major contributions of G.V. Black.

9. Name the first dentist to employ a dental assistant.

10. Name the first female dental assistant.

11. Name the scientist who discovered radiographs.

12. Name the physician who first used nitrous oxide for tooth extractions.

13. Discuss the purpose and activities of the National Museum of Dentistry.

FILL-IN-THE-BLANK STATEMENTS

Select the best term from the list below and complete the following statements.

Commission on Dental Accreditation of the American Dental Association
forensic dentistry
Ida Gray-Rollins
Irene Newman
periodontal disease
preceptorship
Wilhelm Conrad Roentgen

1. _____ was the first dental hygienist.

2. To study under the guidance of one already in the profession is a _____.

3. _____ establishes the identity of an individual on the basis of dental records alone.

4. _____ is a disease of the structures that support the teeth (gums and bone).

5. The _____ accredits dental, dental assisting, dental hygiene, and dental laboratory educational programs.

6. _____ discovered radiographs.

7. _____ was the first African American woman in the United States to earn a formal DDS degree.

MULTIPLE-CHOICE QUESTIONS

Complete each question by circling the best answer.

1. Hesi-Re was _____.
   a. the first female dentist
   b. the earliest recorded dentist
   c. the first dental assistant
   d. the first dental hygienist

2. How long has dental disease existed?
   a. Since the nineteenth century
   b. Since the eighteenth century
   c. Since mankind began
   d. Since the Stone Age

3. Who is referred to as the Father of Medicine?
   a. Hippocrates
   b. G.V. Black
   c. Pierre Fauchard
   d. Paul Revere

4. What does the Hippocratic Oath promise?
   a. To heal all
   b. To treat dental problems in patients of all ages
   c. To act ethically
   d. To include dentistry in medicine

5. What type of dentistry did the Romans provide?
   a. Oral hygiene
   b. Gold crowns
   c. Tooth extraction
   d. All of the above

6. What artist first distinguished molars and premolars?
   a. Claude Monet
   b. Leonardo da Vinci
   c. Vincent van Gogh
   d. Peter Max

7. Who is referred to as the *Father of Modern Surgery?*
   a. Ambroise Paré
   b. Hippocrates
   c. G.V. Black
   d. Pierre Fauchard

8. Who is referred to as the *Father of Modern Dentistry?*
   a. Ambroise Paré
   b. Hippocrates
   c. G.V. Black
   d. Pierre Fauchard

9. Who was John Baker's famous patient?
   a. Paul Revere
   b. George Washington
   c. Leonardo da Vinci
   d. Hippocrates

10. What famous colonial patriot first used forensic evidence?
   a. Paul Revere
   b. George Washington
   c. Abraham Lincoln
   d. Betsy Ross

11. Who was one of the first dentists to travel throughout the colonies?
   a. Paul Revere
   b. George Washington
   c. Abraham Lincoln
   d. Robert Woofendale

12. Who is credited with founding the first dental school in America?
   a. Chapin Harris
   b. Horace Wells
   c. G.V. Black
   d. Edmund Kells

13. Who is referred to as the *Grand Old Man of Dentistry?*
   a. Chapin Harris
   b. Horace Wells
   c. G.V. Black
   d. Edmund Kells

14. Who is credited with employing the first dental assistant?
   a. Chapin Harris
   b. Horace Wells
   c. G.V. Black
   d. Edmund Kells

15. Who was the first dentist to use nitrous oxide in dentistry?
   a. Chapin Harris
   b. Horace Wells
   c. G.V. Black
   d. Edmund Kells

16. Who was the first female dentist in the United States?
   a. Emeline Roberts-Jones
   b. Lucy Beaman Hobbs
   c. G.V. Black
   d. W.B. Saunders

17. Who was the first woman to graduate from dental school?
   a. Emeline Roberts-Jones
   b. Lucy Beaman Hobbs
   c. G.V. Black
   d. W.B. Saunders

18. Where is the National Museum of Dentistry located?
   a. New Orleans, Louisiana
   b. San Francisco, California
   c. Baltimore, Maryland
   d. Seattle, Washington

19. In what year was the first edition of *Modern Dental Assisting* published?
   a. 1982
   b. 1973
   c. 1976
   d. 1981

20. African Americans were first accepted for education in dental schools in what year?
   a. 1867
   b. 1900
   c. 1928
   d. 1865

ACTIVITY

The practice of dentistry has changed dramatically over the past 50 years. To compare the dental experiences of various generations, ask the following questions to one or two people in each of the following age groups: 3 to 10, 11 to 30, 31 to 54, and 55 and older. Compare and analyze their answers to see how dentistry and people's perceptions about dentistry have changed.

Questions to Ask

1. How do you feel about going to the dentist?

2. Do you expect to keep all of your teeth throughout your life? Why or why not?

3. How do you think the practice of dentistry has changed during your life?

4. Are you afraid of going to the dentist? Why or why not?

5. What are your feelings about the profession of dentistry?

2 The Professional Dental Assistant

SHORT-ANSWER QUESTIONS

1. How is being a professional different from having a job?

2. Describe the characteristics of a professional dental assistant.

3. Describe the personal qualities of a dental assistant.

4. Describe how your personal characteristics meet the qualities of a good dental assistant.

5. Identify career opportunities for the educationally qualified dental assistant.

6. Describe the role and purpose of the American Dental Assistants Association.

7. Describe the benefits of membership in the American Dental Assistants Association.

8. Describe the role of the Dental Assisting National Board.

9. Identify the purpose of the Health Insurance Portability and Accountability Act of 1996 (HIPAA).

FILL-IN-THE-BLANK STATEMENTS

Select the best term from the list below and complete the following statements.

American Dental Assistants Association
Certified Dental Assistant
Dental Assisting National Board
HIPAA

1. The professional organization that represents the profession of dental assisting is the _____.

2. The national agency that is responsible for administering the certification examination and issuing certification is the

_____.

3. The credential of an individual who has passed the certification examination and remains current through continuing education is _____.

4. The _____ specifies federal regulations ensuring privacy regarding a patient's healthcare information.

MULTIPLE-CHOICE QUESTIONS

Complete each question by circling the best answer.

1. The essentials of professional appearance are _____.
   a. good health
   b. good grooming
   c. appropriate dress
   d. all of the above

2. How does one demonstrate responsibility?
   a. Arriving on time
   b. Volunteering to help
   c. Showing initiative
   d. All of the above

3. What is the purpose of the ADAA?
   a. To advance the careers of dental assistants
   b. To promote the dental assisting profession
   c. To enhance the delivery of high-quality dental healthcare
   d. All of the above

4. What credential is issued by the DANB?
   a. Registered dental assistant
   b. Certified dental assistant
   c. Licensed dental assistant
   d. Bachelor's degree

5. What is considered confidential information in the dental office?
   a. Financial information only
   b. Treatment information only
   c. Written records only
   d. Everything that is said and done in the dental office

6. HIPAA regulations are designed to protect the patient's _____.
   a. finances
   b. healthcare information
   c. family
   d. employer

ACTIVITIES

1. Go to *Certified Press*, the Dental Assisting National Board's quarterly newsletter, found at http://www.danb.org/About-DANB/News-and-Events/Certified-Press-Newsletter. Review specific topics that are presented for your profession, and give your opinion regarding any new changes.

2. Engage your classmates in a discussion of the personal and professional characteristics they think would be desirable and nondesirable in a dental assistant. Explain why each of the desirable characteristics is important.

3. In the dental office in which you are the patient, what characteristics of the dental assistant impress you the most?

3 The Dental Healthcare Team

1. Identify the members of the dental healthcare team, and explain the role of each in a dental practice.

2. Describe the minimal educational requirements for each dental healthcare team member.

3. Describe the supportive services provided by non–team members.

4. Name and describe each recognized dental specialty.

FILL-IN-THE-BLANK STATEMENTS

Select the best term from the list below and complete the following statements.

dental assistant
dental hygienist
dental laboratory technician
dental public health
dentist
endodontist
oral and maxillofacial radiology

oral and maxillofacial surgery
oral pathology
orthodontics
pediatric dentistry
periodontics
prosthodontics

1. An individual who is trained to provide support to the dentist is a(n) _____.

2. The specialty concerned with the diagnosis and treatment of the supporting structures is _____.

3. The specialty concerned with the diagnosis of disease through various forms of imaging, including radiographs, is _____.

4. A(n) _____ is a legally qualified practitioner of dentistry.

5. An individual who performs technical services specified by a written prescription from the dentist is a(n) _____.

6. A(n) _____ is a licensed auxiliary who provides preventive, therapeutic, and educational services.

7. The specialty of promoting dental health through organized community efforts is _____.

8. _____ is the specialty that is concerned with diseases of the oral structures.

9. A(n) _____ is a dentist who specializes in diseases of the pulp.

10. _____ is the specialty of surgery of the head and neck.

11. _____ is the specialty that is concerned with the correction of malocclusions.

12. _____ is the specialty that is concerned with the restoration and replacement of natural teeth.

13. _____ is the area of dentistry that specializes in children from birth through adolescence.

MULTIPLE-CHOICE QUESTIONS

Complete each question by circling the best answer.

1. Who would not be considered a member of the dental healthcare team?
   a. Dental hygienist
   b. Dental supply person
   c. Dental laboratory technician
   d. Dental assistant

2. What is the minimal length of education for dental hygiene licensure?
   a. 1 academic year
   b. 2 academic years
   c. 3 academic years
   d. 4 academic years

3. What is the minimal length of education for an ADA-accredited dental-assisting program?
   a. 1 academic year
   b. 2 academic years
   c. 3 academic years
   d. 4 academic years

4. What is the minimal length for an ADA-accredited dental laboratory technician program?
   a. 1 academic year
   b. 2 academic years
   c. 3 academic years
   d. 4 academic years

5. What must a dental laboratory technician have in hand before he or she can perform and deliver an indirect restoration or prosthesis?
   a. The patient record
   b. A letter from the dentist
   c. A prescription from the dentist
   d. A drawing of the indirect restoration or prosthesis

ACTIVITY

As a dental-assisting student, you are embarking on an exciting career with many opportunities awaiting you after graduation. It is not too early to think about the career choices you will make. After reading this chapter, answer the following questions to help you formulate long-term career goals.

1. Which of the dental specialties appeals to you as a dental assistant the most? Why?

2. Are you interested in continuing your education to become a dentist or dental specialist? Which specialty and why?

3. Are you more interested in the clinical aspect of dental assisting than in the business office? Why or why not?

4. What attracted you to select dental assisting as a career choice?

5. Would you like to become an expanded function dental assistant? Why or why not?

4 Dental Ethics

SHORT-ANSWER QUESTIONS

1. Explain the basic principles of ethics.

2. Discuss the Code of Ethics of the American Dental Assistants Association.

3. Explain the difference between being "legal" and being "ethical."

4. Identify sources of early learning of ethics.

5. Describe the model for ethical decision making.

6. Give examples of ethical and unethical personal behaviors.

FILL-IN-THE-BLANK STATEMENTS

Select the best term from the list below and complete the following statements.

autonomy
code of ethics
ethics
laws
nonmaleficence

1. _____ are minimal standards of behavior established by statutes.

2. Voluntary standards of behavior established by a profession are a(n) _____.

3. _____ is self-determination.

4. _____ are moral standards of conduct and rules or principles that govern proper conduct.

5. _____ is to do no harm to the patient.

MULTIPLE-CHOICE QUESTIONS

Complete each question by circling the best answer.

1. A basic principle of ethics is _____.
   a. autonomy
   b. justice
   c. nonmaleficence
   d. all of the above

2. What is established as a guide to professional behavior?
   a. Code of conduct
   b. Code of ethics
   c. Code of honor
   d. Code of medicine

3. Ethics are _____.
   a. required by law
   b. open to individual interpretation
   c. settled by court decisions
   d. clear and direct

4. What does the ethical principle of nonmaleficence mean?
   a. The right of privacy
   b. To help others
   c. To treat people fairly
   d. To do no harm

ACTIVITIES

1. Aside from the examples in your textbook, provide an example for each ethical principle, and describe how each example could relate to a situation in your dental-assisting class.
   - Principle of justice
   - Principle of autonomy
   - Principle of well-being
   - Principle of doing no harm

2. Working in small groups, classmates should develop a code of ethics for your dental-assisting class. When the groups have decided on the issues to be included, the entire class should discuss them and agree to abide by the Code of Ethics for the dental assisting class. Do you think this would be a positive experience? Why or why not?

5 Dentistry and the Law

SHORT-ANSWER QUESTIONS

1. Explain the purpose of the state Dental Practice Act.

2. Explain the purpose of licensing dental healthcare professionals.

3. Describe the types of dental auxiliary supervision.

4. Give an example of circumstances that could be considered as patient abandonment.

5. Give an example of the principle of contributory negligence in a dental practice.

6. Give an example of civil law and an example of criminal law.

7. Describe ways to prevent malpractice lawsuits.

8. Describe the difference between written and implied consent.

9. Describe the procedure for obtaining consent for minor patients.

10. Describe the procedure for documenting informed consent.

11. Explain when it is necessary to obtain an informed refusal.

12. Describe the exceptions for disclosure.

13. Give an example of *respondeat superior*.

14. Give an example of *res gestae*.

15. Discuss the indications of child abuse and neglect.

FILL-IN-THE-BLANK STATEMENTS

Select the best term from the list below and complete the following statements.

abandonment
Board of Dentistry
civil law
contract law
criminal law
dental auxiliary
direct supervision
due care
expanded function
expressed contract
general supervision
implied consent

implied contract
licensure
malpractice
mandated reporter
patient of record
reciprocity
res gestae
res ipsa loquitur
respondeat superior
state Dental Practice Act
written consent

1. A(n) _____ can be a dental assistant, a dental hygienist, or a dental laboratory technician.

2. A(n) _____ is an individual who has been examined and diagnosed by the dentist and has had the treatment planned.

3. _____ is a level of supervision in which the dentist is physically present when expanded functions are being performed by the dental auxiliary.

4. A(n) _____ is a specific intraoral function delegated to an auxiliary that requires increased skill and training.

5. _____ is a legal doctrine that holds the employer liable for the acts of the employee.

6. The _____ specifies the legal requirements for an individual to practice dentistry in the state.

7. _____ is an agency that adopts rules and regulations and implements the state Dental Practice Act.

8. _____ gives a person the legal right to practice in a specific state.

9. _____ is the category of law that deals with the relations of individuals or corporations.

10. _____ is a system that allows individuals in one state to obtain a license in another state without retesting.

11. Terminating the dentist-patient relationship without reasonable notice to the patient is _____.

12. _____ is just, proper, and sufficient care or the absence of negligence.

13. _____ deals with a violation against the state or government.

14. _____ is a level of supervision in which the dentist has given instructions but need not be physically present at the time the expanded functions are being performed by the dental auxiliary.

14

15. _____ is a means of professional negligence.

16. _____ is the patient's action indicating consent for treatment.

17. Binding agreements involve _____.

18. A contract that may be verbal or written is a(n) _____.

19. A contract that is established by actions and not words is a(n) _____.

20. _____ involves a written explanation of the diagnostic findings, the prescribed treatment, and the reasonable expectations regarding the results of treatment.

21. _____ is a statement that is made at the time of an alleged negligent act and is admissible as evidence in a court of law.

22. A(n) _____ is a professional who is required by state law to report known or suspected child abuse.

23. _____ means that the act speaks for itself.

MULTIPLE-CHOICE QUESTIONS

Complete each question by circling the best answer.

1. The purpose of being licensed is _____.
   a. to make more money
   b. to protect the public from incompetent practitioners
   c. to keep count of the number of professionals in the field
   d. to have laws to follow

2. Who interprets the state Dental Practice Act?
   a. The governor of the state
   b. The American Dental Association
   c. The state legislature
   d. The Board of Dentistry

3. Reciprocity allows a licensed practitioner to _____.
   a. treat patients from another practice
   b. prescribe drugs
   c. practice in another state
   d. specialize in a field of dentistry

4. *Respondeat superior* states that _____.
   a. a patient can be seen by another dentist without records
   b. an employer is responsible for the actions of his or her employees
   c. a dentist can treat patients in another state
   d. a dentist can specialize and practice that specialty

5. If a dentist is physically present when a dental auxiliary is performing an expanded function, the dentist is providing _____.
   a. direct supervision
   b. physical supervision
   c. general supervision
   d. legal supervision

6. When a dentist discontinues treatment after it has begun, the dentist has performed _____.
   a. a felony
   b. abuse
   c. abandonment
   d. a disservice

7. When can a dentist refuse to treat a patient with HIV infection?
   a. When the staff does not want to treat patients with HIV infection
   b. Under no conditions
   c. When the patient has a dental condition that would be better treated by a specialist
   d. All of the above

8. When a patient receives proper sufficient care, he or she is receiving _____.
   a. poor care
   b. due care
   c. professional care
   d. dental care

9. A category of law is _____.
   a. civil
   b. professional
   c. contract
   d. a and c

10. What are types of contracts?
    a. Professional
    b. Expressed
    c. Implied
    d. b and c

11. How can a professional prevent a malpractice suit?
    a. Have the patient sign a form.
    b. Practice prevention and communication with the patient.
    c. Have a lawyer meet with the patient.
    d. Carry out scheduling and documenting.

12. Which of the following components are necessary for a successful malpractice suit?
    a. Duty to the patient
    b. Dereliction in treatment
    c. Direct cause
    d. All of the above

13. What is the term for a statement that is made at the time of an alleged negligent act and is admissible as evidence in a court of law?
    a. *res ipsa loquitur*
    b. *res gestae*
    c. pro bono
    d. due care

14. The actions of a patient demonstrate _____.
    a. implied consent
    b. verbal consent
    c. written consent
    d. legal consent

15. Where should a broken appointment be recorded?
    a. On a daily schedule
    b. On a ledger
    c. On a patient record
    d. On a recall list

16. What is the purpose of reporting a suspected case of child abuse?
    a. To start legal proceedings
    b. To have documentation
    c. To protect the child from further abuse
    d. To punish the abuser

17. Who are "mandated reporters"?
    a. Professionals required by state law to report known or suspected cases of child abuse
    b. Reporters from a newspaper following a story
    c. Individuals elected to give advice
    d. Written documents on known or suspected cases of child abuse

ACTIVITIES

1. Obtain a copy of your state Dental Practice Act, and review the regulations that are important for dental assistants.

2. Make a list of the functions delegated to the dental assistant, and identify the types of supervision necessary for each delegated function.

3. Describe the practice limitations for a dental assistant in your state.

6 General Anatomy

1. Define and pronounce each of the key terms in this chapter.

2. Explain the difference between anatomy and physiology.

3. Describe the imaginary planes and associated body directions used to divide the body into sections.

4. Name the four levels of organization in the human body.

5. Identify and describe the components of a cell.

6. Identify and describe the four types of tissue in the human body.

7. Name and locate the two major body cavities.

8. Name and locate the regions of the body.

9. Identify the types of stem cells.

FILL-IN-THE-BLANK STATEMENTS

Select the best term from the list below and complete the following statements.

anatomic position	distal	parietal
anatomy	epithelial	physiology
anterior	horizontal plane	proximal
appendicular	medial	stem cells
axial	midsagittal plane	superior
cranial cavity	nucleus	visceral
cytoplasm	organelle	

1. ___anatomy___ is the study of the shape and structure of the human body.

2. ___physiology___ is the study of the functions of the human body.

3. The body is in the ___anatomic position___ when it is erect and facing forward with the arms at the sides and the palms facing up.

4. The ___midsagittal___ is a vertical plane that divides the body into equal left and right halves.

5. The ___horizontal___ divides the body into superior (upper) and inferior (lower) portions.

6. The gel-like fluid inside the cell is ___cytoplasm___.

7. A specialized part of the cell that performs a definite function is the ___organelle___.

8. The center of a cell is the ___nucleus___.

9. The ___cranial cavity___ is a cavity that houses the brain.

10. ___epithelial tissue___ is a type of tissue that forms the covering for all body surfaces.

11. ___superior___ is a part that is above another portion, or closer to the head.

12. ___anterior___ means toward the front surface.

13. ___medial___ means toward, or nearer to, the midline of the body.

14. ___proximal___ means the part is closer to the trunk of the body.

15. ___distal___ is the opposite of proximal, the part that is farther away from the trunk of the body.

16. ___vi___ pertains to internal organs or the covering of organs.

17. The wall of a body cavity is the _____.

18. ___parietal___ refers to the wall of a body cavity.

19. The region of the body that consists of the limbs is the ___appendicular___.

20. ___Stem cells___ are immature, unspecialized cells capable of replication and differentiation into other types of cells or tissues.

MULTIPLE-CHOICE QUESTIONS

Complete each question by circling the best answer.

1. Anatomy is the study of _____.
   a. function
   b. form and structure
   c. internal organs
   d. veins and arteries

2. Physiology is the study of _____.
   a. function
   b. form and structure
   c. internal organs
   d. veins and arteries

3. What imaginary line divides the body into upper and lower portions?
   a. Frontal
   b. Midsagittal
   c. Horizontal
   d. Lateral

4. What imaginary line divides the body into equal right and left halves?
   a. Frontal
   b. Midsagittal
   c. Horizontal
   d. Lateral

5. Name the portion of the cell that carries genetic information.
   a. Cytoplasm
   b. Cell wall
   c. Mitochondria
   d. Nucleus

6. Body tissues that bind and support other tissues are
   _____.
   a. epithelial
   b. muscle
   c. connective
   d. nerve

7. The organizational levels of the body are cells, tissues, organs, and _____.
   a. bones
   b. systems
   c. brain
   d. reproductive

8. The two major cavities in the body are _____.
   a. sagittal and ventral
   b. dorsal and median
   c. cranial and thoracic
   d. dorsal and ventral

9. The axial portion of the body consists of the
   _____.
   a. head
   b. neck
   c. trunk
   d. all of the above

10. The appendicular portion of the body consists of the
    _____.
    a. head
    b. arms
    c. legs
    d. b and c

11. What is the simplest organizational level of the human body?
    a. Tissues
    b. Organs
    c. Body systems
    d. Cells

12. The federal government's lead agency for scientific research on oral, dental, and craniofacial disease is
    the _____.
    a. FDA
    b. EPA
    c. NIDCR
    d. OSHA

1. Label the illustration of the body cavities.

   a. Cranial cavity
   b. Ventral cavity
   c. Dorsal cavity
   d. Pelvic cavity
   e. Thoracic cavity
   f. Spinal cavity
   g. Abdominal cavity
   h. Abdominopelvic cavity

ACTIVITIES

1. With a student partner, discuss why the study of general anatomy is important for a dental assistant. Try to think of at least five reasons.

2. With a student partner, discuss the following:
   a. Each type of tissue and why each is important
   b. The tissues that affect the orofacial part of the body
   c. How and why the health of various tissues affects oral health

7 General Physiology

1. Name and locate each body system.

2. Explain the purpose of each body system.

3. Describe the components of each body system.

4. Explain how each body system functions.

5. Describe the signs and symptoms of common disorders related to each body system.

6. Give examples of conditions that require the interaction of body systems.

FILL-IN-THE-BLANK STATEMENTS

Select the best term from the list below and complete the following statements.

appendicular skeleton	muscle insertion
arteries	muscle origin
articulations	neurons
axial skeleton	osteoblasts
cancellous bone	pericardium
cartilage	periosteum
central nervous system	peripheral nervous system
compact bone	peristalsis
integumentary system	Sharpey fibers
involuntary muscles	veins
joints	

1. The portion of the skeleton that consists of the skull, spinal column, ribs, and sternum is the _____.

2. The portion of the skeleton that consists of the upper extremities and shoulder girdle plus the lower extremities and pelvic girdle is the _____.

3. A specialized connective tissue that covers all bones of the body is the _____.

4. Cells that are associated with bone formation are _____.

5. The _____ anchor the periosteum to the bone.

6. _____ forms the outer layer of bones, where it is needed for strength.

7. The lighter bone that is found in the interior of bones is the _____.

8. _____ is a tough connective, nonvascular, elastic tissue.

9. Structural areas where two or more bones come together are _____.

10. _____ is another term for joints.

11. _____ are muscles that function automatically, without conscious control.

12. The location where the muscle begins is the _____.

13. The location where the muscle ends is the _____.

14. The _____ is a double-walled sac that encloses the heart.

15. Large blood vessels that carry blood away from the heart are _____.

16. Blood vessels that carry blood to the heart are _____.

17. The _____ is composed of the brain and spinal cord.

18. The _____ is composed of the cranial nerves and spinal nerves.

19. _____ are direct nerve impulses.

20. A rhythmic action that moves food through the digestive tract is _____.

21. The _____ involves the skin.

MULTIPLE-CHOICE QUESTIONS

Complete each question by circling the best answer.

1. The skeleton is divided into axial and _____ sections.
   a. peripheral
   b. appendicular
   c. frontal
   d. parietal

2. The connective tissue that covers all bones is _____.
   a. nervous
   b. muscle
   c. epithelial
   d. periosteum

3. The two types of bone are compact and _____.
   a. cortical
   b. trabeculae
   c. cancellous
   d. periosteum

4. Where is cartilage found?
   a. Outside of bones
   b. Where bones join together
   c. Inside of bones
   d. In the teeth

5. What is another term for articulation?
   a. Cartilage
   b. Bone
   c. Bone marrow
   d. Joint

6. Which of the following are type(s) of muscle tissue?
   a. Smooth
   b. Striated
   c. Cardiac
   d. All of the above

7. Which muscle is striated in appearance but resembles smooth muscle in action?
   a. Smooth
   b. Striated
   c. Cardiac
   d. Skeletal

8. Which of the following is a common muscular disorder?
   a. Muscular dystrophy
   b. Endocarditis
   c. Multiple sclerosis
   d. Gout

9. A function of the circulatory system is _____.
   a. to transport nutrients and oxygen to body cells
   b. to provide the body with nutrients
   c. to regulate body temperature and chemical stability
   d. b and c

10. The heart chambers consist of the atria and _____.
    a. pulmonic
    b. aortic
    c. mitral
    d. ventricles

11. Which of the following are function(s) of a blood vessel?
    a. To carry blood away from the heart
    b. To connect the arterial and venous system
    c. To carry blood toward the heart
    d. All of the above

12. The primary function of the lymph system is _____.
    a. to carry blood away from the heart
    b. to provide the body with nutrients
    c. to regulate body temperature and chemical stability
    d. to destroy harmful microorganisms

13. What tissue(s) make up the lymph system?
    a. Lymph vessels
    b. Lymph nodes
    c. Lymph fluid
    d. All of the above

14. What system makes up the nervous system?
    a. Central nervous system
    b. Autonomic nervous system
    c. Peripheral nervous system
    d. a and c

15. The autonomic nervous system is divided into the parasympathetic and _____ nervous systems.
    a. sympathetic
    b. autonomic
    c. peripheral
    d. central

16. The type of neuron that carries impulses toward the brain and spinal cord is _____.
    a. associative
    b. motor
    c. sensory
    d. synapse

17. The main function of the respiratory system is _____.
    a. to carry blood throughout the body
    b. to deliver oxygen to the body
    c. to give the body the ability to move
    d. to contribute to the immune system

18. Which of the following is the role of the digestive system?
    a. To provide nutrition for the body
    b. To deliver oxygen to the body
    c. To give the body the ability to move
    d. To contribute to the immune system

19. Which would *not* be an action of the digestive system?
    a. Ingestion
    b. Sensory function
    c. Movement
    d. Absorption

20. What is the primary function of the endocrine system?
    a. To control growth
    b. To maintain homeostasis
    c. To form and eliminate urine
    d. To regulate the body's activities

21. What is the primary function of the urinary system?
    a. To transport oxygen to cells
    b. To defend against disease
    c. To form and eliminate urine
    d. To regulate body temperature

22. Which body system includes the skin?
    a. Skeletal
    b. Integumentary
    c. Nervous
    d. Muscular

23. Which of the following is an example of an appendage?
    a. Hair
    b. Nails
    c. Glands
    d. All of the above

ACTIVITY

Exercise is an important factor in health. It is recommended that aerobic exercise, which is designed to increase the efficiency of the body's intake of oxygen, should be done for periods of 20 minutes, three to five times a week. To find your optimum level of exertion, subtract your age from the number 220 and then multiply the result by 85%. This gives you the maximum heart rate for your age. To see whether you are achieving the maximum level of exertion, take your pulse for 15 seconds immediately after exercising.

8 Oral Embryology and Histology

1. Define *embryology* and *histology*.

2. Describe the three periods of prenatal development.

3. Explain the types of prenatal influences on dental development.

4. Describe the functions of osteoclasts and osteoblasts.

5. Describe the steps in the formation of the palate.

6. Describe the stages in the development of a tooth.

7. Discuss the genetic and environmental factors that can affect dental development.

8. Explain the difference between the clinical and the anatomic crown.

9. Name and describe the types of tissues within a tooth.

10. Name and describe the three types of dentin.

11. Describe the structure and location of the dental pulp.

12. Name and describe the components of the periodontium.

13. Describe the functions of the periodontal ligaments.

14. Describe the types of oral mucosa, and give an example of each.

Select the best term from the list below and complete the following statements.

ameloblasts
cementoblasts
cementoclasts
conception
embryology
embryonic period
exfoliation
histology

masticatory mucosa
odontoblasts
osteoclasts
periodontium
prenatal development
stratified squamous epithelium
succedaneous

1. _____ is the study of prenatal development.

2. _____ is the study of the structure and function of tissues on a microscopic level.

3. _____ begins at the start of pregnancy and continues until birth.

4. The _____ extends from the beginning of the second week to the end of the eighth week.

5. The union of the male sperm and the ovum of the female is _____.

6. _____ teeth are permanent teeth with primary predecessors; examples are the anterior teeth and premolars.

7. The tissues that support the teeth in the alveolar bone are _____.

8. Enamel-forming cells are _____.

9. _____ are dentin-forming cells.

10. _____ are cementum-forming cells.

11. Cells that resorb cementum are _____.

12. _____ are cells that resorb bone.

13. The normal process of shedding primary teeth is _____.

14. Oral mucosa is made up of _____.

15. Oral mucosa that covers the hard palate, dorsum of the tongue, and gingiva is _____.

MULTIPLE-CHOICE QUESTIONS

Complete each question by circling the best answer.

1. Name the first period of prenatal development.
   a. Embryonic period
   b. Fetal period
   c. Preimplantation period
   d. Embryo

2. Which period of prenatal development is the most critical?
   a. Embryonic period
   b. Fetal period
   c. Preimplantation period
   d. Embryo

3. The embryonic layer that differentiates into cartilage, bones, and muscles is _____.
   a. endoderm
   b. ectoderm
   c. mesoderm
   d. phisoderm

4. Which branchial arch forms the bones, muscles, and nerves of the face and the lower lip?
   a. First
   b. Second
   c. Third
   d. Fourth

5. Which branchial arch forms the side and front of the neck?
   a. First
   b. Second
   c. Third
   d. Fourth

6. The hard and soft palates are formed by the union of the primary and secondary _____.
   a. maxillary processes
   b. premaxilla
   c. palates
   d. palatine processes

7. When does the development of the human face occur?
   a. Second and third weeks
   b. Third and fourth weeks
   c. Fifth to eighth weeks
   d. Ninth to twelfth weeks

8. At birth, how many teeth are in some stage of development?
   a. 20
   b. 32
   c. 44
   d. 52

9. What factor(s) can have a prenatal influence on dental development?
   a. Genetics
   b. Environment
   c. Physical causes
   d. a and b

10. Name the process for the laying down or adding of bone.
    a. Deposition
    b. Discharge
    c. Resorption
    d. Drift

11. Name the process of bone loss or removal.
    a. Deposition
    b. Discharge
    c. Resorption
    d. Drift

12. Growth, calcification, and _____ are the three primary periods in tooth formation.
    a. bud
    b. eruption
    c. cap
    d. bell

13. The final stage in the growth period is the _____.
    a. bud
    b. cap
    c. bell
    d. calcification

14. What is formed in the occlusal surface when multiple cusps join together?
    a. Dentinoenamel junction
    b. Fissure
    c. Pit
    d. b and c

15. What is the name of the process by which teeth move into a functional position in the oral cavity?
    a. Eruption
    b. Exfoliation
    c. Development
    d. Resorption

16. The portion of a tooth that is visible in the mouth is the _____.
    a. anatomic crown
    b. enamel crown
    c. facial crown
    d. clinical crown

17. The cementoenamel junction is located _____.
    a. on the occlusal surface
    b. between the dentin and the enamel
    c. between the pulp and the cementum
    d. between the cementum and the enamel

18. The hardest substance in the human body is _____.
    a. bone
    b. enamel
    c. dentin
    d. cartilage

19. What is the name of the largest mineral component in enamel?
    a. Calcium
    b. Magnesium
    c. Iron
    d. Palladium

20. Pain is transmitted through dentin by way of

    _____.
    a. dentinal tubules
    b. dentinal fibers
    c. odontoblasts
    d. nerves

21. The type of dentin that is also known as *reparative*

    dentin is _____.
    a. primary dentin
    b. secondary dentin
    c. tertiary dentin
    d. odontoblasts

22. The pulp is made up of _____.
    a. blood vessels
    b. bone
    c. nerves
    d. a and c

23. What types of cells form the intercellular substance of the pulp?
    a. Odontoblasts
    b. Fibroblasts
    c. Cementoblasts
    d. Dentinoblasts

24. The primary function of the periodontal ligament is

    _____.
    a. to support the tooth
    b. to maintain the tooth
    c. to retain the tooth
    d. all of the above

25. Which type of oral mucosa forms the inside of the cheeks, lips, and soft palate?
    a. Masticatory mucosa
    b. Specialized mucosa
    c. Lining mucosa
    d. Gingival mucosa

LABELING EXERCISES

1. Label the illustration of a dental pulp.

    a. Coronal pulp
    b. Pulp horns
    c. Accessory canal
    d. Apical foramen
    e. Radicular pulp

2. Label the illustration of the periodontium.

a. Cementum
b. Alveolar bone
c. Periodontal ligament

TOPICS FOR DISCUSSION

Expectant parents wonder whether their child will be male or female, will be tall or short, or will have brown eyes or blue. Many expectant parents do not realize that all of these attributes are determined at the instant of conception. All expectant parents want a healthy baby to be born. Ask your friends or relatives who have children the following questions. If they cannot answer them, perhaps you can answer for them.

Questions to Ask

1. Which trimester is the most critical for the development of the baby?

2. By which week of pregnancy are all of the primary teeth developed?

3. Is it safe to take drugs or alcohol during pregnancy?

4. What does the baby look like 1 month after conception?

5. What is the rule of thumb in determining a delivery date?

9 Head and Neck Anatomy

SHORT-ANSWER QUESTIONS

1. Identify the regions of the head.

2. Identify the bones of the cranium and face.

3. Locate and identify the muscles of the head and neck.

4. Identify and trace the routes of the blood vessels in the head and neck.

5. Identify the components of the temporomandibular joint.

6. Describe the action of the temporomandibular joint.

7. Describe locations of the major and minor salivary glands and associated ducts.

8. Describe and locate the divisions of the trigeminal nerve.

9. Identify the location of the major lymph node sites of the body.

10. Identify and locate the paranasal sinuses of the skull.

11. Integrate the knowledge about head and neck anatomy into clinical practice.

Select the best term from the list below and complete the following statements.

abducens nerve	masseter muscle
anterior jugular vein	occipital region
articular space	parotid duct
buccal	salivary glands
circumvallate lingual papillae	sternocleidomastoid
cranium	temporomandibular disorder
greater palatine nerve	temporomandibular joint
infraorbital region	trapezius
lacrimal bones	xerostomia

1. A vein that begins below the chin, descends near the midline, and drains into the external jugular vein is the
   _____.

2. The eight bones that cover and protect the brain are the _____.

3. The _____ serves the posterior hard palate and the posterior lingual gingiva.

4. _____ pertains to structures that are closest to the inner cheek.

5. Large papillae on the tongue are the _____.

6. The region of the head that is located below the orbital region is the _____.

7. Paired facial bones that help form the medial wall of the orbit are the _____.

8. The _____ is the strongest and most obvious muscle of mastication.

9. The _____ is the region of the head overlying the occipital bone and covered by the scalp.

10. The _____ produce saliva.

11. One of the cervical muscles that divide the neck region into anterior and posterior cervical triangles is the
    _____.

12. The space between the capsular ligament and between the surfaces of the glenoid fossa and the condyle is the
    _____.

13. The _____ is the sixth cranial nerve, which serves the eye muscle.

14. A joint on each side of the head that allows for movement of the mandible is the _____.

15. _____ is a disease process associated with the temporomandibular joint.

16. The _____ is one of the cervical muscles that lift the clavicle and scapula to shrug the shoulder.

17. _____ is a term for decreased production of saliva.

18. The _____ is associated with the parotid salivary gland, which opens into the oral cavity at the parotid
    papilla.

MULTIPLE-CHOICE QUESTIONS

Complete each question by circling the best answer.

1. The regions of the head include the frontal, parietal, occipital, temporal, orbital, nasal, infraorbital, and
   _____.
   a. mandible
   b. maxilla
   c. zygomatic
   d. lacrimal

2. What bone forms the forehead?
   a. Occipital
   b. Frontal
   c. Parietal
   d. Zygomatic

3. What bone forms the back and base of the cranium?
   a. Parietal
   b. Temporal
   c. Occipital
   d. Frontal

4. Which bones form the cheek?
   a. Sphenoid
   b. Zygomatic
   c. Temporal
   d. Nasal

5. Which bones form the upper jaw and hard palate?
   a. Zygomatic
   b. Sphenoid
   c. Mandible
   d. Maxilla

6. Name the only movable bone of the skull.
   a. Coronoid process
   b. Temporal
   c. Mandible
   d. Maxilla

7. Where is the mental foramen located?
   a. Maxilla
   b. Coronoid process
   c. Mandible
   d. Glenoid process

8. What are the basic types of movement by the temporomandibular joint?
   a. Up and down
   b. Hinge and glide
   c. Side to side
   d. Back and forth

9. What type of sign or symptom may a patient who is experiencing temporomandibular disorder exhibit?
   a. Migraine
   b. Nausea
   c. Fever
   d. Pain

10. Which cranial nerve innervates all muscles of mastication?
    a. Third
    b. Fourth
    c. Fifth
    d. Sixth

11. What is the name of the horseshoe-shaped bone where the muscles of the tongue and the floor of the mouth attach?
    a. Hyoid
    b. Sphenoid
    c. Mandible
    d. Vomer

12. Which of the major salivary glands is the largest?
    a. Submandibular
    b. Sublingual
    c. Parotid
    d. Submaxillary

13. What is another name for the parotid duct?
    a. Duct of Rivinus
    b. von Ebner's salivary gland
    c. Wharton's duct
    d. Stensen duct

14. Which artery is behind the ramus with five branches?
    a. Infraorbital artery
    b. Facial artery
    c. Inferior alveolar artery
    d. Lingual artery

15. Which artery supplies the maxillary molars, premolar teeth, and gingiva?
    a. Inferior alveolar artery
    b. Posterior superior alveolar artery
    c. Facial artery
    d. Lingual artery

16. How many pairs of cranial nerves are connected to the brain?
    a. 4 pairs
    b. 6 pairs
    c. 10 pairs
    d. 12 pairs

17. Which division of the trigeminal nerve subdivides into the buccal, lingual, and inferior alveolar nerves?
    a. Mandibular division
    b. Facial division
    c. Lingual division
    d. Maxillary division

18. In which type of dental examination would lymph nodes be palpated?
    a. Physical examination
    b. Intraoral examination
    c. Extraoral examination
    d. Radiographic examination

19. What is the term for enlarged or palpable lymph nodes?
    a. Lymphadenopathy
    b. Xerostomia
    c. Parkinson's disease
    d. Lymphitis

TOPICS FOR DISCUSSION

One of the most important responsibilities of the clinical assistant is to control moisture during a dental procedure. Moisture can contaminate the operative site, prevent a dental material from setting, cause a dental sealant to fail, or be a reason to restart a procedure.

1. What type of moisture could interfere with a dental procedure?

2. How is saliva produced?

3. Locate where in the mouth saliva would be produced.

4. Describe ways that you can control moisture during a procedure.

10 Landmarks of the Face and Oral Cavity

SHORT-ANSWER QUESTIONS

1. Name and identify the landmarks of the face.

2. Name and identify the landmarks of the oral cavity.

3. Describe the structures found in the vestibular region of the oral cavity.

4. Describe the area of the oral cavity proper.

5. Describe the characteristics of normal gingival tissue.

6. Describe the functions of the taste buds.

FILL-IN-THE-BLANK STATEMENTS

Select the best term from the list below and complete the following statements.

ala of the nose
anterior naris
canthus
commissure
Fordyce's spots
gingiva
glabella
labial frenum

mental protuberance
nasion
philtrum
septum
tragus of the ear
vermilion border
vestibule

1. The _____ is the fold of tissue at the corner of the eyelids.

2. The winglike tip of the outer side of each nostril is the _____.

3. The _____ is the rectangular area from under the nose to the midline of the upper lip.

4. The _____ is the cartilage projection anterior to the external opening of the ear.

5. The _____ is the midpoint between the eyes, just below the eyebrows.

6. The _____ is the smooth surface of the frontal bone directly above the root of the nose.

7. The tissue that divides the nasal cavity into two nasal fossae is the _____.

8. The _____ is also referred to as the *nostril*.

9. The part of the mandible that forms the chin is the _____.

10. The _____ is the darker-colored border around the lips.

11. The _____ is the angle at the corner of the mouth where the upper and lower lips join.

12. The space between the teeth and the inner mucosa lining of the lips and cheeks is the _____.

13. _____ are normal variations that sometimes appear on the buccal mucosa.

14. The _____ is a band of tissue that passes from the facial oral mucosa at the midline of the arch to the midline of the inner surface of the lip.

15. The masticatory mucosa that covers the alveolar processes of the jaws and surrounds the necks of the teeth is the _____.

MULTIPLE-CHOICE QUESTIONS

Complete each question by circling the best answer.

1. What region of the face extends from the eyebrows to the hairline?
   a. Temple
   b. Zygomatic malar
   c. Forehead
   d. Nose

2. The line that marks a color change from your face to your lips is referred to as the _____.
   a. commissure
   b. vermilion border
   c. Fordyce
   d. labial frenum

3. What type of tissue covers the oral cavity?
   a. Mucous membrane
   b. Epithelia
   c. Squamous
   d. Stratified

4. Besides the oral cavity proper, name the other region of the oral cavity.
   a. Gingiva
   b. Tongue
   c. Lips
   d. Vestibule

5. The structure that passes from the oral mucosa to the facial midline of the mandibular arch is the _____.
   a. tongue
   b. frenum
   c. uvula
   d. incisive papilla

6. What is the proper term for the "gums"?
   a. Epithelia
   b. Incisive
   c. Skin
   d. Gingiva

7. What is another term for unattached gingiva?
   a. Interdental gingiva
   b. Gingival groove
   c. Free gingiva
   d. Attached gingiva

8. What is another term for interdental gingiva?
   a. Interdental papilla
   b. Gingival groove
   c. Free gingiva
   d. Attached gingiva

9. What is the name of the pear-shaped pad of tissue behind the maxillary incisors?
   a. Palatine rugae
   b. Incisive papilla
   c. Palatine raphe
   d. Uvula

10. What is the name of the hanging pear-shaped projection of tissue at the border of the soft palate?
   a. Palatine rugae
   b. Free gingiva
   c. Uvula
   d. Incisive papilla

11. What is the correct term for the upper surface of the tongue?
   a. Frontal
   b. Dorsum
   c. Ventral
   d. Apex

12. The thin fold of mucous membrane that extends from the floor of the mouth to the underside of the tongue is the _____.
   a. sublingual fold
   b. sublingual caruncle
   c. lingual frenum
   d. incisive frenum

LABELING EXERCISE

1. Label the features of the face.

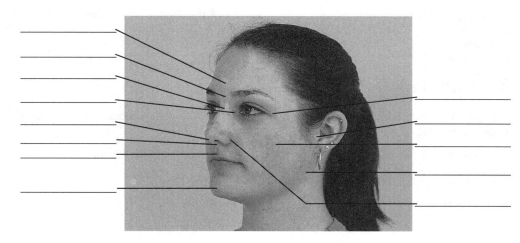

1. Canthus
2. Inner canthus
3. Ala
4. Philtrum
5. Tragus
6. Nasion
7. Glabella
8. Root
9. Septum
10. Anterior naris
11. Mental protuberance
12. Angle of the mandible
13. Zygomatic arch

ACTIVITIES

1. Identify the features of the face. To do this activity, you will need the following:
   - Student partner
   - Cotton-tipped applicator

   Using the cotton-tipped applicator, point to each of the following structures on your partner's face:

   1. Ala of the nose
   2. Inner canthus and outer canthus of the eye
   3. Commissure of the lips
   4. Tragus
   5. Nasion
   6. Glabella
   7. Philtrum
   8. Bridge of the nose
   9. Vermilion border
   10. Zygomatic arch
   11. Septum
   12. Anterior naris
   13. Mental protuberance
   14. Angle of the mandible

2. Identify the major landmarks, structures, and normal tissues of the mouth. To do this activity, you will need the following:
   - Student partner
   - Mask, gloves, gown
   - Mouth mirror
   - Cotton-tipped applicator

   Using the mouth mirror for vision and retraction, point to each of following structures in your partner's mouth with the cotton-tipped applicator:

   1. Dorsum of tongue
   2. Area of gag reflex
   3. Hard and soft palates
   4. Gingival margin
   5. Incisive papilla
   6. Mandibular labial frenum
   7. Maxillary labial frenum
   8. Sublingual frenum
   9. Vestibule of the mouth
   10. Wharton's duct
   11. Uvula
   12. Palatal rugae
   13. Attached gingivae
   14. Ventral surface of the tongue
   15. Interdental gingivae
   16. Mucogingival junction

3. Throughout the ages, women have applied makeup to enhance their natural facial features. Look at some of the cosmetic advertisements in current magazines or newspapers, and identify the facial features that are enhanced by the application of various shades of foundation, lipstick, eyeliner, and blush.

   1. What natural landmark is enhanced by the use of lip liner?

   2. Blush is applied over which structure of the face?

   3. How can the use of eyeliner change the appearance of the eyes?

11 Overview of the Dentitions

SHORT-ANSWER QUESTIONS

1. Explain how the size and shape of teeth determine their functions.

2. Describe the various functions of different types of teeth.

3. Name and identify the location of each of the tooth surfaces.

4. Name and describe the types of teeth.

5. Explain the differences among primary, mixed, and permanent dentitions.

6. Define occlusion, centric occlusion, and malocclusion.

7. Name and describe Angle's classification of malocclusion.

8. Name and describe the three primary systems of tooth numbering.

FILL-IN-THE-BLANK STATEMENTS

Select the best term from the list below and complete the following statements.

anterior	malocclusion
centric occlusion	mandible
curve of Spee	masticatory surface
deciduous	maxilla
dentition	mesial surface
distal surface	occlusion
embrasure	quadrant
functional occlusion	sextant
interproximal space	succedaneous teeth

1. Natural teeth in the dental arch are the _____.

2. Baby or primary teeth are called _____.

3. The natural contact of the maxillary and mandibular teeth in all positions is termed _____.

4. Permanent teeth that replace primary teeth are _____.

5. The teeth in the front of the mouth are called the _____.

6. The upper jaw is the _____.

7. The lower jaw is the _____.

8. A _____ is one fourth of the dentition.

9. A _____ is one sixth of the dentition.

10. The _____ is the surface of the tooth toward the midline.

11. The _____ is the surface of the tooth distant from the midline.

12. The chewing surface of the teeth is the _____.

13. The _____ is the area between adjacent tooth surfaces.

14. A(n) _____ is a triangular space in the gingival direction between the proximal surfaces of two adjoining teeth in contact.

15. Teeth are in _____ when there is maximum contact between the occluding surfaces of the maxillary and mandibular teeth.

16. Teeth are in _____ when the teeth make contact during biting and chewing movements.

17. _____ is an abnormal or malpositioned relationship of the maxillary teeth to the mandibular teeth when they are in centric occlusion.

18. The _____ is the curvature formed by the maxillary and mandibular arches in occlusion.

MULTIPLE-CHOICE QUESTIONS

Complete each question by circling the best answer.

1. Name the set(s) of teeth humans have in their lifetime.
   a. Mixed
   b. Primary
   c. Permanent
   d. b and c

2. How many teeth are in the primary dentition?
   a. 10
   b. 20
   c. 28
   d. 32

3. What is the term for the four sections of the divided dental arches?
   a. Sextant
   b. Maxillary
   c. Mandibular
   d. Quadrant

4. What term is used for the front teeth?
   a. Maxillary
   b. Anterior
   c. Mandibular
   d. Posterior

5. Name the most posterior teeth.
   a. Centrals
   b. Laterals
   c. Premolars
   d. Molars

6. Which tooth is referred to as the "cornerstone" of the dental arch?
   a. Lateral
   b. Central
   c. Canine
   d. Molar

7. Name the surface of the tooth that faces the tongue.
   a. Lingual
   b. Facial
   c. Mesial
   d. Distal

8. What is the name for the space between adjacent teeth?
   a. Occlusion
   b. Bite
   c. Interproximal
   d. Facial

9. The name of the area where adjacent teeth physically touch is the _____.
   a. embrasure
   b. contact area
   c. occlusion
   d. interproximal

10. The name of the triangular space between adjacent teeth is the _____.
    a. embrasure
    b. contact area
    c. occlusion
    d. interproximal

11. The junction of two tooth surfaces is a _____.
    a. margin
    b. proximal surface
    c. line angle
    d. pit

12. Which one-third portion of a tooth's surface is positioned toward the end of the root?
    a. Occlusal one third
    b. Middle one third
    c. Apical one third
    d. Proximal one third

13. The term for the position of teeth during chewing is _____.
    a. functional occlusion
    b. malocclusion
    c. mastication
    d. distoclusion

14. An individual who has an incorrect bite is given a diagnosis of _____.
    a. functional occlusion
    b. malocclusion
    c. mastication
    d. neutroclusion

15. What is the technical term for class III occlusion?
    a. Functional occlusion
    b. Distocclusion
    c. Malocclusion
    d. Mesiocclusion

16. What classification is neutroclusion?
    a. Class I
    b. Class II
    c. Class III
    d. Class IV

17. What is the name for the curve of the occlusal plane?
    a. Curve of occlusion
    b. Curve of Spee
    c. Curve of molars
    d. Curve of Otho

1. Label the surfaces of the teeth.

a. Mesial surface
b. Distal surface
c. Palatal surface
d. Occlusal surface
e. Proximal surface with contact area
f. Incisal surface
g. Lingual surface
h. Facial surfaces (buccal/labial)

2. Label the occlusal view of the permanent dentition as shown using the Universal/National system.

a. Maxillary incisors
b. Maxillary canine
c. Maxillary premolars
d. Maxillary molars
e. Mandibular incisors
f. Mandibular canine
g. Mandibular premolars
h. Mandibular molars

43

Fill in the number of each tooth using the Universal, Palmer Notation, and ISO/FDI numbering systems. You may wish to refer to a typodont or a study model of the adult and primary dentitions.

	Universal	Palmer Notation	ISO/FDI
Maxillary right second molar			
Maxillary right first molar			
Maxillary right first premolar			
Maxillary right canine			
Maxillary right lateral			
Maxillary right central			
Maxillary left central			
Maxillary left canine			
Maxillary left second premolar			
Maxillary left first molar			
Maxillary left third molar			
Mandibular left second molar			
Mandibular left first molar			
Mandibular left canine			
Mandibular left lateral			
Mandibular left central			
Mandibular right central			
Mandibular right canine			
Mandibular right second premolar			
Mandibular right second molar			

12 Tooth Morphology

SHORT-ANSWER QUESTIONS

1. Identify each tooth using the correct terms and Universal/National System code numbers.

2. Identify the location of each permanent tooth.

3. Use the correct terminology when discussing features of the permanent dentition.

4. Describe the general and specific features of each tooth in the permanent dentition.

5. Discuss clinical considerations of each tooth in the permanent dentition.

6. Compare and contrast the features of the primary and permanent dentitions.

7. Describe the general and specific features of the primary dentition.

8. Discuss clinical considerations with the primary dentition.

FILL-IN-THE-BLANK STATEMENTS

Select the best term from the list below and complete the following statements.

canine eminence
central groove
cingulum
cusp
fossa
furcation
imbrication lines

incisal edge
inclined cuspal planes
mamelon
marginal ridge
morphology
nonsuccedaneous

1. The _____ is a major elevation on the masticatory surface of canines and posterior teeth.

2. A wide, shallow depression on the lingual surface of anterior teeth is the _____.

3. _____ is an area between two or more root branches.

4. _____ is the external vertical bony ridge on the labial surface of the canines.

5. The most prominent developmental groove on posterior teeth is the _____.

6. The _____ is a raised, rounded area on the cervical third of the lingual surface.

7. Slight ridges that run mesiodistally in the cervical third of teeth are _____.

8. The rounded enamel extension on the incisal ridge of incisors is the _____.

9. A rounded, raised border on the mesial and distal portions of the lingual surface of anterior teeth and the occlusal table of posterior teeth is the _____.

10. A ridge on the permanent incisors that appears flattened on the labial, lingual, or incisal view after tooth eruption is the _____.

11. _____ are the sloping areas between cusp ridges.

12. _____ refers to a tooth that does not replace a primary tooth.

13. _____ is the study of the form and shape of teeth.

MULTIPLE-CHOICE QUESTIONS

Complete each question by circling the best answer.

1. How many anterior teeth are in the permanent dentition?
   a. 10
   b. 12
   c. 28
   d. 32

2. What term is given to a permanent tooth that replaces a primary tooth of the same type?
   a. Implant
   b. Crown
   c. Succedaneous
   d. Molar

3. What is the rounded, raised area on the cervical third of the lingual surface of anterior teeth?
   a. Cingulum
   b. Mamelon
   c. Ridge
   d. Edge

4. What feature do newly erupted central and lateral incisors have on their incisal ridge?
   a. Cingulum
   b. Mamelon
   c. Ridge
   d. Cusp

5. Which teeth are the longest ones in the permanent dentition?
   a. Molars
   b. Central incisors
   c. Premolars
   d. Canines

6. Which teeth are the smallest ones in the permanent dentition?
   a. Maxillary molars
   b. Maxillary laterals
   c. Mandibular premolars
   d. Mandibular centrals

7. What is the name for the developmental horizontal lines on anterior teeth?
   a. Imbrication lines
   b. Marginal lines
   c. Oblique lines
   d. Incisal lines

8. What feature borders the occlusal table of a posterior tooth?
   a. Oblique ridges
   b. Triangular ridges
   c. Marginal ridges
   d. Incisal ridges

9. What is the pinpoint depression where two or more grooves meet?
   a. Fossa
   b. Sulcus
   c. Ridge
   d. Pit

10. Which teeth are frequently extracted as part of orthodontic treatment?
    a. Lateral incisors
    b. First premolars
    c. Third molars
    d. Canines

11. What occlusal form does the mandibular second premolar resemble?
    a. Incisal edge
    b. Two cusps
    c. Three cusps
    d. b and c

12. Which term is given to the area at which three roots divide?
    a. Furcation
    b. Bifurcation
    c. Trifurcation
    d. Quadrifurcation

13. What term is given to a tooth that does not replace a primary tooth?
    a. Succedaneous
    b. Nonsuccedaneous
    c. Supernumerary
    d. Developmental

14. What is the name of the fifth cusp on a maxillary first molar?
    a. Cingulum
    b. Fossa
    c. Mamelon
    d. Cusp of Carabelli

15. How many roots do mandibular molars have?
    a. One
    b. Two
    c. Three
    d. b or c

16. Which teeth are referred to as the "wisdom" teeth?
    a. Central incisors
    b. Canines
    c. First molars
    d. Third molars

17. How thick is the enamel covering on a primary tooth?
    a. Thin
    b. Medium
    c. Thick
    d. Twice as thick as the enamel on a permanent tooth

18. What method of identification is used in the Universal/National System for the primary dentition?
    a. Numeric
    b. Italicized
    c. Alphabetic
    d. Pictorial

19. Which primary tooth has an H-shaped groove pattern on its occlusal surface?
    a. Maxillary premolar
    b. Mandibular molar
    c. Mandibular premolar
    d. Maxillary molar

20. Which primary tooth is the largest?
    a. Maxillary central
    b. Mandibular molar
    c. Maxillary molar
    d. Mandibular canine

LABELING EXERCISES

1. Label the features on the occlusal surface on a permanent posterior tooth.
   a. Cusp ridge
   b. Cusp tip
   c. Inclined cuspal plane
   d. Marginal ridge
   e. Marginal ridge

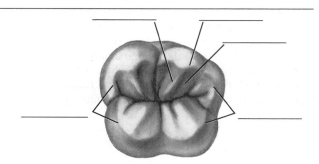

Chapter **12** **Tooth Morphology**

2. Label the features of a lingual view of a permanent maxillary canine.
   a. Cingulum
   b. Lingual ridge
   c. Lingual fossae
   d. Cusp tip
   e. Marginal ridges

ACTIVITIES

1. Look in your mouth and determine whether your mandibular second premolar is a three-cusp or a two-cusp type.

2. From a selection of all permanent teeth (sterilized extracted teeth or models), determine which are first and second premolars.

3. From a selection of all permanent teeth (sterilized extracted teeth or models), determine which are first, second, third, maxillary, and mandibular molars.

4. Examine the teeth of your classmates and note the variation in the cusp of Carabelli.

5. Identify the surfaces and landmarks of the anterior and posterior permanent teeth. To do this activity, you will need the following materials:
   ■ Typodonts or study models of the permanent dentition
   ■ Cotton-tipped applicator or explorer

   Use your cotton-tipped applicator or explorer to point to each of the following surfaces and landmarks of the permanent dentition:

   a. Incisal surface of the maxillary left canine
   b. Labial surface of the mandibular right lateral incisor
   c. Lingual surface of the mandibular left central incisor
   d. Mesial surface of the maxillary right central incisor
   e. Distal surface of the mandibular left lateral incisor
   f. Occlusal surface of the mandibular left first premolar
   g. Lingual surface of the maxillary left first molar
   h. Buccal surface of the mandibular left second molar
   i. Mesial surface of the maxillary right first premolar
   j. Distal surface of the mandibular right second molar
   k. Buccal cusp on a mandibular right second premolar
   l. Occlusal pit on the maxillary right second molar
   m. Marginal ridge on the mandibular left first molar
   n. Cingulum on the maxillary right canine
   o. Lingual fossa on the mandibular left canine
   p. Cusp tip on the maxillary right canine

13 Dental Caries

SHORT-ANSWER QUESTIONS

1. Explain why dental caries is an infectious disease.

2. Describe the process of dental caries.

3. Name the risk factors for dental caries.

4. Explain the purpose of caries activity tests.

5. Describe possible methods of transmission of oral bacteria.

6. Name the infective agents in the caries process.

7. Describe the role of saliva in oral health.

8. Explain the causes and effects of diet on dental caries.

9. Explain the remineralization process.

10. Distinguish the difference between root caries and smooth surface caries.

11. Describe the methods of detecting dental caries.

12. Name the most common chronic disease in children.

13. What is the purpose of CAMBRA?

14. Demonstrate or describe the technique for using a caries detection device.

FILL-IN-THE-BLANK STATEMENTS

Select the best term from the list below and complete the following statements.

caries
cavitation
CAMBRA
demineralization
fermentable carbohydrates
incipient caries
lactobacillus

mutans streptococci
pellicle
plaque
rampant caries
remineralization
xerostomia

1. Another name for tooth decay is _____.

2. _____ is the loss of minerals from the tooth.

3. _____ is the replacement of minerals in the tooth.

4. The type of bacteria primarily responsible for caries is _____.

5. _____ is a type of bacteria that produces lactic acid from carbohydrates.

6. _____ is a colorless sticky mass of microorganisms that adheres to tooth surfaces.

7. The formation of a cavity or hole is _____.

8. _____ is tooth decay that is beginning to form.

9. Decay that develops rapidly and is widespread throughout the mouth is termed _____.

10. _____ is dryness of the mouth caused by abnormal reduction in the amount of saliva.

11. The thin coating of salivary materials that are deposited on tooth surfaces is a _____.

12. Simple carbohydrates such as sucrose, fructose, lactose, and glucose are _____.

13. Managing dental caries by risk assessment is known as _____.

MULTIPLE-CHOICE QUESTIONS

Complete each question by circling the best answer.

1. What bacterium causes dental caries?
   a. Spirochetes
   b. Mutans streptococci
   c. Staphylococci
   d. Monocytes

2. What is the soft, sticky, bacterial mass that adheres to teeth?
   a. Decay
   b. Lactobacillus
   c. Plaque
   d. Carbohydrates

3. What mineral in the enamel makes the crystal easier to dissolve?
   a. Carbonated apatite
   b. Iron
   c. Calcium
   d. Magnesium

4. The three factors necessary for the formation of dental caries are bacteria, fermentable carbohydrates, and

   _____.
   a. saliva
   b. poor toothbrushing habits
   c. a susceptible tooth
   d. nonfluoridated water

5. What is the term for the dissolving of calcium and phosphate from a tooth?
   a. Demineralization
   b. Resorption
   c. Remineralization
   d. Absorption

6. A patient with rapid and extensive formation of caries

   is given a diagnosis of _____.
   a. malocclusion
   b. xerostomia
   c. rampant caries
   d. temporomandibular disorder

7. Dental caries that occurs under or adjacent to existing

   dental restorations is termed _____.
   a. gingivitis
   b. periodontitis
   c. rampant caries
   d. recurrent caries

8. How does saliva protect the teeth from dental caries?
   a. Physical actions
   b. Chemical actions
   c. Antibacterial actions
   d. All of the above

CASE STUDY

Jeremy Allen is a 13-year-old patient of the practice. To date, he has undergone nine restorations and is scheduled to come back to have another restoration placed. In reviewing his patient record, you notice that most of his restorations are on the chewing surface of his teeth.

1. Do you think it is normal for a 13-year-old to have this many restorations?

2. What might be the cause for Jeremy's high rate of caries?

3. What term is used to describe the surface of the teeth mentioned with restorations?

4. What could be done to help lower Jeremy's caries rate?

5. How would you educate Jeremy to help reduce his rate of caries?

COMPETENCY 13-1: PERFORMING CARIES DETECTION USING THE KAVO DIAGNODENT CARIES DETECTION DEVICE (EXPANDED FUNCTION)

Performance Objective

By following a routine procedure that meets stated protocols, the student will perform a caries detection procedure using an electronic caries detection device.

Evaluation and Grading Criteria

3   Student competently met the stated criteria without assistance.
2   Student required assistance in order to meet the stated criteria.
1   Student showed uncertainty when performing the stated criteria.
0   Student was not prepared and needs to repeat the step.
N/A   No evaluation of this step.
Instructor shall define grades for each point range earned on completion of each performance-evaluated task.

Performance Standards

The minimum number of satisfactory performances required before final evaluation is _____.

Instructor shall identify by * those steps considered critical. If a step is missed or minimum competency is not met, the evaluated procedure fails and must be repeated.

PERFORMANCE CRITERIA	*	SELF	PEER	INSTRUCTOR	COMMENTS
1. Personal protective equipment placed according to procedure.					
Establish Zero Baseline					
2. Before scanning, selected an anatomic reference point on a healthy nonrestored tooth.					
3. Held the probe tip against the tooth at right angles to the surface.					
4. Gently squeezed the gray ring switch of the handpiece.					
5. Successfully established the zero baseline. (Display shows "Set 0," also confirmed by an audible beep.)					
6. Recorded the anatomic location where the zero baseline was established in the patient's dental record for future reference.					
Scanning Procedure					
7. Cleaned and dried the teeth using a prophy brush or other acceptable means.					
8. Identified surfaces of the tooth to be tested.					
9. During examination of suspicious sites, used light contact when touching the tip of the handpiece to the surface of the tooth.					

Continued

10. Placed the probe tip directly on the pits and fissures, making sure the tip was in contact with the long axis of the tooth.				
11. Slowly rotated or rocked the handpiece in a pendulum-like manner when the tip was in contact with the fissure.				
12. Recorded the readings.				
13. After the scan was completed, held the tip in the air and held the gray ring switch until "Set 0" appeared on the display.				
14. Procedure documented in patient record.				

ADDITIONAL COMMENTS

Total number of points earned _____

Grade _____ Instructor's initials _____

COMPETENCY 13-2: PERFORMING CARIES RISK ASSESSMENT (EXPANDED FUNCTION)

Performance Objective

By following a routine procedure that meets stated protocols, the student will perform a caries risk assessment using the caries risk test (CRT, Ivoclar) and comparing the density of mutans streptococci (MS) and lactobacilli (LB) colonies with the corresponding evaluation pictures.

Evaluation and Grading Criteria

__3__ Student competently met the stated criteria without assistance.
__2__ Student required assistance in order to meet the stated criteria.
__1__ Student showed uncertainty when performing the stated criteria.
__0__ Student was not prepared and needs to repeat the step.
__N/A__ No evaluation of this step.
Instructor shall define grades for each point range earned on completion of each performance-evaluated task.

Performance Standards

The minimum number of satisfactory performances required before final evaluation is _____.

Instructor shall identify by * those steps considered critical. If a step is missed or minimum competency is not met, the evaluated procedure fails and must be repeated.

PERFORMANCE CRITERIA	*	SELF	PEER	INSTRUCTOR	COMMENTS
1. Personal protective equipment placed according to procedure.					
2. Explained the procedure to the patient.					
3. Instructed the patient to chew the paraffin wax pellet.					
4. Instructed the patient to expectorate into the paper cup.					
5. Removed the agar carrier from the test vial, and placed an $NaHCO_3$ tablet at the bottom of the vial.					
6. Carefully removed the protective foils from the two agar surfaces without touching the agar.					
7. Thoroughly wet both agar surfaces using a pipette. Avoided scratching the agar surface. Held the carrier at an angle while wetting.					
8. Slid the agar carrier back into the vial, and closed the vial tightly.					
9. Used a waterproof pen to note the name of the patient and the date on the lid of the vial.					

Continued

10. Placed the test vial upright in the incubator and incubated at 37° C (99° F) for 49 hours.				
11. Removed the vial from the incubator.				
12. Compared the density of MS and LB colonies with the corresponding evaluation pictures on a chart. *Tip: Hold the agar carrier at a slight angle under a light source to see the colonies clearly.*				
13. Procedure documented in patient record.				

Total number of points earned _____

Grade _____ Instructor's initials _____

14 Periodontal Disease

1. Name and describe the tissues of the periodontium.

2. Describe the prevalence of periodontal disease.

3. Name the structures that make up the periodontium.

4. Identify systemic factors that influence periodontal disease.

5. Identify and describe the two main types of periodontal disease.

6. Explain the significance of plaque and calculus in periodontal disease.

7. Identify the risk factors that contribute to periodontal disease.

8. Describe the systemic conditions that are linked to periodontal disease.

9. Describe the clinical characteristics of gingivitis.

10. Describe the progression of periodontitis.

FILL-IN-THE-BLANK STATEMENTS

Select the best term from the list below and complete the following statements.

calculus	periodontium
gingivitis	plaque
periodontal diseases	subgingival
periodontitis	supragingival

1. A soft deposit on teeth that consists of bacteria and bacterial by-products is _____.

2. _____ is made up of calcium and phosphate salts in saliva that become mineralized and adhere to the tooth surface.

3. The _____ are structures that surround, support, and are attached to the teeth.

4. Diseases of the periodontium are _____.

5. _____ refers to the area above the gingiva.

6. _____ refers to the area below the gingiva.

7. Inflammation of the gingival tissue is _____.

8. _____ is an inflammatory disease of the supporting tissues of the teeth.

MULTIPLE-CHOICE QUESTIONS

Complete each question by circling the best answer.

1. Gingivitis is defined as _____.
   a. inflammation of the periodontium
   b. inflammation of the alveolar process
   c. inflammation of the gingival tissue
   d. inflammation of the oral mucosa

2. Which of the following is a clinical sign of gingivitis?
   a. Caries
   b. Redness
   c. Fever
   d. Ulcers

3. Which of the following can be done to reverse gingivitis?
   a. Improve brushing and flossing techniques.
   b. Take antibiotics.
   c. Undergo root planing.
   d. Nothing will reverse gingivitis.

4. Periodontitis is defined as _____.
   a. inflammation of the supporting tissues of the teeth
   b. inflammation of the alveolar process
   c. inflammation of the gingiva
   d. inflammation of the oral mucosa

5. Which of the following systemic diseases is related to periodontal disease?
   a. Cardiovascular disease
   b. Preterm low birth weight
   c. Respiratory disease
   d. All of the above

CASE STUDY

You are working for an orthodontist, and Sally Hunter is a 14-year-old patient of the practice. Sally is wearing appliances on her teeth and has returned to your office for her 6-week checkup. While removing elastics from her appliances, you note that her gingiva is red and slightly inflamed. You look at her patient record, and there is no indication of this condition at her last checkup.

1. What do you think could cause the redness and inflammation of Sally's gingival tissue?

2. Could there be any other reason for this gingival appearance?

3. Why should there be a note in the patient's chart regarding the oral tissues?

4. What would likely be the orthodontist's diagnosis for Sally's gingiva?

5. How can this problem be alleviated?

INTERACTIVE DENTAL OFFICE PATIENT CASE EXERCISE Θvolve
learning system

Access the Interactive Dental Office on Evolve and click on the patient case for Louisa Van Doren.
- Review Mrs. Van Doren's record.
- Mount her radiographs.
- Answer the following questions.

1. Does Mrs. Van Doren's health history contain any information regarding a condition that could lead to periodontal complications?

2. While viewing Mrs. Van Doren's radiographs, what did you notice about the level of bone?

15 Preventive Dentistry

SHORT-ANSWER QUESTIONS

1. Explain the goal of preventive dentistry.

2. Name and describe the components of a preventive dentistry program.

3. Identify sources of systemic fluoride.

4. Discuss techniques for educating patients in preventive care.

5. Name and discuss three methods of administering fluoride therapy.

6. Describe the effects of excessive amounts of fluoride.

7. Describe the purpose of a fluoride needs assessment.

8. Compare and contrast various methods of toothbrushing.

9. Describe the process for cleaning a denture.

FILL-IN-THE-BLANK STATEMENTS

Select the best term from the list below and complete the following statements.

dental sealants   **systemic fluoride**
disclosing agent   **topical fluoride**
preventive dentistry

1. _____ includes proper nutrition and a plaque control program.

2. A _____ is a coloring agent that is applied to teeth to make plaque visible.

3. A coating that covers the occlusal pits and fissures is _____.

4. Fluoride that is ingested and circulated throughout the body is _____.

5. _____ is fluoride that is applied directly to the teeth.

MULTIPLE-CHOICE QUESTIONS

Complete each question by circling the best answer.

1. What is the goal of preventive dentistry?
   a. To save money
   b. To limit visits to the dentist
   c. To have a healthy mouth
   d. To eliminate the need for dental insurance

2. What is one of the most common dental diseases?
   a. Crooked teeth
   b. Dental caries
   c. Missing teeth
   d. Impacted teeth

3. What is the goal of a patient education program?
   a. To teach patients how to take care of their teeth and develop sound dental habits
   b. To eliminate visits to the dentist
   c. To teach patients how to educate family members
   d. To save money on dental bills

4. What is the initial step in a patient education program?
   a. Insurance approval
   b. Intraoral examination
   c. Listening to the patient
   d. Radiographs

5. Dental sealants _____.
   a. take the place of restorations
   b. hold restorative materials in place
   c. are a type of desensitizer
   d. are made of a hard covering that is placed in the pits and fissures of teeth

6. Fluoride combats decay by _____.
   a. slowing remineralization
   b. sealing the teeth
   c. enhancing remineralization
   d. both a and c

7. What technique is used in the dental office to provide fluoride treatment?
   a. Ingestion
   b. Topical
   c. Systemic
   d. Intravenous

8. What dental condition is the result of too much fluoide?
   a. Caries
   b. Gingivitis
   c. Fluorosis
   d. Periodontitis

9. What precaution is necessary for children who are using fluoridated toothpaste?
   a. Making sure the child does not swallow the toothpaste
   b. Having the child drink water after brushing
   c. Using the toothpaste only before bedtime
   d. Using only twice a day

10. What is the key dietary factor that relates to dental caries?
    a. Proteins
    b. Fats
    c. Carbohydrates
    d. Sugar

11. What information must a patient include in a food diary?
    a. Time the food was eaten
    b. Quantity
    c. Amount of sugar that was added
    d. All of the above

12. How do sugar-free sodas relate to dental caries?
    a. Decrease acidity
    b. Increase saliva production
    c. Increase acidity
    d. Decrease saliva production

13. What can patients do daily to remove plaque?
    a. Brush
    b. Rinse with water
    c. Floss
    d. a and c

14. Which type of toothbrush bristles are usually recommended?
    a. Soft
    b. Medium
    c. Hard
    d. Natural

15. Which method of toothbrushing is generally recommended?
    a. Modified Stillman
    b. Modified Bass
    c. Circular
    d. Back and forth

16. What is dental tape?
    a. An oral irrigation dental aid
    b. A flat-type interproximal dental aid
    c. A rounded-type interproximal dental aid
    d. Tape used for removal of calculus

17. What type(s) of dental floss is most effective?
    a. Flavored
    b. Waxed
    c. Unwaxed
    d. b and c

18. What can be used to clean dentures?
    a. Commercial denture cleaner
    b. Mild soap
    c. Dishwashing liquid
    d. All of the above

19. Which of the following is recommended after meals and snacks when toothbrushing and flossing are not possible?
    a. Rinse with mouthwash.
    b. Eat an apple.
    c. Rinse with water.
    d. Run your tongue around your teeth.

20. Fluoride varnish is used with which group of patients?
    a. Children
    b. Patients of any age
    c. Adults
    d. Elderly patients

TOPICS FOR DISCUSSION

When you are working in a dental practice, you will see a wide variety of patients with varying ages, personalities, habits, and oral health issues. You want to provide good preventive oral healthcare. How would you deal with the following situations?

1. A 10-year-old boy does not think he should give up eating sweets all day long.

2. A 62-year-old woman says she cannot floss because of her arthritis.

3. A mother is afraid to allow her children to have a fluoride treatment because she heard that fluoride is poison.

4. A 50-year-old man with poor oral hygiene is also a heavy smoker.

5. A 45-year-old woman who just had a denture placed is wondering how to take care of it.

MULTIMEDIA PROCEDURES RECOMMENDED REVIEW

- Applying Topical Fluoride Gel or Foam
- Flossing Techniques
- Toothbrushing Methods

COMPETENCY 15-1: APPLYING TOPICAL FLUORIDE GEL OR FOAM (EXPANDED FUNCTION)

Performance Objective

By following a routine procedure that meets stated protocols, the student will demonstrate the proper technique for applying a topical fluoride gel or foam.

Evaluation and Grading Criteria

_3_ Student competently met the stated criteria without assistance.
_2_ Student required assistance in order to meet the stated criteria.
_1_ Student showed uncertainty when performing the stated criteria.
_0_ Student was not prepared and needs to repeat the step.
N/A No evaluation of this step.
Instructor shall define grades for each point range earned on completion of each performance-evaluated task.

Performance Standards

The minimum number of satisfactory performances required before final evaluation is _____.

Instructor shall identify by * those steps considered critical. If a step is missed or minimum competency is not met, the evaluated procedure fails and must be repeated.

PERFORMANCE CRITERIA	*	SELF	PEER	INSTRUCTOR	COMMENTS
1. Selected the appropriate tray and other materials.					
2. Personal protective equipment placed according to procedure.					
3. Checked to see if calculus was present; and if so requested it be removed by the hygienist or dentist.					
4. Positioned the patient and provided patient instructions.					
5. Dispensed the appropriate amount of fluoride material into the tray.					
6. Dried the teeth.					
7. Inserted the tray and placed cotton rolls between the arches.					
8. Promptly placed the saliva ejector and tilted the patient's head forward.					
9. Removed the tray without allowing the patient to rinse or swallow.					

Continued

10. Used the saliva ejector or HVE tip to remove excess saliva and solution.				
11. Instructed the patient not to rinse, eat, drink, or brush the teeth for at least 30 minutes.				
12. Procedure documented in patient record.				

ADDITIONAL COMMENT

Total number of points earned _____

Grade _____ Instructor's initials _____

COMPETENCY 15-2: APPLYING FLUORIDE VARNISH (EXPANDED FUNCTION)

Performance Objective

By following a routine procedure that meets stated protocols, the student will competently and effectively apply fluoride varnish on a patient.

Evaluation and Grading Criteria

 3 Student competently met the stated criteria without assistance.
 2 Student required assistance in order to meet the stated criteria.
 1 Student showed uncertainty when performing the stated criteria.
 0 Student was not prepared and needs to repeat the step.
N/A No evaluation of this step.

Instructor shall define grades for each point range earned on completion of each performance-evaluated task.

Performance Standards

The minimum number of satisfactory performances required before final evaluation is _____.

Instructor shall identify by * those steps considered critical. If step is missed or minimum competency is not met, the evaluated procedure fails and must be repeated.

PERFORMANCE CRITERIA	*	SELF	PEER	INSTRUCTOR	COMMENTS
1. Obtained informed consent from the patient, or parent or legal guardian in the case of a minor patient.					
2. Gathered supplies and single unit dose for application.					
3. Personal protective equipment placed according to procedure.					
4. Reclined the patient to an ergonomically correct position.					
5. Wiped the teeth to be varnished with the gauze or cotton roll, and inserted saliva ejector.					
6. Used a cotton-tip applicator, brush, or syringe-style applicator to apply 0.3 to 0.5 mL of varnish (unit dose) to clinical crown of teeth.					
7. Used dental floss as needed to draw the varnish interproximally.					
8. Allowed the patient to rinse after the procedure was completed.					
9. Reminded the patient to avoid eating hard foods, drinking hot or alcoholic beverages, brushing, and flossing for at least 4 to 6 hours, or preferably until the day after the application.					

Continued

10. Reminded the patient to drink through a straw for the first few hours after application.					
11. Procedure documented in patient record.					

ADDITIONAL COMMENT

Total number of points earned: _____

Grade _____ Instructor's initials _____

COMPETENCY 15-3: ASSISTING THE PATIENT WITH DENTAL FLOSS (EXPANDED FUNCTION)

Performance Objective

By following a routine procedure that meets stated protocols, the student will demonstrate the proper technique for assisting a patient in learning how to use dental floss.

Evaluation and Grading Criteria

__3__   Student competently met the stated criteria without assistance.

__2__   Student required assistance in order to meet the stated criteria.

__1__   Student showed uncertainty when performing the stated criteria.

__0__   Student was not prepared and needs to repeat the step.

__N/A__   No evaluation of this step.

Instructor shall define grades for each point range earned on completion of each performance-evaluated task.

Performance Standards

The minimum number of satisfactory performances required before final evaluation is _____.

Instructor shall identify by * those steps considered critical. If step is missed or minimum competency is not met, the evaluated procedure fails and must be repeated.

PERFORMANCE CRITERIA	*	SELF	PEER	INSTRUCTOR	COMMENTS
1. Dispensed the appropriate amount of dental floss; wrapped the excess around middle or index fingures.					
2. Stretched the floss tightly between the fingers, and used the thumb and index finger to guide the floss into place.					
3. Held the floss tightly between the thumb and forefinger of each hand.					
4. Passed the floss gently between the teeth using a sawing motion. Guided the floss to the gumline.					
5. Curved the floss into a C-shape against each tooth, and wiped up and down against tooth surfaces.					
6. Repeated these steps on each side of all teeth in both arches.					
7. Moved a fresh piece of floss into the working position as the floss became frayed or soiled.					
8. Used a bridge threader to floss under any fixed bridges.					

Continued

9. Procedure accurately documented in the patient record.					
ADDITIONAL COMMENT					

Total number of points earned _____

Grade _____ Instructor's initials _____

16 Nutrition

SHORT-ANSWER QUESTIONS

1. What are the goals of the Healthy People 2020 report, and why are they important?

2. Explain how diet and nutrition can affect oral conditions.

3. Explain why the study of nutrition is important to the dental assistant.

4. List the five areas of the MyPlate food guide.

5. Describe the difference between recommended dietary allowance (RDA) and Dietary Reference Intake (DRI).

6. Describe the difference between vitamins and minerals.

7. Describe the role and sources of carbohydrates in the daily diet.

8. Explain the need for minerals in the diet.

9. Describe the types of eating disorders.

10. Explain how to interpret food labels.

11. Discuss the requirement for labeling food products.

12. Explain the criteria that must be met for a food to be considered "organic."

13. What foods are considered to be cariogenic?

14. Name several sources of antioxidants.

FILL-IN-THE-BLANK STATEMENTS

Select the best term from the list below and complete the following statements.

amino acids   nutrients
anorexia nervosa   organic
bulimia   MyPlate

1. Compounds in proteins used by the body to build and repair tissue are _____.

2. _____ is an eating disorder that is caused by an altered self-image.

3. An eating disorder characterized by binge eating and self-induced vomiting is _____.

4. _____ are organic and inorganic chemicals in food that supply energy.

5. Food products that have been grown without the use of any chemical pesticides, herbicides, or fertilizers are labeled as _____.

6. The current nutrition guide published by the United States Department of Agriculture is the _____.

MULTIPLE-CHOICE QUESTIONS

Complete each question by circling the best answer.

1. Nutrients provide a body _____.
   a. growth
   b. energy
   c. maintenance
   d. all of the above

2. The three types of carbohydrates are simple sugars, complex carbohydrates, and _____.
   a. fats
   b. proteins
   c. dietary fiber
   d. water

3. The term used for a food that is capable of causing tooth decay is _____.
   a. nutrient
   b. cariogenic
   c. vitamin
   d. sugar

4. What key nutrients help build and repair the human body?
   a. Fats
   b. Vitamins
   c. Minerals
   d. Proteins

5. How many of the amino acids are essential?
   a. 2
   b. 4
   c. 8
   d. 12

6. Sources of proteins are _____.
   a. breads
   b. nuts
   c. pasta
   d. apples

7. Which systemic disease is related to having too much fat in the diet?
   a. Cardiovascular disease
   b. Allergies
   c. Multiple sclerosis
   d. Parkinson's disease

8. Which cholesterol is the "good cholesterol"?
   a. HDL
   b. LDL
   c. DDS
   d. ADA

9. Which vitamins are not destroyed by cooking and are stored in the body?
   a. Organic vitamins
   b. Water-soluble vitamins
   c. Fat-soluble vitamins
   d. Inorganic vitamins

10. Which vitamins are referred to as the *B-complex vitamins?*
    a. Organic vitamins
    b. Water-soluble vitamins
    c. Fat-soluble vitamins
    d. Inorganic vitamins

11. Which vitamin is fat soluble?
    a. Calcium
    b. Riboflavin
    c. Vitamin D
    d. Magnesium

12. Which vitamin is water soluble?
    a. Vitamin A
    b. Vitamin C
    c. Vitamin D
    d. Vitamin K

13. Which nutrient is often called "the forgotten nutrient"?
    a. Calcium
    b. Vitamin C
    c. Iron
    d. Water

14. Which governmental agency regulates the labeling of food products?
    a. FDA
    b. USDA
    c. ADA
    d. OSHA

15. What criteria are used to determine whether a product is "organic"?
    a. Grown without the use of chemical pesticides
    b. Grown without the use of herbicides
    c. Grown without the use of fertilizers
    d. All of the above

16. What eating disorder is diagnosed when people starve themselves?
    a. Anorexia nervosa
    b. Fasting
    c. Bulimia
    d. Dieting

TOPICS FOR DISCUSSION

As a healthcare provider, you are involved in educating your patients about many health issues. Nutrition is one area that cannot be ignored. Not only will lack of proper nutrition contribute to poor health, but it can also contribute to dental disease. Obesity in children has become an epidemic in today's society.

1. What do you think contributes to children's being overweight?

2. Describe a commercial that contributes to children's wanting to eat more.

3. Is there one eating habit that contributes to children's being overweight?

4. What should be the role of the dental team in educating families and their children?

5. How can poor nutrition habits affect a person's oral health?

Mrs. Diane Hernandez is an active 76-year-old woman. Because she is on a fixed income, her diet is lacking in dairy products, fruits, and vegetables. She tends to eat soft foods that consist mainly of simple carbohydrates. She also enjoys between-meal snacks, also high in carbohydrates.

1. What types of between-meal snacks would be healthy alternatives?

2. How could she increase her intake of dairy products, fruits, and vegetables and stay within her budget?

Oral Pathology

SHORT-ANSWER QUESTIONS

1. Explain why the dental assistant needs to study oral pathology.

2. List and define the categories of diagnostic information.

3. Describe the warning signs of oral cancer.

4. Describe the types of oral lesions.

5. Name the five lesions associated with HIV/AIDS.

6. Describe the appearance of lesions associated with the use of smokeless tobacco.

7. Differentiate between chronic and acute inflammation.

8. Identify two oral conditions related to nutritional factors.

9. Recognize developmental disorders of the dentition.

10. List and define three anomalies that affect the number of teeth.

11. List and define five anomalies that affect the shape of teeth.

12. Define, describe, and identify the developmental anomalies discussed in this chapter.

13. Describe the oral conditions of a patient with bulimia.

Select the best term from the list below and complete the following statements.

abscess
biopsy
candidiasis
carcinoma
cellulitis
congenital disorder
cyst
ecchymosis
erosion
glossitis
granuloma

hematoma
lesion
leukemia
leukoplakia
lichen planus
metastasize
meth mouth
pathology
sarcoma
xerostomia

1. _____ is the study of disease.

2. A pathologic site is considered a(n) _____.

3. _____ is the wearing away of tissue.

4. A(n) _____ is a closed cell or pouch with a definite wall.

5. A(n) _____ is a localized collection of pus anywhere in the body.

6. A swelling or mass of blood collected in one area or organ is a(n) _____.

7. _____ is the medical term for bruising.

8. A granular tumor or growth is a _____.

9. _____ is the formation of white spots or patches on the mucosa.

10. A benign, chronic disease that affects the skin and oral mucosa is _____.

11. _____ is a superficial infection that is caused by a yeastlike fungus.

12. _____ is the inflammation of cellular or connective tissue.

13. _____ is a general term used to describe inflammation of the tongue.

14. _____ is a malignant tumor in epithelial tissue.

15. _____ is a malignant tumor in connective tissue such as muscle or bone.

16. A malignant disease of the blood-forming organs is _____.

17. _____ is dryness of the mouth caused by reduction of saliva.

18. A disorder that is present at birth is a(n) _____.

19. A(n) _____ is the removal of tissue from living patients for diagnostic examination.

20. _____ is the spreading of disease from one part of the body to another.

21. _____ is the term for the advanced tooth decay caused by the heavy use of methamphetamine.

MULTIPLE-CHOICE QUESTIONS

Complete each question by circling the best answer.

1. What types of lesions are below the surface?
   a. Ulcers
   b. Plaque
   c. Blisters
   d. Bruises

2. What types of lesions are above the surface?
   a. Ulcers
   b. Cysts
   c. Blisters
   d. Bruises

3. What types of lesions are even with the surface?
   a. Ulcers
   b. Cysts
   c. Plaque
   d. Bruises

4. What condition appears as a white patch or area?
   a. Ulcer
   b. Candidiasis
   c. Leukoplakia
   d. Blister

5. What condition results from an infection caused by a yeastlike fungus?
   a. Plaque
   b. Ulcer
   c. Leukoplakia
   d. Candidiasis

6. What is another term for "canker sore"?
   a. Aphthous ulcer
   b. Cellulitis
   c. Leukoplakia
   d. Plaque

7. What is the condition in which inflammation causes severe pain and high fever?
   a. Glossitis
   b. Cellulitis
   c. Bruxism
   d. Candidiasis

8. What is the term for inflammation of the tongue?
   a. Aphthous ulcer
   b. Bruxism
   c. Glossitis
   d. Cellulitis

9. What is the condition in which a pattern on the tongue changes?
   a. Pseudomembranosus
   b. Candidiasis
   c. Glossitis
   d. Geographic tongue

10. What is the condition in which the body does not absorb vitamin B_{12}?
    a. Pernicious anemia
    b. Leukemia
    c. Periodontitis
    d. AIDS

11. What type of cancer affects the blood-forming organs?
    a. Carcinoma
    b. Sarcoma
    c. Leukemia
    d. Lymphoma

12. What is a common precancerous lesion among users of smokeless tobacco?
    a. Carcinoma
    b. Leukoplakia
    c. Lymphoma
    d. Leukemia

13. What is the term for a malignant lesion in the epithelial tissue of the oral cavity?
    a. Gingivitis
    b. Lymphoma
    c. Carcinoma
    d. Leukoplakia

14. What causes radiation caries?
    a. Heat
    b. Harmful rays
    c. Cold
    d. Lack of saliva

15. What is the condition frequently seen on the lateral border of the tongue of patients with HIV/AIDS?
    a. Hairy leukoplakia
    b. Kaposi's sarcoma
    c. Lymphadenopathy
    d. Herpes labialis

16. What opportunistic infection is seen as purplish-colored lesions on the skin or oral mucosa of patients with HIV/AIDS?
    a. Leukoplakia
    b. Kaposi's sarcoma
    c. Lymphadenopathy
    d. Herpes labialis

17. What is the malignant condition that involves the lymph nodes of patients with HIV/AIDS?
    a. Leukoplakia
    b. Kaposi's sarcoma
    c. Lymphadenopathy
    d. Herpes labialis

18. What is the term for abnormally large jaws?
    a. Macrognathia
    b. Micrognathia
    c. Lymphoma
    d. Trismus

19. What is the name for bony growths in the palate?
    a. Periodontitis
    b. Candidiasis
    c. Hyperplasia
    d. Torus palatinus

20. What is a more common term for ankyloglossia?
    a. Lisp
    b. Cleft palate
    c. Tongue-tie
    d. Warts

21. What is the dental term for "tooth within a tooth"?
    a. Macrognathia
    b. Dens in dente
    c. Torus
    d. Exostosis

22. What is the term used for abnormally small teeth?
    a. Anodontia
    b. Microdontia
    c. Supernumerary teeth
    d. Gemination

23. What term is used to describe two teeth joining together?
    a. Macrodontia
    b. Dens in dente
    c. Twinning
    d. Fusion

24. Name the hereditary abnormality in which there are hypoplasia-type defects in the enamel formation.
    a. Anodontia
    b. Ameloblastoma
    c. Amelogenesis imperfecta
    d. Dentinogenesis imperfecta

25. Which of the following is a potential complication of oral-facial piercing?
    a. Infection
    b. Chipped teeth
    c. Broken teeth
    d. All of the above

26. What factor(s) can cause meth mouth?
    a. Consumption of sugary soft drinks
    b. Lack of saliva caused by the drug
    c. Clenching and grinding of the teeth
    d. a and c
    e. All of the above

CASE STUDY

Tom Evans, one of your long time patients, just discovered a large bump on his palate. He points to a torus palatinus. He is certain that it just appeared. However, you notice on Tom's chart a notation that he has a large torus palatinus. How do you respond to Tom when he asks you these questions?

1. Could it be from something I ate?

2. Could it be caused by stress?

3. Is it harmful?

4. Why did it just appear?

18 Microbiology

SHORT-ANSWER QUESTIONS

1. Name the contributions of the early pioneers in microbiology.

2. Explain why the study of microbiology is important for the dental assistant.

3. Identify the types of bacteria according to their shape.

4. List the major groups of microorganisms.

5. Describe the differences among aerobes, anaerobes, and facultative anaerobes.

6. Identify diseases caused by *Chlamydia*.

7. Identify the most resistant forms of life known, and explain how they survive.

8. Discuss specificity in relation to viruses.

9. Compare viruses with bacteria, and name diseases caused by each.

10. Describe how prions differ from viruses and bacteria.

11. Name two diseases caused by prions.

12. Explain how West Nile virus is spread.

13. Explain how the H1N1 virus is spread.

14. Explain how each type of hepatitis is transmitted.

15. Describe the effects of HIV on the immune system.

16. Identify the methods of HIV transmission.

17. Identify the method of transmission of methicillin-resistant *Staphylococcus aureus* (MRSA) and describe its characteristics.

FILL-IN-THE-BLANK STATEMENTS

Select the best term from the list below and complete the following statements.

aerobes	**nonpathogenic**
anaerobes	**oral candidiasis**
Creutzfeldt-Jakob disease	**pathogenic**
facultative anaerobes	**prions**
H1N1 flu virus	**protozoa**
HAV	**provirus**
HBV	**spore**
microbiology	**virulent**
MRSA	**West Nile virus**

1. The study of microorganisms is _____.

2. Disease-producing microorganisms are termed _____.

3. _____ are non–disease-producing microorganisms.

4. _____ is capable of causing a serious disease.

5. _____ are a variety of bacteria that require oxygen to grow.

6. Bacteria that grow in the absence of oxygen and are destroyed by oxygen are _____.

7. Organisms that can grow in the presence or the absence of oxygen are _____.

8. A(n) _____ is a single-celled microscopic animal without a rigid cell wall.

9. A(n) _____ is a hidden virus during the latency period.

10. Very tiny infectious agents that do not contain DNA or RNA are _____.

11. Some bacteria can change into a highly resistant form called _____.

80

12. _____ is a rare chronic brain disease with onset in middle to late life (40 to 60 years).

13. _____ is a yeast infection of the oral mucosa.

14. _____ is a virus necessary for co-infection with HDV.

15. _____ is a virus that is spread by the fecal-oral route.

16. _____ is spread by mosquitoes.

17. _____ is a virus caused by A type viruses.

18. _____ is a bacterium that is resistant to some antibiotics.

MULTIPLE-CHOICE QUESTIONS

Complete each question by circling the best answer.

1. Why is microbiology important to the dental assistant?
   a. The dental assistant learns how to use a microscope.
   b. The dental assistant gains an enhanced understanding of infection control.
   c. The dental assistant better understands higher-level science courses.
   d. The dental assistant learns about the background of dental materials.

2. Who is referred to as the Father of Microbiology?
   a. Pierre Fauchard
   b. Joseph Lister
   c. Louis Pasteur
   d. G.V. Black

3. Who was the first to record that microorganisms were responsible for hospital-acquired infections?
   a. Pierre Fauchard
   b. Joseph Lister
   c. Louis Pasteur
   d. Lucy Hobbs

4. Who is credited for discovering the rabies vaccine?
   a. Pierre Fauchard
   b. Joseph Lister
   c. Louis Pasteur
   d. G.V. Black

5. Which is a primary shape of bacteria?
   a. Circular
   b. Bacillus-like
   c. Spiral
   d. All of the above

6. What is the name of the staining process for separating bacteria?
   a. Pathology test
   b. Biopsy
   c. Scratch test
   d. Gram test

7. What is the term for bacteria that require oxygen to grow?
   a. Aerobes
   b. Anaerobes
   c. Aerated
   d. Aerial

8. What is the most resistant form of bacterial life?
   a. Rickettsiae
   b. Viruses
   c. Spores
   d. Fungi

9. How are prions different from other microorganisms?
   a. They contain only fat and one nucleic acid.
   b. They contain only protein and no nucleic acids.
   c. They contain no protein and only nucleic acids.
   d. They contain only carbohydrates and no phosphoric acids.

10. Bacteria cause which of the following oral diseases?
    a. Dental caries
    b. Periodontal disease
    c. Malocclusion
    d. Both a and b

11. Which of the following forms of hepatitis is blood-borne?
    a. Hepatitis C
    b. Hepatitis D
    c. Hepatitis B
    d. All of the above

12. Pontiac fever is a type of which disease?
    a. Tuberculosis
    b. Legionnaires' disease
    c. HIV
    d. Herpes simplex

13. Bacteria cause which of the following diseases?
    a. Tetanus
    b. Syphilis
    c. Tuberculosis
    d. All of the above

14. The first oral indicator of syphilis is _____.
    a. a cold sore
    b. inflamed gingivae
    c. a chancre
    d. all of the above

15. Herpes simplex type 2 is also known as _____.
    a. genital herpes
    b. oral herpes
    c. chickenpox
    d. all of the above

TOPICS FOR DISCUSSION

Newspaper headlines and announcements at your school state that a severe case of influenza virus is going around. Your younger sister is concerned and asks you the following questions. How do you answer her?

1. Why can't everyone take an antibiotic and not get sick?

2. Why do we have to get a different flu vaccination every year?

3. Why can't doctors make one extra strong vaccination?

4. How is the influenza virus spread?

19 Disease Transmission and Infection Prevention

SHORT-ANSWER QUESTIONS

1. Describe the roles of the CDC and OSHA in infection control.

2. Explain the difference between Universal Precautions and Standard Precautions.

3. Describe the differences between a chronic infection and an acute infection.

4. Describe the types of immunities, and give examples of each.

5. Give an example of a latent infection.

6. Identify the links in the chain of infection.

7. Describe the methods of disease transmission in a dental office.

8. Describe the infection control considerations for use of high-tech equipment.

9. Describe the components of an OSHA Exposure Control Plan.

10. Explain the rationale for Standard Precautions.

11. Identify the OSHA categories of risk for occupational exposure.

12. Describe the first aid necessary after an exposure incident.

13. Discuss the rationale for hepatitis B vaccination for dental assistants.

14. Explain the importance of hand care for dental assistants.

15. Explain proper hand hygiene for dental assistants.

16. Explain the advantages of alcohol-based hand rubs.

17. Discuss the types of personal protective equipment (PPE) needed for dental assistants.

18. Demonstrate the proper sequence for donning and removal of PPE.

19. Identify the various types of gloves used in a dental office.

20. Explain the types and symptoms of latex reactions.

21. Describe the proper handling and disposal methods for each type of waste generated in dentistry.

22. Explain the CDC recommendations regarding the use of a saliva ejector.

23. Describe the rationale for the CDC recommendations regarding Creutzfeldt-Jakob disease and other prion-related diseases.

24. Describe the rationale for the CDC recommendations regarding laser plumes.

25. Explain the precautions necessary when one is treating a patient with active tuberculosis.

FILL-IN-THE-BLANK STATEMENTS

Select the best term from the list below and complete the following statements.

acquired immunity
acute infection
anaphylaxis
artificially acquired immunity
chronic infection
communicable diseases

contaminated waste
direct contact
droplet infection
hazardous waste
indirect contact
infection prevention

infectious waste
inherited immunity
latent infection
natural acquired immunity
occupational exposure
OSHA Blood-borne Pathogens Standard

percutaneous
permucosal
personal protective equipment
sharps
Standard Precautions

1. A(n) _____ is a persistent infection in which the symptoms come and go.

2. A(n) _____ has symptoms that are quite severe and of short duration.

3. An infection of long duration is called a(n) _____.

4. The _____ is designed to protect employees against occupational exposure to blood-borne pathogens.

5. _____ is touching or contact with a patient's blood or saliva.

6. _____ is touching or contact with a contaminated surface or instrument.

7. A(n) _____ exposure enters the mucosal surfaces of the eyes, nose, or mouth.

8. A(n) _____ exposure enters through the skin, such as through needle sticks, cuts, and human bites.

9. A(n) _____ exposure contacts mucous membranes, such as the eye or the mouth.

10. _____ is any reasonably anticipated skin, eye, or mucous membrane contact, or percutaneous injury with blood or any other potentially infectious materials, that occurs during work hours.

11. _____ is a standard of care that is designed to protect healthcare providers from pathogens that can be spread by blood or any other body fluid, excretion, or secretion.

12. Items such as protective clothing, masks, gloves, and eyewear to protect employees are considered _____.

13. _____ is waste that presents a danger to humans or to the environment.

14. _____ is waste that is capable of transmitting an infectious disease.

15. Contaminated needles, scalpel blades, orthodontic wires, and endodontic instruments are considered _____.

16. _____ are contaminated items that may contain the body fluids of patients, such as gloves and patient napkins.

17. The most severe form of immediate allergic reaction is _____.

18. Infections that can be spread from another person or through contact with body fluids are called _____.

19. _____ is immunity that is present at birth.

20. _____ is immunity that develops during a person's lifetime.

21. _____ occurs when a person has contracted and is recovering from a disease.

22. _____ occurs as the result of a vaccination.

23. _____ is the ultimate goal of all infection control procedures and policies.

MULTIPLE-CHOICE QUESTIONS

Complete each question by circling the best answer.

1. What is the most common route of contamination?
   a. Air
   b. Direct contact
   c. Water
   d. Indirect contact

2. The term for acquiring an infection through mucosal tissues is

   _____.
   a. airborne
   b. spatter
   c. droplet infection
   d. parenteral

3. What infection control measures help prevent disease transmission from the dental team to the patient?
   a. Gloves
   b. Handwashing
   c. Masks
   d. All of the above

4. The purpose of the OSHA Blood-borne Pathogens

   Standard is to _____.
   a. protect patients
   b. protect the community
   c. protect employees
   d. protect the Red Cross

5. How often must the Exposure Control Plan be reviewed and updated?
   a. Weekly
   b. Monthly
   c. Bimonthly
   d. Annually

6. Standard Precautions are used to _____.
   a. protect healthcare providers from pathogens that can be spread by blood or any other body fluid, excretion, or secretion
   b. perform specific steps in instrument processing
   c. treat only patients without disease
   d. follow a specific routine in sterilization

7. What agency has recently released infection control guidelines?
   a. Centers for Disease Control and Prevention (CDC)
   b. Occupational Safety and Health Administration (OSHA)
   c. U.S. Food and Drug Administration (FDA)
   d. Environmental Protection Agency (EPA)

8. Which of the following statements about latex allergies is TRUE?
   a. The primary cause of death associated with latex allergies is anaphylaxis.
   b. There is no specific cure for latex allergies.
   c. Persons who suspect they have a latex allergy should see a physician.
   d. All of the above

9. Irritant dermatitis does not involve the immune system.
   a. True
   b. False

10. What must an employee do if he or she does not want the hepatitis B vaccine?
    a. Get a signature from his or her personal doctor.
    b. Sign an informed refusal form.
    c. Have a contract drawn up by his or her lawyer.
    d. All of the above

11. Long, artificial nails and rings should be avoided when one is working in a dental office because

    _____.
    a. they can stab/scratch a patient
    b. they can harbor pathogens
    c. they can contaminate items
    d. All of the above

12. An example of PPE is _____.
    a. a dental dam
    b. gloves
    c. a patient napkin
    d. a suction tip

13. What determines the type of PPE that should be worn?
    a. Risk of exposure
    b. Time of day
    c. Whether an advanced function is being performed
    d. Whether a patient has been premedicated

14. An example of protective eyewear is

_____.
    a. contact lenses
    b. sunglasses
    c. side shields
    d. a magnifying glass

15. What is perhaps the most critical piece of PPE?
    a. Eyewear
    b. Mask
    c. Protective clothing
    d. Gloves

16. Sterile gloves are most commonly worn for a

_____.
    a. prosthodontic procedure
    b. orthodontic procedure
    c. surgical procedure
    d. pediatric procedure

17. When should utility gloves be worn?
    a. When taking out the trash
    b. When disinfecting the treatment area
    c. When preparing instruments for sterilization
    d. b and c

18. What type of gloves should be worn to open drawers during a dental procedure?
    a. Sterile gloves
    b. Overgloves
    c. Powder-free latex gloves
    d. Utility gloves

19. An example of contaminated waste is _____.
    a. patient napkins
    b. paper towels
    c. used barriers
    d. a and c

20. Another term for infectious waste is _____.
    a. contaminated waste
    b. disposable waste
    c. regulated waste
    d. general waste

CASE STUDY

Sheila is a dental assistant in your office who has been in the profession for 15 years. She constantly neglects to wear PPE when working in the laboratory and when breaking down and disinfecting treatment rooms. Sheila says that she never wore PPE during her first 15 years as a dental assistant and she did not get any diseases.

1. Why should Sheila start wearing PPE when she didn't wear any for 15 years?

2. Why has dentistry made such a change in its standards?

3. What type of PPE should you wear when working in the laboratory?

4. What type of PPE should you wear when breaking down and disinfecting a treatment room?

5. How should the dentist handle this situation with Sheila?

MULTIMEDIA PROCEDURES RECOMMENDED REVIEW

■ Handwashing Techniques

COMPETENCY 19-1: APPLYING FIRST AID AFTER AN EXPOSURE INCIDENT

Performance Objective

By following a routine procedure that meets stated protocols, the student will role-play the proper technique for administering first aid after an exposure incident.

Evaluation and Grading Criteria

3   Student competently met the stated criteria without assistance.
2   Student required assistance in order to meet the stated criteria.
1   Student showed uncertainty when performing the stated criteria.
0   Student was not prepared and needs to repeat the step.
N/A   No evaluation of this step.

Performance Standards

The minimum number of satisfactory performances required before final evaluation is _____.

Instructor shall identify by * those steps considered critical. If step is missed or minimum competency is not met, the evaluated procedure fails and must be repeated.

PERFORMANCE CRITERIA	*	SELF	PEER	INSTRUCTOR	COMMENTS
1. Stopped operations immediately.					
2. Removed gloves.					
3. If the area of broken skin was bleeding, gently squeezed the site to express a small amount of visible blood.					
4. Washed hands thoroughly, using antimicrobial soap and warm water.					
5. Dried hands.					
6. Applied a small amount of antiseptic to the affected area.					
7. Applied an adhesive bandage to the area.					
8. Completed applicable postexposure follow-up steps.					
9. Notified the employer of the injury immediately after first aid was provided.					

ADDITIONAL COMMENTS

Total number of points earned _____

Grade_____   Instructor's initials _____

COMPETENCY 19-2: HANDWASHING BEFORE GLOVING

Performance Objective
The student will demonstrate the proper technique for handwashing before gloving.

Evaluation and Grading Criteria
 3   Student competently met the stated criteria without assistance.
 2   Student required assistance in order to meet the stated criteria.
 1   Student showed uncertainty when performing the stated criteria.
 0   Student was not prepared and needs to repeat the step.
 N/A   No evaluation of this step.

Performance Standards
The minimum number of satisfactory performances required before final evaluation is _____.

Instructor shall identify by * those steps considered critical. If step is missed or minimum competency is not met, the evaluated procedure fails and must be repeated.

PERFORMANCE CRITERIA	*	SELF	PEER	INSTRUCTOR	COMMENTS
1. Removed all jewelry, including watch and rings.					
2. Used the foot or electronic control to regulate the flow of water. (If this was not available, used a paper towel to grasp the faucets to turn them on and off. Discarded the towel after use.)					
3. Used liquid soap, dispensed with a foot-activated or electronic device.					
4. Vigorously rubbed lathered hands together under a stream of water to remove surface debris.					
5. Dispensed additional soap, and vigorously rubbed lathered hands together for a minimum of 10 seconds under a stream of water.					
6. Rinsed the hands with cool water.					
7. Used a paper towel to thoroughly dry the hands and then the forearms.					
ADDITIONAL COMMENTS					

Total number of points earned _____

Grade_____ Instructor's initials _____

COMPETENCY 19-3: APPLYING AN ALCOHOL-BASED HAND RUB

Performance Objective

The student will demonstrate the proper technique for applying an alcohol-based hand rub.

Evaluation and Grading Criteria

3   Student competently met the stated criteria without assistance.
2   Student required assistance in order to meet the stated criteria.
1   Student showed uncertainty when performing the stated criteria.
0   Student was not prepared and needs to repeat the step.
N/A   No evaluation of this step.

Performance Standards

The minimum number of satisfactory performances required before final evaluation is _____.

Instructor shall identify by * those steps considered critical. If step is missed or minimum competency is not met, the evaluated procedure fails and must be repeated.

PERFORMANCE CRITERIA	*	SELF	PEER	INSTRUCTOR	COMMENTS
1. Washed and dried hands thoroughly with soap and water if they were visibly soiled or contaminated with organic matter.					
2. Read the directions carefully to determine the proper amount of product to dispense.					
3. Dispensed the proper amount of the product into the palm of one hand.					
4. Rubbed the palms of the hands together.					
5. Rubbed the product in between the fingers.					
6. Rubbed the product over the backs of the hands.					
ADDITIONAL COMMENTS					

Total number of points earned _____

Grade _____ Instructor's initials _____

Chapter **19** Disease Transmission and Infection Prevention

COMPETENCY 19-4: PUTTING ON PERSONAL PROTECTIVE EQUIPMENT

Performance Objective
The student will demonstrate the proper technique for putting on personal protective equipment prior to providing patient care.

Evaluation and Grading Criteria
<u>3</u>   Student competently met the stated criteria without assistance.
<u>2</u>   Student required assistance in order to meet the stated criteria.
<u>1</u>   Student showed uncertainty when performing the stated criteria.
<u>0</u>   Student was not prepared and needs to repeat the step.
<u>N/A</u>   No evaluation of this step.

Performance Standards
The minimum number of satisfactory performances required before final evaluation is _____.

Instructor shall identify by * those steps considered critical. If step is missed or minimum competency is not met, the evaluated procedure fails and must be repeated.

PERFORMANCE CRITERIA	*	SELF	PEER	INSTRUCTOR	COMMENTS
1. Put on protective clothing over the uniform, street clothes, or scrubs.					
2. Put on a surgical mask and adjusted the fit.					
3. Put on protective eyewear.					
4. Thoroughly washed and dried the hands. (If hands were not visibly soiled, used an alcohol-based hand rub.)					
5. Held one glove at the cuff, placed the opposite hand inside the glove, and pulled it onto the hand. Repeated the procedure with a new glove for the other hand.					

Note: The sequence of 2 and 3 may be interchangeable. Most important is that the gloves are put on last to avoid contaminating them before they are placed in the patient's mouth.

ADDITIONAL COMMENTS

Total number of points earned _____

Grade_____ Instructor's initials _____

COMPETENCY 19-5: REMOVING PERSONAL PROTECTIVE EQUIPMENT

Performance Objective

By following a routine procedure that meets stated protocols, the student will demonstrate the proper technique for removing personal protective equipment.

Evaluation and Grading Criteria

3   Student competently met the stated criteria without assistance.
2   Student required assistance in order to meet the stated criteria.
1   Student showed uncertainty when performing the stated criteria.
0   Student was not prepared and needs to repeat the step.
N/A   No evaluation of this step.

Instructor shall define grades for each point range earned on completion of each performance-evaluated task.

Performance Standards

The minimum number of satisfactory performances required before final evaluation is _____.

Instructor shall identify by * those steps considered critical. If step is missed or minimum competency is not met, the evaluated procedure fails and must be repeated.

PERFORMANCE CRITERIA	*	SELF	PEER	INSTRUCTOR	COMMENTS
Gloves					
1. Used a gloved hand to grasp the opposite glove at the outside cuff. Pulled downward, turning the glove inside out while pulling it away from the hand.					
2. For the other hand, used ungloved fingers to grasp the inside (uncontaminated area) of the cuff of the remaining glove. Pulled downward to remove the glove, turning it inside out.					
3. Discarded the gloves into the waste receptacle.					
4. Washed and thoroughly dried hands. *Note:* If no visible contamination exists and if gloves have not been torn or punctured during the procedure, an alcohol-based hand rub may be used in place of handwashing.					

Continued

Chapter **19 Disease Transmission and Infection Prevention**

Eyewear					
5. Removed the eyewear by touching it only on the ear rests.					
6. Placed the eyewear on a disposable towel for proper cleaning and disinfecting.					
Masks					
7. Slid fingers on each hand under the elastic strap in front of ears and removed the mask, ensuring that fingers contacted only the mask's ties or elastic strap.					
8. Discarded the mask into the waste receptacle.					
Protective Clothing					
9. Pulled the gown off, turning it inside out during removal.					
10. Ensured that the contaminated outside surface of the gown did not touch underlying clothes or skin during removal.					

Total number of points earned _____

Grade _____ Instructor's initials _____

COMPETENCY 19-6: DISINFECTING AN ALGINATE IMPRESSION

Performance Objective
By following a routine procedure that meets stated protocols, the student will demonstrate the proper technique for disinfecting an alginate impression.

Evaluation and Grading Criteria
3   Student competently met the stated criteria without assistance.
2   Student required assistance in order to meet the stated criteria.
1   Student showed uncertainty when performing the stated criteria.
0   Student was not prepared and needs to repeat the step.
N/A   No evaluation of this step.
Note: Disinfecting applies to many aspects of dental care.
Instructor shall define grades for each point range earned on completion of each performance-evaluated task.

Performance Standards
The minimum number of satisfactory performances required before final evaluation is _____.

Instructor shall identify by * those steps considered critical. If step is missed or minimum competency is not met, the evaluated procedure fails and must be repeated.

PERFORMANCE CRITERIA	*	SELF	PEER	INSTRUCTOR	COMMENTS
1. Rinsed the impression to clean it and removed excess water.					
2. Personal protective equipment placed according to procedure.					
3. Disinfected the impression using an intermediate-level hospital disinfectant.					
a. If spraying technique used, impression sprayed thoroughly and wrapped in moist paper towel for recommended time.					
b. If immersion technique used, impression immersed in disinfectant and removed after recommended contact time.					
4. Impression rinsed under tap water to remove residual disinfectant.					
5. Impression shaken to remove excess water.					
ADDITIONAL COMMENTS					

Total number of points earned _____

Grade _____   Instructor's initials _____

20 Principles and Techniques of Disinfection

SHORT-ANSWER QUESTIONS

1. Explain why dental treatment room surfaces need barriers or disinfection.

2. List the types of surfaces in the dental office that are commonly covered with barriers.

3. Describe two methods for dealing with surface contamination.

4. Explain the differences between disinfection and sterilization.

5. Explain the differences between a disinfectant and an antiseptic.

6. Name the government agency that is responsible for registering disinfectants.

7. Identify chemical products commonly used for intermediate- and low-level surface disinfection, and explain the advantages and disadvantages of each.

8. Explain the process of cleaning and disinfecting a treatment room.

9. Describe the process of precleaning contaminated dental instruments.

10. Explain the precautions that should be taken when one is using chemical sterilants or disinfectants.

11. Describe the CDC Guidelines for disinfecting clinical contact surfaces.

12. Describe the CDC Guidelines for disinfecting housekeeping surfaces.

FILL-IN-THE-BLANK STATEMENTS

Select the best term from the list below and complete the following statements.

bioburden
broad-spectrum
chlorine dioxide
disinfectant
greener infection control
glutaraldehyde
intermediate-level disinfectant
iodophor

low-level disinfectant
precleaning
residual activity
splash, spatter, and droplet surfaces
surface barrier
synthetic phenol compound
transfer surfaces
tuberculocidal

1. A(n) _____ is a fluid-impervious material that is used to cover surfaces that are likely to become contaminated.

2. _____ are surfaces that are not directly touched but often are touched by contaminated instruments.

3. _____ are surfaces that do not contact the members of the dental team or the contaminated instruments or supplies.

4. _____ is the removal of bioburden before disinfection.

5. A chemical to reduce or lower the number of microorganisms is a(n) _____.

6. _____ is the action that continues long after initial application.

7. Blood, saliva, and other body fluids are considered _____.

8. A(n) _____ agent is capable of inactivating *Mycobacterium tuberculosis.*

9. A disinfectant that is capable of killing a wide range of microbes is labeled _____.

10. An EPA-registered intermediate-level hospital disinfectant is an _____.

11. A(n) _____ is an EPA-registered intermediate-level hospital disinfectant with broad-spectrum disinfecting action.

12. _____ is classified as a high-level disinfectant or sterilant.

13. _____ is an effective rapid-acting environmental surface disinfectant or chemical sterilant.

14. A(n) _____ destroys *M. tuberculosis,* viruses, fungi, and vegetative bacteria and is used for disinfecting dental operatory surfaces.

15. A(n) _____ destroys certain viruses and fungi and can be used for general housecleaning purposes (e.g., walls, floors).

16. Minimizing the environmental impact of infection control products and procedures is called _____.

MULTIPLE-CHOICE QUESTIONS

Complete each question by circling the best answer.

1. Why must surfaces in dental treatment rooms be disinfected or protected with barriers?
   a. To prevent you from injuring yourself
   b. To prevent patient-to-patient transmission of microorganisms
   c. To prevent dentist-to-patient transmission of microorganisms
   d. To prevent hygienist-to-assistant transmission of microorganisms

2. Which of the following is used to prevent surface contamination?
   a. Sterilization
   b. Disinfection
   c. Barriers
   d. b and c

3. What is the purpose of surface barriers?
   a. To prevent cross-contamination
   b. To protect surfaces from dental materials
   c. To cover the instruments
   d. To keep water from touching the unit

4. What should you do if a barrier becomes torn?
   a. Tape it.
   b. Replace it.
   c. Clean and disinfect the surface under the barrier.
   d. b and c

5. Which regulatory agency requires the use of surface disinfection?
   a. OSHA
   b. FDA
   c. ADA
   d. all of the above

6. Why must surfaces be precleaned?
   a. To remove the bioburden
   b. To remove the barrier
   c. To remove spilled dental materials
   d. To remove stains

7. Which would most commonly have a barrier placed instead of being disinfected?
   a. Operator's stool
   b. Light switch
   c. Countertop
   d. Dental assistant's stool

8. Where are antiseptics used?
   a. On surfaces
   b. On instruments
   c. On skin
   d. On equipment

9. Which agency regulates disinfectants?
   a. OSHA
   b. FDA
   c. CDC
   d. EPA

10. Which of the following chemical solutions is recommended for heat-resistant items?
    a. Glutaraldehyde
    b. Alcohol
    c. Iodophors
    d. All of the above

11. What is the name of the disinfectant that can leave a reddish or yellowish stain?
    a. Glutaraldehyde
    b. Alcohol
    c. Iodophors
    d. Sodium hypochlorite

12. What is a disadvantage of synthetic phenols?
    a. They leave a reddish stain.
    b. They can leave a residual film on surfaces.
    c. They evaporate quickly on surfaces.
    d. They are highly toxic.

13. What is a common term for sodium hypochlorite?
    a. Ammonia
    b. Vinegar
    c. Oil
    d. Bleach

14. Which disinfectant is not effective if blood or saliva is present?
    a. Alcohol
    b. Glutaraldehyde
    c. Chlorine dioxide
    d. Sodium hypochlorite

15. What is a common use of chlorine dioxide?
    a. Instruments
    b. Surface disinfectant
    c. Sterilant
    d. b and c

16. Which is a way to practice greener infection control?
    a. Conserve water and energy.
    b. Use products with recyclable packaging.
    c. Use digital radiography.
    d. All of the above

TOPICS FOR DISCUSSION

The dentist in your office has a habit of talking too much to patients, which always puts you behind. Today you are running 30 minutes behind, and you still have not prepared the treatment room for the next patient.

1. What corners can you cut to get the room ready quickly?

2. Because this scenario happens quite frequently, would the use of disinfectants or barriers work better in this office? Why?

3. What items need to be replaced for the next patient on the dental-assisting unit?

4. What items need to be replaced for the next patient on the dental unit?

5. What personal protective equipment items need to be replaced?

MULTIMEDIA PROCEDURES RECOMMENDED REVIEW

- Placing and Removing Surface Barriers
- Treatment Room Cleaning and Disinfection

COMPETENCY 20-1: PLACING AND REMOVING SURFACE BARRIERS

Performance Objective

By following a routine procedure that meets stated protocols, the student will demonstrate the proper technique for placing and removing surface barriers.

Evaluation and Grading Criteria

3   Student competently met the stated criteria without assistance.
2   Student required assistance in order to meet the stated criteria.
1   Student showed uncertainty when performing the stated criteria.
0   Student was not prepared and needs to repeat the step.
N/A No evaluation of this step.
Instructor shall define grades for each point range earned on completion of each performance-evaluated task.

Performance Standards

The minimum number of satisfactory performances required before final evaluation is _____.

Instructor shall identify by * those steps considered critical. If step is missed or minimum competency is not met, the evaluated procedure fails and must be repeated.

PERFORMANCE CRITERIA	*	SELF	PEER	INSTRUCTOR	COMMENTS
Placement of Surface Barriers					
1. Washed and dried hands.					
2. Assembled the appropriate setup.					
3. Personal protective equipment placed according to procedure.					
4. Selected the appropriate surface barriers.					
5. Placed each barrier over the entire surface to be protected.					
Removal of Surface Barriers					
6. Wore utility gloves to remove contaminated surface barriers.					
7. Very carefully removed each cover.					
8. Discarded the used covers into the regular waste receptacle.					
9. Washed, disinfected, and removed utility gloves.					
10. Washed and dried hands.					
ADDITIONAL COMMENTS					

Total number of points earned _____

Grade _____ Instructor's initials _____

COMPETENCY 20-2: PERFORMING TREATMENT ROOM CLEANING AND DISINFECTION

Performance Objective
By following a routine procedure that meets stated protocols, the student will demonstrate the proper technique for precleaning and disinfecting a dental treatment room and equipment surfaces.

Evaluation and Grading Criteria
 3   Student competently met the stated criteria without assistance.
 2   Student required assistance in order to meet the stated criteria.
 1   Student showed uncertainty when performing the stated criteria.
 0   Student was not prepared and needs to repeat the step.
 N/A   No evaluation of this step.
Instructor shall define grades for each point range earned on completion of each performance-evaluated task.

Performance Standards
The minimum number of satisfactory performances required before final evaluation is _____.

Instructor shall identify by * those steps considered critical. If step is missed or minimum competency is not met, the evaluated procedure fails and must be repeated.

PERFORMANCE CRITERIA	*	SELF	PEER	INSTRUCTOR	COMMENTS
1. Assembled the appropriate setup.					
2. Personal protective equipment placed according to procedure.					
3. Checked to see that the precleaning and disinfecting product had been prepared correctly and was fresh. Read and followed the manufacturer's instructions.					
4. Sprayed the paper towel or gauze pad with the product and vigorously wiped the surface.					
5. Sprayed a fresh paper towel or gauze pad with the product.					
6. Allowed the surface to remain moist for the manufacturer's recommended time.					
7. Wiped off any excess moisture from disinfectant before seating next patient.					
8. Used water to rinse any residual disinfectant from surfaces that could come in contact with the patient's skin or mouth.					
ADDITIONAL COMMENTS					

Total number of points earned _____

Grade _____   Instructor's initials _____

107

21 Principles and Techniques of Instrument Processing and Sterilization

SHORT-ANSWER QUESTIONS

1. Describe and discuss the seven steps involved in processing dental instruments.

2. Describe the three most common methods of heat sterilization, and list the advantages and disadvantages of each.

3. Describe the precautions necessary when materials are packaged for sterilization.

4. Describe the steps required for sterilization of a high-speed dental handpiece.

5. Explain the differences between process indicators and process integrators.

6. Describe when and how biologic monitoring is done.

7. Explain the primary disadvantage of "flash" sterilization.

8. Describe the three forms of sterilization monitoring.

9. Explain how sterilization failures can occur.

10. Explain the limitations of liquid chemical sterilants.

11. Describe the classification of instruments used to determine the type of processing that should be used.

12. Explain the purpose of using a holding solution before instrument processing.

13. Describe the safety precautions necessary when one is operating an ultrasonic cleaner.

14. Describe the CDC Guidelines for sterilization and disinfection of patient care items.

15. Describe the CDC Guidelines for cleaning and decontamination of instruments.

16. Describe the CDC Guidelines for preparation and packaging of instruments for sterilization.

FILL-IN-THE-BLANK STATEMENTS

Select the best term from the list below and complete the following statements.

autoclave

biologic indicators

biologic monitor

chemical vapor sterilizer

clean area

contaminated area

critical instrument

dry heat sterilizer

endospore

event-related packaging

multi-parameter indicator

noncritical instruments

semicritical instruments

single-parameter indicator

sterilant

ultrasonic cleaner

use-life

1. _____ means that it is assumed the contents of a package will remain sterile indefinitely unless the packaging is compromised.

2. A(n) _____ is an agent capable of killing all microorganisms.

3. The _____ is a piece of equipment that is used for sterilizing by means of moist heat under pressure.

4. _____ are vials or strips, also known as *spore tests,* that contain harmless bacterial spores and are used to determine whether a sterilizer is working.

5. The _____ is a piece of equipment that is used for sterilizing by means of hot formaldehyde vapors under pressure.

6. An instrument used to penetrate soft tissue or bone is identified as a(n) _____.

7. Instruments that come in contact with oral tissues but do not penetrate soft tissue or bone are identified as

   _____.

8. _____ are instruments that come into contact with intact skin only.

9. In the _____ of the sterilization center, sterilized instruments, fresh disposable supplies, and prepared trays are stored.

10. The _____ of the sterilization center is where contaminated items are brought for precleaning.

11. A piece of equipment used for sterilization by means of heated air is the _____.

12. _____ is the length of time that a germicidal solution is effective after it has been prepared for use.

13. The _____ verifies sterilization by confirming that all spore-forming microorganisms have been destroyed.

14. Tapes, strips, and tabs with heat-sensitive chemicals that change color when exposed to a certain temperature are examples of a(n) _____.

15. A(n) _____ is a resistant, dormant structure that is formed inside of some bacteria and can withstand adverse conditions.

16. The _____ is a device that loosens and removes debris with the use of sound waves traveling through a liquid.

17. A(n) _____ is an indicator that reacts to time, temperature, and the presence of steam.

MULTIPLE-CHOICE QUESTIONS

Complete each question by circling the best answer.

1. The instrument classifications used to determine the method of sterilization and disinfection are _____.
   a. critical
   b. semicritical
   c. noncritical
   d. All of the above

2. What type of personal protective equipment is necessary when one is processing instruments?
   a. Goggle-type eyewear
   b. Sterile gloves
   c. Surgical scrubs
   d. Hairnet

3. The basic rule of the workflow pattern in an instrument-processing area is _____.
   a. triangular
   b. square
   c. single-loop
   d. double-loop

4. If instruments cannot be processed immediately, what should be done with them?
   a. They should be kept in the dental treatment area.
   b. They should be wrapped in aluminum foil.
   c. They should be covered with a patient napkin.
   d. They should be placed in a holding solution.

5. Which are methods of precleaning instruments?
   a. By hand scrubbing
   b. By ultrasonic cleaning
   c. With a thermal washer and disinfector
   d. All of the above

6. Which method of precleaning instruments is LEAST desirable?
   a. Hand scrubbing
   b. Ultrasonic cleaning
   c. Thermal washer
   d. Microwave

7. The ultrasonic cleaner works _____.
   a. by microwaves
   b. by sound waves
   c. by ultraviolet waves
   d. by light waves

8. Kitchen dishwashers cannot be used to preclean instruments because they are _____.
   a. not ADA approved
   b. not CDC approved
   c. not FDA approved
   d. not OSHA approved

9. Rusting of instruments can be prevented by _____.
   a. use of a disinfectant
   b. use of lubrication
   c. use of proper wrapping
   d. use of wax

10. Instruments should be packaged for sterilization to _____.
    a. maintain sterility
    b. identify them
    c. maintain organization
    d. make setup easier

11. Which of the following is a reason why pins, staples, and paper clips are not used on instrument packaging?
    a. The package becomes too hot to touch.
    b. You cannot record information on the package.
    c. They will damage the sterilizer.
    d. They will cause holes in the packaging.

12. Which is a form of sterilization monitoring?
    a. Physical
    b. Chemical
    c. Biologic
    d. All of the above

13. Where do you place a process indicator?
    a. Inside the package
    b. Outside the package
    c. Inside the sterilizer
    d. Outside the sterilizer

14. Another term for spore testing is _____.
    a. biologic monitoring
    b. single-parameter indicator
    c. multi-parameter indicator
    d. All of the above

15. Do multi-parameter indicators ensure that an item is sterile?
    a. Yes
    b. No

16. What is the best way to determine whether sterilization has occurred?
    a. Check the sterilizer.
    b. Use a process multi-parameter indicator.
    c. Use biologic monitoring.
    d. Use a single-parameter indicator.

17. What causes sterilization failures?
    a. Improper contact of sterilizing agent
    b. Improper temperature
    c. Overloading of the sterilizer
    d. All of the above

18. What are commonly used forms of heat sterilization?
    a. Steam
    b. Chemical vapor
    c. Dry heat
    d. All of the above

19. What is a primary disadvantage of "flash" sterilization?
    a. Type of sterilizer
    b. Inability to wrap items
    c. Temperature
    d. Sterilizing agent used

20. What is a major advantage of chemical vapor sterilization?
    a. Sterilizing time is faster.
    b. More instruments can be sterilized at one time.
    c. Instruments will not rust.
    d. The instrument does not have to be wrapped.

21. An example of dry heat sterilization is

    _____.

    a. static air
    b. chemical vapor
    c. autoclave
    d. microwave

22. How do you rinse instruments that have been processed in a liquid chemical sterilant?
    a. With hot water
    b. With cold water
    c. With sterile water
    d. With carbonated water

23. How do you prepare a high-speed handpiece for sterilization?
    a. Place it in a holding bath.
    b. Flush water through it.
    c. Soak it in soapy water.
    d. Take it apart.

24. What type of heat sterilization is appropriate for high-speed handpieces?
    a. Steam
    b. Chemical vapor
    c. Liquid chemical sterilant
    d. a and b

TOPICS FOR DISCUSSION

You are the only clinical assistant in the practice, and your morning has been very hectic. None of the contaminated instruments have been processed for the afternoon. When you finally get a break and get back to the sterilization center, your dirty instruments are in the ultrasonic, and the trays and paper products are on the counter.

1. How could this backup have been prevented?

2. You have five trays of instruments in the ultrasonic. What can you do?

3. What could you have done immediately after performing a procedure to change this circumstance?

4. Is there anyone else in the dental office who could help keep this under control? If so, how could you work through this circumstance?

5. Should you discuss this with the dentist?

MULTIMEDIA PROCEDURES RECOMMENDED REVIEW

- Autoclaving Instruments
- Operating the Ultrasonic Cleaner

COMPETENCY 21-1: OPERATING THE ULTRASONIC CLEANER

Performance Objective
By following a routine procedure that meets stated protocols, when provided with the appropriate materials, the student will demonstrate the proper technique for precleaning instruments before sterilization using the ultrasonic cleaner.

Evaluation and Grading Criteria
<u>3</u>   Student competently met the stated criteria without assistance.
<u>2</u>   Student required assistance in order to meet the stated criteria.
<u>1</u>   Student showed uncertainty when performing the stated criteria.
<u>0</u>   Student was not prepared and needs to repeat the step.
<u>N/A</u>   No evaluation of this step.
Instructor shall define grades for each point range earned on completion of each performance-evaluated task.

Performance Standards
The minimum number of satisfactory performances required before final evaluation is _____.

Instructor shall identify by * those steps considered critical. If step is missed or minimum competency is not met, the evaluated procedure fails and must be repeated.

PERFORMANCE CRITERIA	*	SELF	PEER	INSTRUCTOR	COMMENTS
1. Personal protective equipment placed according to procedure.					
2. Removed the lid from the container and checked the level of solution.					
3. Placed instruments or cassette into the basket.					
4. Replaced the lid and turned the cycle to ON.					
5. After the cleaning cycle, removed the basket and rinsed the instruments.					
6. Emptied the basket onto the towel.					
7. Replaced the lid on the ultrasonic cleaner.					
ADDITIONAL COMMENTS					

Total number of points earned _____

Grade _____ Instructor's initials _____

COMPETENCY 21-2: AUTOCLAVING INSTRUMENTS

Performance Objective

By following a routine procedure that meets stated protocols, when provided with the appropriate materials, the student will demonstrate the proper technique for preparing and autoclaving instruments.

Evaluation and Grading Criteria

<u>3</u>   Student competently met the stated criteria without assistance.
<u>2</u>   Student required assistance in order to meet the stated criteria.
<u>1</u>   Student showed uncertainty when performing the stated criteria.
<u>0</u>   Student was not prepared and needs to repeat the step.
<u>N/A</u>   No evaluation of this step.
Instructor shall define grades for each point range earned on completion of each performance-evaluated task.

Performance Standards

The minimum number of satisfactory performances required before final evaluation is _____.

Instructor shall identify by * those steps considered critical. If step is missed or minimum competency is not met, the evaluated procedure fails and must be repeated.

PERFORMANCE CRITERIA	*	SELF	PEER	INSTRUCTOR	COMMENTS
1. Personal protective equipment placed according to procedure.					
2. Properly cleaned and prepared the instruments for autoclaving.					
3. Placed the process integrator into the package.					
4. Packaged, sealed, and labeled the instruments.					
5. Placed, bagged, and sealed items in the autoclave.					
6. Tilted glass or metal canisters at an angle.					
7. Placed larger packs at the bottom of the chamber.					
8. Did not overload the autoclave.					
9. Followed the manufacturer's instructions.					
10. Checked the level of water. (If necessary, added more distilled water.)					
11. Set the autoclave controls for the appropriate time, temperature, and pressure.					
12. At the end of the sterilization cycle, vented the steam into the room and allowed the contents of the autoclave to dry and cool.					

Continued

13. Checked the external process indicator for color change.					
14. Removed the instruments when they were cool and dry.					
ADDITIONAL COMMENTS					

Total number of points earned _____

Grade _____ Instructor's initials _____

COMPETENCY 21-3: STERILIZING INSTRUMENTS WITH UNSATURATED CHEMICAL VAPOR

Performance Objective

By following a routine procedure that meets stated protocols, when provided with the appropriate materials, the student will demonstrate the proper technique for preparing and sterilizing instruments with chemical vapor.

Evaluation and Grading Criteria

3   Student competently met the stated criteria without assistance.
2   Student required assistance in order to meet the stated criteria.
1   Student showed uncertainty when performing the stated criteria.
0   Student was not prepared and needs to repeat the step.
N/A   No evaluation of this step.

Instructor shall define grades for each point range earned on completion of each performance-evaluated task.

Performance Standards

The minimum number of satisfactory performances required before final evaluation is _____.

Instructor shall identify by * those steps considered critical. If step is missed or minimum competency is not met, the evaluated procedure fails and must be repeated.

PERFORMANCE CRITERIA	*	SELF	PEER	INSTRUCTOR	COMMENTS
Wrapping the Instruments					
1. Personal protective equipment placed according to procedure.					
2. Ensured that the instruments are clean and dry.					
3. Wrapped the instruments.					
4. Ensured that packages were not too large.					
Loading and Operating the Chemical Vapor Sterilizer					
5. Read and followed the manufacturer's instructions.					
6. Read the information on the MSDS for the chemical liquid.					
7. Loaded the sterilizer according to manufacturer's instructions.					
8. Set the controls for the proper time and temperature.					
9. Followed the manufacturer's instructions for venting and cooling.					

Continued

Chapter **21 Principles and Techniques of Instrument Processing and Sterilization**

10. Checked the external process indicator for color change.					
11. Removed the instruments when they were cool and dry.					

ADDITIONAL COMMENTS

Total number of points earned _____

Grade _____ Instructor's initials _____

Performance Objective

By following a routine procedure that meets stated protocols, when provided with the appropriate materials, the student will demonstrate the proper technique for preparing and sterilizing instruments with dry heat.

Evaluation and Grading Criteria

3   Student competently met the stated criteria without assistance.
2   Student required assistance in order to meet the stated criteria.
1   Student showed uncertainty when performing the stated criteria.
0   Student was not prepared and needs to repeat the step.
N/A   No evaluation of this step.

Instructor shall define grades for each point range earned on completion of each performance-evaluated task.

Performance Standards

The minimum number of satisfactory performances required before final evaluation is _____.

Instructor shall identify by * those steps considered critical. If step is missed or minimum competency is not met, the evaluated procedure fails and must be repeated.

PERFORMANCE CRITERIA	*	SELF	PEER	INSTRUCTOR	COMMENTS
Wrapping the Instruments					
1. Personal protective equipment placed according to procedure.					
2. Cleaned and dried the instruments before wrapping.					
3. Opened hinged instruments.					
4. Wrapped instruments.					
Loading and Operating the Dry Heat Sterilizer					
5. Read and followed the manufacturer's instructions.					
6. Inserted the process integrator into the test load package.					
7. Loaded the instruments into the dry heat chamber.					
8. Set the time and temperature.					
9. Did not place additional instruments in the load once the sterilization cycle had begun.					
10. Allowed the packs to cool before handling.					
11. Checked the indicators for color change.					
ADDITIONAL COMMENTS					

Total quantity of points earned _____

Grade _____ Instructor's initials _____

COMPETENCY 21-5: STERILIZING INSTRUMENTS WITH CHEMICAL LIQUID STERILANTS

Performance Objective

By following a routine procedure that meets stated protocols, when provided with the appropriate materials, the student will demonstrate the proper technique for preparing and sterilizing instruments with a chemical sterilant.

Evaluation and Grading Criteria

3   Student competently met the stated criteria without assistance.
2   Student required assistance in order to meet the stated criteria.
1   Student showed uncertainty when performing the stated criteria.
0   Student was not prepared and needs to repeat the step.
N/A   No evaluation of this step.
Instructor shall define grades for each point range earned on completion of each performance-evaluated task.

Performance Standards

The minimum number of satisfactory performances required before final evaluation is _____.

Instructor shall identify by * those steps considered critical. If step is missed or minimum competency is not met, the evaluated procedure fails and must be repeated.

PERFORMANCE CRITERIA	*	SELF	PEER	INSTRUCTOR	COMMENTS
Preparing the Solution					
1. Personal protective equipment placed according to procedure.					
2. Followed the manufacturer's instructions for preparing and activating, using, and disposing of the solution.					
3. Prepared the solution for use as a sterilant. Labeled the containers with the name of the chemical, date of preparation, and any other information relating to the hazards of the product.					
4. Covered the container and kept it closed unless putting instruments in or taking them out.					
Using the Solution					
5. Precleaned, rinsed, and dried items to be processed.					
6. Placed the items in a perforated tray or pan. Placed the pan in the solution and covered the container. Or as an alternative, used tongs.					
7. Ensured that all items were fully submerged in the solution for the entire contact time.					

Continued

8. Rinsed processed items thoroughly with water and dried. Placed items in a clean package.				
Maintaining the Solution				
9. Tested the glutaraldehyde concentration of the solution with a chemical test kit (available from the manufacturer).				
10. Replaced the solution as indicated on the instructions, or when the level of the solution became low or the solution became visibly dirty.				
11. When replacing the used solution, discarded all of the used solution, cleaned the container with a detergent, rinsed with water, dried, and filled the container with fresh solution.				

ADDITIONAL COMMENTS

Total number of points earned _____

Grade _____ Instructor's initials _____

COMPETENCY 21-6: PERFORMING BIOLOGIC MONITORING

Performance Objective
By following a routine procedure that meets stated protocols, the student will demonstrate the proper technique for performing biologic monitoring.

Evaluation and Grading Criteria
3   Student competently met the stated criteria without assistance.
2   Student required assistance in order to meet the stated criteria.
1   Student showed uncertainty when performing the stated criteria.
0   Student was not prepared and needs to repeat the step.
N/A   No evaluation of this step.
Instructor shall define grades for each point range earned on completion of each performance-evaluated task.

Performance Standards
The minimum number of satisfactory performances required before final evaluation is _____.

Instructor shall identify by * those steps considered critical. If step is missed or minimum competency is not met, the evaluated procedure fails and must be repeated.

PERFORMANCE CRITERIA	*	SELF	PEER	INSTRUCTOR	COMMENTS
1. Personal protective equipment placed according to procedure.					
2. Placed the Biologic Indicator (BI) strip in the bundle of instruments and sealed the package.					
3. Placed the pack with the BI strip in the center of the sterilizer load.					
4. Placed the remainder of the packaged instruments into the sterilizer and processed the load through a normal sterilization cycle.					
5. Removed utility gloves, mask, and eyewear. Washed and dried hands.					
6. Recorded the date of the test; the type of sterilizer; the cycle, temperature, and time; and the name of the person operating the sterilizer.					
7. Removed and processed BI strip after the load was sterilized.					
8. Mailed the processed spore test strips and the control BI strip to the monitoring service.					

ADDITIONAL COMMENTS

Total number of points earned _____

Grade _____ Instructor's initials _____

Chapter **21** **Principles and Techniques of Instrument Processing and Sterilization**

COMPETENCY 21-7: STERILIZING THE DENTAL HANDPIECE

Performance Objective
By following a routine procedure that meets stated protocols, when provided with the appropriate materials, the student will demonstrate the proper technique for preparing, cleaning, and sterilizing the dental handpiece.

Evaluation and Grading Criteria
3   Student competently met the stated criteria without assistance.
2   Student required assistance in order to meet the stated criteria.
1   Student showed uncertainty when performing the stated criteria.
0   Student was not prepared and needs to repeat the step.
N/A   No evaluation of this step.
Instructor shall define grades for each point range earned on completion of each performance-evaluated task.

Performance Standards
The minimum number of satisfactory performances required before final evaluation is _____.

Instructor shall identify by * those steps considered critical. If step is missed or minimum competency is not met, the evaluated procedure fails and must be repeated.

PERFORMANCE CRITERIA	*	SELF	PEER	INSTRUCTOR	COMMENTS
1. Personal protective equipment placed according to procedure.					
2. With the bur still in the chuck, wiped any visible debris from the handpiece. Operated the handpiece for approximately 10 to 20 seconds.					
3. Removed the bur from the handpiece and then removed the handpiece from the hose.					
4. Used a handpiece cleaner recommended by the manufacturer to remove internal debris and lubricated the handpiece according to the manufacturer's recommendations.					
5. Reattached the handpiece to an air hose, inserted a bur, and operated the handpiece to blow out the excess lubricant from the rotating parts.					
6. Used a cotton-tipped applicator dampened with isopropyl alcohol to remove all excess lubricant from fiberoptic interfaces and exposed optical surfaces.					
7. Dried the handpiece and packaged it for sterilization.					
ADDITIONAL COMMENTS					

Total number of points earned _____

Grade _____ Instructor's initials _____

22 Regulatory and Advisory Agencies

1. Explain the difference between regulations and recommendations.

2. List four professional sources for dental information.

3. Name the premier resource for safety and infection prevention information in dentistry.

4. Describe the role of the Centers for Disease Control and Prevention.

5. Explain the primary difference between OSHA and NIOSH.

6. Describe the role of the Environmental Protection Agency in relation to dentistry.

7. Describe the role of the U.S. Food and Drug Administration in relation to dentistry.

8. Describe the role of the National Institutes of Health.

9. Describe the role of the National Institute of Dental and Craniofacial Research.

10. Describe the role of the Public Health Agency of Canada.

FILL-IN-THE-BLANK STATEMENTS

Select the best term from the list below and complete the following statements.

ADA	**NIOSH**
CDC	**OSAP**
EPA	**OSHA**
FDA	**PHAC**

1. The _____ is a federal regulatory agency that is concerned with the regulation of sterilization equipment.

2. The federal nonregulatory agency that issues recommendations on health and safety is the _____.

3. The _____ is the professional organization for dentists.

4. The federal regulatory agency that enforces regulations that pertain to employee safety is _____.

5. _____ is the premier resource for safety and infection prevention information in dentistry.

6. _____ is the federal agency that is responsible for conducting research and making recommendations for the prevention of work-related disease and injury.

7. The _____ is the federal regulatory agency that deals with issues of concern to the environment or public safety.

8. The _____ is the main federal agency responsible for public health in Canada.

MULTIPLE-CHOICE QUESTIONS

Complete each question by circling the best answer.

1. What is the primary role of the CDC in dentistry?
   a. Public health
   b. Research
   c. Drugs
   d. Employees

2. What is a primary role of the FDA?
   a. Fund research projects
   b. Provide public health information
   c. Regulate medical and dental devices
   d. Protect employees

3. What is the primary role of the EPA?
   a. Research
   b. Public health
   c. Employees
   d. Environment

4. What is the primary focus of OSHA in dentistry?
   a. Public health
   b. Employees
   c. Environment
   d. Research

TOPICS FOR DISCUSSION

The dentist in your office asks you to be responsible for maintaining OSHA compliance in the office and to provide training on infection prevention to the new employees. A high school student will be coming in to help with sterilization, and you must provide her with appropriate training. Where will you get the latest information, and how will you find the newest OSHA regulations?

23 Chemical and Waste Management

SHORT-ANSWER QUESTIONS

1. Describe potential long-term and short-term effects of exposure to chemicals.

2. Explain the components of the OSHA Hazard Communication Standard.

3. Describe three common methods of chemical exposure.

4. Describe the components of a Hazard Communication Program.

5. Explain the purpose of a material safety data sheet.

6. Describe the difference between chronic and acute chemical exposure.

7. Identify four methods of personal protection against chemical exposure.

8. Describe how chemicals should generally be stored.

9. Discuss the record keeping requirements of the Hazard Communication Standard.

10. Identify types of regulated waste generated in a dental office.

11. Identify types of toxic waste generated in a dental office.

12. Discuss the packaging of regulated waste for transport.

FILL-IN-THE-BLANK STATEMENTS

Select the best term from the list below and complete the following statements.

acute exposure
chemical inventory
chronic exposure
contaminated waste
Hazard Communication Standard

hazardous waste
infectious waste
material safety data sheet (MSDS)
regulated waste
toxic waste

1. The _____ is an OSHA standard regarding an employee's right to know about chemicals in the workplace.

2. A form that provides health and safety information regarding materials that contain chemicals is a _____.

3. _____ is repeated exposures, generally of lower levels, over a long period.

4. _____ exposure pertains to high levels of exposure over a short period of time.

5. Waste that has certain properties or contains chemicals that could pose a danger to human health and the environment after it is discarded is _____.

6. A(n) _____ is a comprehensive list of every product used in the office that contains chemicals.

7. Items that have had contact with blood, saliva, or other body secretions are called _____.

8. Waste that is capable of causing an infectious disease is _____.

9. _____ is infectious waste that requires special handling, neutralization, and disposal.

10. Waste that is capable of having a poisonous effect is _____.

MULTIPLE-CHOICE QUESTIONS

Complete each question by circling the best answer.

1. What body systems could develop health-related problems as a result of inhalation exposure to chemicals in the dental office?
   a. Neurologic
   b. Senses
   c. Respiratory
   d. Endocrine

2. What is (are) primary method(s) of chemical exposure?
   a. Inhalation
   b. Ingestion
   c. Skin contact
   d. All of the above

3. Acute chemical exposure involves _____.
   a. short-term exposure in large quantity
   b. repeated exposure in small quantity
   c. short-term exposure in small quantity
   d. long-term exposure in small quantity

4. What is a method of personal protection against chemical exposure?
   a. Ventilation
   b. Disinfected surfaces
   c. Inhalation protection
   d. Hair protection

132

Chapter **23** **Chemical and Waste Management**

5. What are the OSHA requirements regarding an eye-wash unit?
   a. Eyewash unit in every treatment room
   b. Eyewash unit in areas where chemicals are used
   c. Eyewash unit in the building
   d. Eyewash unit on each floor

6. What could be the most likely effects of exposure to radiographic processing solutions kept in a poorly ventilated area?
   a. Cardiac problems
   b. Reproductive problems
   c. Respiratory problems
   d. Urinary problems

7. In general, how should chemicals be stored?
   a. In a cool, dry, dark place
   b. In a locked cabinet
   c. Under water
   d. In a hot, moist place

8. Chemicals are determined to be hazardous if they are
   _____.
   a. ignitable
   b. corrosive
   c. reactive
   d. All of the above

9. What is another term for the Hazard Communication Standard?
   a. Employee beware law
   b. Employee right-to-know law
   c. Hazardous chemical law
   d. Chemical safety law

10. What chemicals must be included in a chemical inventory?
    a. Over-the-counter drugs
    b. Prescription drugs
    c. All chemicals
    d. Dental materials

11. What is an MSDS?
    a. Material subscribed dental sheet
    b. Material safety data sheet
    c. Materials for sterilization and dental surgery
    d. Microbiology standards and disease standards

12. What materials are exempt from labeling requirements?
    a. Food
    b. Drugs
    c. Cosmetics
    d. All of the above

13. Which dental professional must receive training about hazardous chemicals?
    a. Dental laboratory technician
    b. Dental hygienist
    c. Dental assistant
    d. All of the above

14. How long must training records be kept on file?
    a. 1 year
    b. 5 years
    c. 10 years
    d. 20 years

15. An example of regulated waste is a _____.
    a. patient napkin
    b. contaminated needle
    c. dental dam
    d. 2- × 2-inch gauze

CASE STUDY

Pamela is a dental assistant who is in charge of preparing chemical labels for containers in the office. She needs to prepare a label for a product that is highly flammable, reactive, and toxic. Pamela is also missing some material safety data sheets for other products in the office.

1. What types of containers will Pamela need to label?

2. What number will Pamela write in the blue triangle?

3. What number will Pamela write in the red triangle?

4. What number will Pamela write in the yellow triangle?

5. Where can Pamela get a material safety data sheet for other products in the office?

COMPETENCY 23-1: CREATING AN APPROPRIATE LABEL FOR A SECONDARY CONTAINER

Performance Objective

By following a routine procedure that meets stated protocols, the student will demonstrate the proper technique for using information from a material safety data sheet (MSDS) to complete a chemical label for a secondary container.

Evaluation and Grading Criteria

<u>3</u>   Student competently met the stated criteria without assistance.
<u>2</u>   Student required assistance in order to meet the stated criteria.
<u>1</u>   Student showed uncertainty when performing the stated criteria.
<u>0</u>   Student was not prepared and needs to repeat the step.
<u>N/A</u>   No evaluation of this step.
Instructor shall define grades for each point range earned on completion of each performance-evaluated task.

Performance Standards

The minimum number of satisfactory performances required before final evaluation is _____.

Instructor shall identify by * those steps considered critical. If step is missed or minimum competency is not met, the evaluated procedure fails and must be repeated.

PERFORMANCE CRITERIA	*	SELF	PEER	INSTRUCTOR	COMMENTS
1. Wrote the manufacturer's name and address on the label.					
2. Wrote the name of the chemical(s) and the "target organ" on the label.					
3. Wrote the appropriate health hazard code in the blue diamond.					
4. Wrote the appropriate flammability and explosion hazard code in the red diamond.					
5. Wrote the appropriate reactivity code in the yellow diamond.					
6. Wrote the appropriate specific hazard warning in the white diamond.					
ADDITIONAL COMMENTS					

Total number of points earned _____

Grade _____ Instructor's initials _____

24 Dental Unit Waterlines

SHORT-ANSWER QUESTIONS

1. Discuss why dental units have more bacteria than faucets do.

2. Explain the role of biofilm in dental unit waterline contamination.

3. Discuss why there is a renewed interest in dental unit waterline contamination.

4. Explain the factors in bacterial contamination of dental unit water.

5. Identify the primary source of microorganisms in dental unit water.

6. Describe methods to reduce bacterial contamination in dental unit waterlines.

FILL-IN-THE-BLANK STATEMENTS

Select the best term from the list below and complete the following statements.

biofilm
colony-forming units
dental unit waterlines
Legionella

microfiltration
planktonic bacteria
retraction
self-contained water reservoir

1. _____ are slime-producing bacterial communities that may also harbor fungi, algae, and protozoa.

2. The bacterium responsible for the disease legionellosis is _____.

3. _____ is the use of membrane filters to trap microorganisms suspended in water.

4. _____ are the minimum number of separable cells on the surface of a semisolid agar medium that create a visible colony.

5. _____ are made of small-bore plastic tubing and are used to deliver dental treatment water through a dental unit.

6. A(n) _____ is a container that is used to hold and supply water or other solutions to handpieces and air-water syringes attached to a dental unit.

137

7. _____ is the entry of fluids and microorganisms into waterlines as a result of negative water pressure. Also referred to as "suck back."

8. Bacteria that are floating in water are _____.

MULTIPLE-CHOICE QUESTIONS

Complete each question by circling the best answer.

1. Are waterborne diseases limited to dentistry?
   a. Yes
   b. No

2. When was the presence of bacteria first reported in dental unit waterlines?
   a. 5 years ago
   b. 10 years ago
   c. 20 years ago
   d. 30 years ago

3. What type of public health problem exists regarding contaminated dental water?
   a. Widespread
   b. Localized
   c. No problem at this time
   d. Epidemic

4. What bacteria cause the disease legionellosis?
   a. Streptococci
   b. *Legionella* bacteria
   c. Bacilli
   d. Staphylococci

5. Where is biofilm found?
   a. Suction tips
   b. Handpiece waterlines
   c. Air-water syringe waterlines
   d. b and c

6. Should water be heated in the dental units to kill the bacteria?
   a. Yes
   b. No
   c. It doesn't matter.

7. Can biofilm in dental unit waterlines be completely eliminated?
   a. Yes
   b. No

8. If sterile water is used in a self-contained reservoir, will the water that enters the patient's mouth be sterile?
   a. Yes
   b. No

9. How often should microfilters in waterlines be changed?
   a. Daily
   b. Weekly
   c. Bimonthly
   d. According to manufacturer directions

10. According to CDC guidelines, whom should you contact when selecting a chemical for the dental unit?
    a. ADA
    b. Equipment manufacturer
    c. OSHA
    d. CDC

11. According to CDC guidelines, what type of water must be used as an irrigant for surgery involving bone?
    a. Saline water
    b. Tap water
    c. Sterile water
    d. Carbonated water

12. Will flushing dental unit waterlines remove biofilm?
    a. Yes
    b. No

13. When should the high-volume evacuator be used to minimize aerosol?
    a. With the high-speed handpiece
    b. With the ultrasonic scaler
    c. With the air-water syringe
    d. All of the above

14. Will the use of a rubber dam totally eliminate the dental assistant's exposure to microorganisms?
    a. Yes
    b. No

15. What type of personal protective equipment (PPE) is especially critical when aerosol is being generated?
    a. Eyewear
    b. Mask
    c. Gloves
    d. a and b

A patient of the practice comments on a news program she saw on television regarding transmission of diseases from water in the dental office. She confides in you that she is not sure she wants to continue her treatment plan. How would you answer the following questions from your patient?

1. Is HIV transmitted from dental unit water?

2. What does the practice do to make the water safe?

3. What type of water does the practice use for surgery?

4. Is it safe to have dental treatment that requires water?

Performance Objective

By following a routine procedure that meets stated protocols, the student will demonstrate the proper technique for obtaining a water sample and preparing it for shipping.

Evaluation and Grading Criteria

 3 Student competently met the stated criteria without assistance.
 2 Student required assistance in order to meet the stated criteria.
 1 Student showed uncertainty when performing the stated criteria.
 0 Student was not prepared and needs to repeat the step.
 N/A No evaluation of this step.
Instructor shall define grades for each point range earned on completion of each performance-evaluated task.

Performance Standards

The minimum number of satisfactory performances required before final evaluation is _____.

Instructor shall identify by * those steps considered critical. If step is missed or minimum competency is not met, the evaluated procedure fails and must be repeated.

PERFORMANCE CRITERIA	*	SELF	PEER	INSTRUCTOR	COMMENTS
1. Personal protective equipment placed according to procedure.					
2. Placed the refrigerant pack in the Styrofoam lid and placed it in the freezer overnight.					
3. Flushed waterlines for a minimum of 2 minutes before taking samples.					
4. Filled sterile collection vials to approximately three-fourths full. *Did not touch the outlet of the waterline or the interior of the collection vial.*					
5. Used a permanent marker to label each water sample. Indicated the sample location and the type. For example, Operatory 3, air-water syringe (Op3, a-w).					
6. Filled out the sample submission form and enclosed it with the samples.					
7. Placed refrigerant pack and water samples in Styrofoam shipper.					
8. Placed Styrofoam shipper in mailer box.					
9. Completed U.S. Express Mail shipping label and affixed to box.					
ADDITIONAL COMMENTS					

Total number of points earned _____

Grade _____ Instructor's initials _____

25 Ergonomics

SHORT-ANSWER QUESTIONS

1. Describe the goal of ergonomics.

2. Discuss exercises that can reduce muscle fatigue and strengthen muscles.

3. Describe the neutral working position.

4. Describe exercises to reduce eyestrain.

5. Describe exercises to reduce neck strain.

6. Identify common symptoms of musculoskeletal disorders.

7. Identify three categories of risk factors that contribute to increased risk of injury.

8. Describe the symptoms of carpal tunnel syndrome.

FILL-IN-THE-BLANK STATEMENTS

Select the best term from the list below and complete the following statements.

carpal tunnel syndrome
cumulative trauma disorders
ergonomics
maximum horizontal reach
maximum vertical reach
musculoskeletal disorders

neutral position
normal horizontal reach
sprains
strains
thenar eminence

1. _____ is the adaptation of the work environment to the human body.

2. Pain that results from ongoing stresses to muscles, tendons, nerves, and joints is _____.

3. _____ are disorders of the muscles and skeleton such as neck and shoulder pain, back pain, and carpal tunnel syndrome.

4. _____ is the reach created by the sweep of the forearm with the upper arm held at the side.

143

5. The reach created by the vertical sweep of the forearm while keeping the elbow at mid-torso level is the _____.

6. _____ is the reach created when the upper arm is fully extended.

7. Injuries caused by extreme stretching of muscles or ligaments are _____.

8. _____ are injuries caused by a sudden twisting or wrenching of a joint with stretching or tearing of ligaments.

9. _____ is the fleshy elevation of the palm side of the hand.

10. Pain associated with continued flexion and extension of the wrist is _____.

11. _____ is the position in which the body is properly aligned and the distribution of weight throughout the spine is equal.

MULTIPLE-CHOICE QUESTIONS

Complete each question by circling the best answer.

1. Ergonomics is the _____.
   a. prevention of air pollution
   b. adaptation of the work environment to the human body
   c. adaptation of the human body to its exercise routine
   d. foundation of team dentistry

2. The goal of ergonomics is to _____.
   a. learn proper exercises
   b. help people stay healthy
   c. perform work more effectively
   d. b and c

3. What types of disorders are considered to be musculoskeletal disorders?
   a. Headaches
   b. Heartburn
   c. Eating
   d. Neurologic disorders

4. What is the most common risk factor that contributes to musculoskeletal disorders?
   a. Short dental procedures
   b. Working on the maxillary arch
   c. Poor posture
   d. Infectious patients

5. What is "neutral position"?
   a. Sitting upright
   b. Keeping weight evenly distributed
   c. Being ready for instrument transfer
   d. a and b

6. A reach that is created by the sweep of the forearm with the upper arm held at the side is _____.
   a. normal vertical reach
   b. normal horizontal reach
   c. abnormal vertical reach
   d. abnormal horizontal reach

7. What types of gloves are most likely to aggravate carpal tunnel syndrome?
   a. Sterile gloves
   b. Overgloves
   c. Ambidextrous gloves
   d. Utility gloves

8. How can you reduce eyestrain?
   a. Wear prescription glasses.
   b. Change your visual distance from short to long distance.
   c. Wear side shields.
   d. Use better lighting.

9. What exercise relieves neck strain?
   a. Sit-ups
   b. Jumping jacks
   c. Jogging
   d. Full back releases

10. What is one of the most important factors in preventing carpal tunnel syndrome?
    a. Resting the eyes
    b. Resting the back
    c. Resting the hands
    d. Resting the legs

TOPICS FOR DISCUSSION

You started working as a dental assistant in Dr. Cardono's office 2 weeks ago. Last Monday you were the only chairside assistant, and you assisted on several crown and bridge appointments in a row. On Tuesday, you noticed that your neck and shoulders were stiff and sore. It hurt to turn your head, and your back ached.

1. Is it likely that sleeping in an awkward position caused your stiff neck?

2. What else could have caused your pain?

3. Is there anything you can do to prevent the pain from getting worse?

4. Is there anything you can suggest to the person who schedules the patients?

5. What exercises could you do to help loosen your neck and shoulders?

MULTIMEDIA PROCEDURES RECOMMENDED REVIEW

- Body Strengthening Exercises

26 The Patient Record

SHORT-ANSWER QUESTIONS

1. Describe the rationale for why each patient has his or her own patient record.

2. Name four information-gathering forms that would be completed by the patient before any treatment is provided.

3. Discuss the importance of the patient's medical and dental health history as it relates to a patient's dental treatment.

FILL-IN-THE-BLANK STATEMENTS

Select the best term from the list below and complete the following statements.

alert
assessment
chronic
chronologic

demographic
forensics
litigation
registration

1. _____ is the act of conducting legal proceedings such as a lawsuit or trial.

2. The process of evaluating a patient's condition is known as_____.

3. A patient's illness is classified as _____ if it persists for a long time.

4. A(n) _____ time period is one that is arranged in order of occurrence.

5. _____ information can include a person's address, phone number, and work information.

6. A(n) _____ sticker is placed on the inside of a patient record to bring attention to a medical condition or allergy.

7. A new patient will complete a(n) _____ form, which includes personal information, information regarding the party responsible for payment, and insurance information.

8. _____ can be used to establish the identity of an individual on the basis of scientific methods.

147

MULTIPLE-CHOICE QUESTIONS

Complete each question by circling the best answer.

1. What specific information must the dental team receive from the patient before it can provide dental treatment?
   a. Medical history, financial status, and treatment plan
   b. Patient registration, medical history, and informed consent
   c. Financial status, radiographs, and treatment plan
   d. Treatment plan, progress notes, and informed consent

2. Which term describes the collection of data to help the dentist make a correct diagnosis?
   a. Assessment
   b. Decision
   c. Recall
   d. Prescription

3. The patient record is a permanent document of whom?
   a. The patient
   b. The dentist
   c. A court of law
   d. The dental practice

4. Quality assurance is an important asset of a practice because _____.
   a. it describes how qualified the dental staff is
   b. it describes the financial stability of the dental practice
   c. it describes the type of care a patient is receiving
   d. it describes the location of a dental practice for a specific patient population

5. The patient should be instructed to enter his or her name on the registration form as _____.
   a. first initial and last name only
   b. first name and last initial only
   c. first initial of the first, middle, and last names
   d. full first, last name, and middle initial

6. Where would you file the patient's registration form?
   a. In the front section of the patient record
   b. In a secured file cabinet
   c. With the patient's clinical information
   d. With the patient's ledger

7. When a medical-dental history form is being completed, the patient must verify that the entered information is accurate by including a _____.
   a. chart number
   b. signature and date
   c. Social Security number
   d. insurance number

8. The dental history section of a health history form provides the dental team with information regarding _____.
   a. dental procedures that are legal for the dental assistant to complete
   b. previous dental treatment and care
   c. necessary dental treatment and care
   d. information about the previous dentist

9. Which medical condition would require an alert sticker to be placed on the inside of a patient record?
   a. The patient with migraines
   b. The patient has a toothache
   c. The patient with an allergy to penicillin
   d. The patient with a broken leg

10. What additional form would a patient complete and sign if he or she were having extensive surgical treatment completed by a specialist?
    a. Progress notes
    b. Treatment plan form
    c. Clinical examination form
    d. Informed consent form

CASE STUDY

Jenny Stewart is a new patient to the practice and has been asked to arrive 15 minutes before her scheduled appointment to complete new-patient forms. As you go to introduce yourself and call her back to the treatment area, Ms. Stewart points to a specific tooth that has been bothering her for a couple of weeks. You seat Ms. Stewart in the operatory and begin reviewing the medical-dental health history with her. You see that she has checked "yes" for having high blood pressure and is taking medication for this. She also noted that she is allergic to penicillin.

1. What forms would have been handed to Ms. Stewart to complete in the reception area?

2. Ms. Stewart indicated that she takes medication for high blood pressure. Where on the medical-dental history form would the type of medication she is taking be noted, and what additional information will the dentist want to know about her high blood pressure?

3. Are there any medical alerts that should be indicated on the patient record? If so, what are they, and how would these be indicated on the patient record?

4. Why would there be a question on the dental history section about who her previous dentist was and how often she saw that dentist?

5. The dentist is ready to examine the patient clinically. What form will be used to chart existing dental conditions?

6. Complete the progress notes for Ms. Stewart's dental visit in the following space.

7. The next time Ms. Stewart returns to the office, what form would be used to inquire about changes in her health?

DENTRIX EXERCISES

Before you can begin this exercise it will be necessary to download the Dentrix G4 Learning Edition to your computer. Please review the step-by-step installation instructions posted on the companion Evolve website (//evolve.elsevier.com/Bird/modern).

Practice Setup

Before you work through any Dentrix exercises, refer to the **Practice Setup** instructions posted on the Evolve website. Also refer to the Dentrix *User's Guide,* Chapter 2.

Patient Record

An important component of the practice management system is electronic storage and filing of patient records. In Dentrix, this is completed in the Family File. The Family File manages and stores both patient and family information, such as address, phone number, insurance coverage, and important health information. For additional information, refer to the Dentrix *User's Guide,* Chapter 3.

Exercise 1: Selecting a Patient of Record

Please refer to the information on the Evolve website on **Selecting a Patient** and **Editing a Patient's File.** Then answer the following questions for each patient listed below:

1. Sally Hayes

   a. What is her marital status?

   b. Does she have children?

   c. What is her date of birth?

   d. Does she have insurance? If so, with which provider(s)?

   e. Does she have any medical alerts? If yes, please specify.

2. Lawrence Schow

   a. What is his marital status?

   b. Does he have children?

   c. What is his date of birth?

   d. Does he have insurance? If so, with which provider(s)?

   e. Does he have any medical alerts? If yes, please specify.

3. Randall Young

   a. What is his marital status?

   b. Does he have children?

   c. What is his date of birth?

   d. Does he have insurance? If so, with which provider(s)?

   e. Does he have any medical alerts? If yes, please specify.

Exercise 2: Creating a New Patient/Family

Please refer to the information on the Evolve website on **Creating a New Family.** Then complete the following exercise:
   Prepare a Family File for the Brooks family.
   - Assign Gregory as the head of house.
   - Add Jessica as a new family member.
   - Add Christopher as a new family member.

Gregory H. Brooks

DOB	10/11/1978
Social Security #	231-47-4956
Home Address	3871 South Dockside Dr.
	Southside, NV 33333

Occupation:	Sales rep for Verizon Wireless
	250 Westwood Ave.
	Southside, NV 33333
Phone	213-555-7290 (home)
	213-555-4199 (cell)
	213-972-4300 (work)
Dental Insurance	Blue Cross Blue Shield
	Group#21774
Medical Alerts	N/A
Dentist	Dennis Smith

Jessica Brooks

DOB	5/20/1984
Social Security #	342-11-7843
Home Address	3871 South Dockside Dr.
	Southside, NV 33333
Occupation	Stay at home mother
Phone	213-555-7290 (home)
	213-586-4198 (cell)
Dental Insurance	Blue Cross Blue Shield
	(under husband's policy) 21774
Medical Alerts	Pregnant
Dentist	Maria Cook

Christopher L. Brooks

DOB	1/22/2005
Social Security #	N/A
Home Address	3871 South Dockside Dr.
	Southside, NV 33333
Dental Insurance	Blue Cross Blue Shield
	(under father's policy) 21774
Medical Alerts	Allergic to penicillin
Dentist	Brenda Childs

PATIENT INFORMATION (CONFIDENTIAL)

NAME _____ FIRST _____ MI _____ LAST _____ DATE _____
ADDRESS _____ CITY _____ STATE/PROV. _____ ZIP/P.C. _____
E-MAIL _____ CELL PHONE _____ HOME PHONE _____
SS#/SIN _____ BIRTHDATE _____
CHECK APPROPRIATE BOX: ☐ MINOR ☐ SINGLE ☐ MARRIED ☐ DIVORCED ☐ WIDOWED ☐ SEPARATED
IF COLLEGE STUDENT, F.T. / P.T., NAME OF SCHOOL _____ CITY _____ STATE/PROV. _____
PATIENT'S OR PARENT'S/GUARDIAN'S EMPLOYER _____ WORK PHONE _____
BUSINESS ADDRESS _____ CITY _____ STATE/PROV. _____ ZIP/P.C. _____
SPOUSE OR PARENT'S/GUARDIAN'S NAME _____ EMPLOYER _____ WORK PHONE _____
WHOM MAY WE THANK FOR REFERRING YOU? _____
PERSON TO CONTACT IN CASE OF AN EMERGENCY _____ PHONE _____

RESPONSIBLE PARTY

NAME OF PERSON RESPONSIBLE FOR THIS ACCOUNT _____ RELATIONSHIP TO PATIENT _____
ADDRESS _____ HOME PHONE _____
DRIVER'S LICENSE # _____ BIRTHDATE _____ SS#/SIN _____
EMPLOYER _____ WORK PHONE _____
IS THIS PERSON CURRENTLY A PATIENT IN OUR OFFICE? ☐ YES ☐ NO

INSURANCE INFORMATION

NAME OF INSURED _____ RELATIONSHIP TO PATIENT _____
BIRTHDATE _____ SS#/SIN _____ DATE EMPLOYED _____
NAME OF EMPLOYER _____ UNION OR LOCAL # _____ WORK PHONE _____
EMPLOYER ADDRESS _____ CITY _____ STATE/PROV. _____ ZIP/P.C. _____
INSURANCE CO. _____ TEL. # _____ GRP # _____ POLICY / I.D. # _____
INS. CO. ADDRESS _____ CITY _____ STATE/PROV. _____ ZIP/P.C. _____
HOW MUCH IS YOUR DEDUCTIBLE? _____ HOW MUCH HAVE YOU USED? _____ MAX ANNUAL BENEFIT? _____

DO YOU HAVE ANY ADDITIONAL INSURANCE? ☐ YES ☐ NO   IF YES, COMPLETE THE FOLLOWING:

NAME OF INSURED _____ RELATIONSHIP TO PATIENT _____
BIRTHDATE _____ SS#/SIN _____ DATE EMPLOYED _____
NAME OF EMPLOYER _____ UNION OR LOCAL # _____ WORK PHONE _____
EMPLOYER ADDRESS _____ CITY _____ STATE/PROV. _____ ZIP/P.C. _____
INSURANCE CO. _____ TEL. # _____ GRP # _____ POLICY / I.D. # _____
INS. CO. ADDRESS _____ CITY _____ STATE/PROV. _____ ZIP/P.C. _____
HOW MUCH IS YOUR DEDUCTIBLE? _____ HOW MUCH HAVE YOU USED? _____ MAX ANNUAL BENEFIT? _____

X _____
SIGNATURE OF PATIENT OR PARENT/GUARDIAN IF MINOR   PATIENT NUMBER

REGISTRATION

Dentrix Dental Practice
727 E Utah Valley Drive, # 500
American Fork UT 84003
(801)555-9300

Patient Information

Please take a moment to enter or update your information to help us ensure the quality of your care is excellent.

Chart #: _____ FOR OFFICE USE ONLY

Patient Name: _____ (Last) _____ (First) _____ (MI) _____ (Preferred Name)

Title: _____ (Mr/Ms/Mrs/Jr/Sr)   Gender: ○ Male ○ Female   Family Status: ○ Married ○ Single ○ Child ○ Other

Birth Date: _____   Prev. Visit: _____   Email Address: _____

Phone: _____ (Home) _____ (Work) _____ (Ext) _____ (Mobile)   Best time to call: _____

Address: _____
_____ (City) _____ (State) _____ (Zip Code)

Preferred appointment times:
☐ Mon ☐ Tue ☐ Wed ☐ Thur ☐ Fri ☐ Sat
☐ Morning ☐ Afternoon ☐ Evening ☐ Any time

Whom may we thank for referring you to our practice?
☐ Dental Office ☐ Yellow Pages ☐ Internet
☐ Newspaper ☐ School ☐ Work
☐ Other (name below):

Name of person, office, or other source referring you to our practice:
_____

page 1

Examples of Registration Forms. Print form courtesy Patterson Office Supplies, Champaign, IL. Dentrix screen shot courtesy Henry Schein Practice Solutions, American Fork, UT.

PATIENT'S MEDICAL HISTORY

PATIENT'S NAME _____ DATE OF BIRTH _____

ALTHOUGH DENTAL PERSONNEL PRIMARILY TREAT THE AREA IN AND AROUND YOUR MOUTH, YOUR MOUTH IS A PART OF YOUR ENTIRE BODY. HEALTH PROBLEMS THAT YOU MAY HAVE, OR MEDICATION THAT YOU MAY BE TAKING, COULD HAVE AN IMPORTANT INTERRELATIONSHIP WITH THE DENTISTRY THAT YOU WILL BE RECEIVING. THANK YOU FOR ANSWERING THE FOLLOWING QUESTIONS.

	YES	NO
1. ARE YOU IN GOOD HEALTH	☐	☐
2. HAVE THERE BEEN ANY CHANGES IN YOUR GENERAL HEALTH WITHIN THE PAST YEAR	☐	☐
3. DATE OF YOUR LAST PHYSICAL EXAM:		
4. PHYSICIAN'S NAME		
ADDRESS		
PHONE NO.		
5. ARE YOU NOW UNDER THE CARE OF A PHYSICIAN	☐	☐
6. HAVE YOU EVER BEEN HOSPITALIZED FOR ANY SURGICAL OPERATION OR SERIOUS ILLNESS PLEASE EXPLAIN.		
7. ARE YOU TAKING ANY MEDICINE(S) INCLUDING NON-PRESCRIPTION MEDICINE IF YES, WHAT MEDICINE(S) ARE YOU TAKING	☐	☐
8. HAVE YOU HAD ANY ABNORMAL BLEEDING	☐	☐
9. DO YOU BRUISE EASILY	☐	☐
10. HAVE YOU EVER REQUIRED A BLOOD TRANSFUSION	☐	☐
11. HAVE YOU HAD A RECENT WEIGHT LOSS	☐	☐

	YES	NO
12. HAVE YOU EVER TAKEN FEN-PHEN/REDUX	☐	☐
13. HAVE YOU EVER TAKEN FOSAMAX, BONIVA, ACTONEL OR ANY CANCER MEDICATIONS CONTAINING BISPHOSPHONATES	☐	☐
14. HAVE YOU TAKEN VIAGRA, REVATIO, CIALIS OR LEVITRA IN THE LAST 24 HOURS	☐	☐
15. DO YOU USE TOBACCO	☐	☐
16. DO YOU OR HAVE YOU USED CONTROLLED SUBSTANCES	☐	☐
17. ARE YOU WEARING CONTACT LENSES	☐	☐
18. DO YOU HAVE A PERSISTENT COUGH OR THROAT CLEARING NOT ASSOCIATED WITH A KNOWN ILLNESS (LASTING MORE THAN 3 WEEKS)	☐	☐
19. DO YOU HAVE ANY DISEASE, CONDITION OR PROBLEM NOT LISTED ABOVE THAT YOU THINK I SHOULD KNOW ABOUT	☐	☐

WOMEN ONLY:

	YES	NO
ARE YOU PREGNANT OR THINK YOU MAY BE PREGNANT	☐	☐
ARE YOU NURSING	☐	☐
ARE YOU TAKING BIRTH CONTROL PILLS	☐	☐

ARE YOU ALLERGIC TO OR HAVE YOU HAD REACTIONS TO:

	YES	NO
LOCAL ANESTHETICS LIKE NOVOCAINE	☐	☐
PENICILLIN OR OTHER ANTIBIOTICS	☐	☐
SULFA DRUGS	☐	☐
BARBITURATES, SEDATIVES OR SLEEPING PILLS	☐	☐
ASPIRIN	☐	☐
IODINE	☐	☐
ANY METALS (E.G., NICKEL, MERCURY, ETC.)	☐	☐
LATEX / RUBBER	☐	☐
OTHER (PLEASE LIST)		

DO YOU HAVE OR HAVE YOU EVER HAD THE FOLLOWING:

	YES	NO
RHEUMATIC HEART DISEASE OR RHEUMATIC FEVER	☐	☐
SCARLET FEVER	☐	☐
HEART DEFECT OR HEART MURMUR	☐	☐
HEART TROUBLE, HEART ATTACK, OR ANGINA	☐	☐
CHEST PAIN	☐	☐
SHORTNESS OF BREATH	☐	☐
PACEMAKER	☐	☐
HEART SURGERY	☐	☐
HIGH/LOW BLOOD PRESSURE	☐	☐
CONGENITAL HEART PROBLEM	☐	☐
SWELLING OF FEET, ANKLES, HANDS	☐	☐
HEPATITIS, JAUNDICE OR LIVER DISEASE	☐	☐
STROKE	☐	☐
SINUS TROUBLE	☐	☐
LUNG OR BREATHING PROBLEMS	☐	☐
ASTHMA OR HAY FEVER	☐	☐

	YES	NO
HIVES OR SKIN RASH	☐	☐
FAINTING OR DIZZY SPELLS	☐	☐
DIABETES	☐	☐
AIDS OR HIV INFECTION	☐	☐
THYROID PROBLEMS	☐	☐
ALLERGIES	☐	☐
ARTHRITIS OR RHEUMATISM	☐	☐
JOINT REPLACEMENT OR IMPLANT	☐	☐
STOMACH ULCER	☐	☐
KIDNEY TROUBLE	☐	☐
TUBERCULOSIS	☐	☐
PERSISTENT COUGH	☐	☐
COUGH THAT PRODUCES BLOOD	☐	☐
CHEMOTHERAPY (CANCER, LEUKEMIA)	☐	☐
SEXUALLY TRANSMITTED DISEASE	☐	☐
EPILEPSY OR SEIZURES	☐	☐
ANEMIA	☐	☐
GLAUCOMA	☐	☐
NERVOUSNESS	☐	☐
TONSILLITIS	☐	☐
TUMORS	☐	☐
MENTAL HEALTH CARE	☐	☐
BACK PROBLEMS	☐	☐
CHEMICAL DEPENDENCY	☐	☐
MITRAL VALVE PROLAPSE	☐	☐
CORTISONE TREATMENT	☐	☐
COLD SORES/FEVER BLISTERS	☐	☐
HYPOGLYCEMIA	☐	☐
EATING DISORDERS	☐	☐

PATIENT'S NUMBER _____

HEALTH HISTORY

Medical & Dental History Form

Patient Name: [_____] [_____] [__] [_____]
              Last   First   MI   Preferred Name

Please take a moment to let us know about your medical and dental history so we may serve you more effectively and in a way that watches out for your overall health and well-being.

Would you consider yourself to be in fairly good health?
◯ Yes   ◯ No

Within the past year, have there been any changes in your general health?
◯ Yes   ◯ No

What is the date (or approximate date) of your last medical exam?
[_____]

Your Primary Care Physician's name, address, & phone number:
[_____]

Please mark any of the following to indicate Yes in response to the question:

☐ Have you ever had complications following dental treatment?
☐ Are you currently under the care of a physician due to a specific condition?
☐ Have you been hospitalized within the last 5 years due to a surgery or illness?
☐ Are you currently taking any prescription or non-prescription medications?
☐ Do you use tobacco (smoking or chewing)?
☐ Do you require the use of corrective lenses (contacts or glasses)?
☐ Do you have any other conditions, diseases, etc., not listed above that we should be aware of?

If any of the previous questions are marked, please explain:
[_____]

page 1

Examples of Registration Forms. Print form courtesy Patterson Office Supplies, Champaign, IL. Dentrix screen shot courtesy Henry Schein Practice Solutions, American Fork, UT.

Continued

PATIENT'S DENTAL HISTORY

PATIENT'S NAME _____ DATE OF BIRTH _____

REASON FOR THIS VISIT _____

WHEN WAS YOUR LAST DENTAL VISIT _____ WHAT WAS DONE THEN _____

HOW OFTEN DID YOU VISIT THE DENTIST BEFORE THEN _____

PREVIOUS DENTIST (NAME AND LOCATION) _____

HAVE YOU HAD A COMPLETE SERIES OF DENTAL FILMS (X-RAYS) TAKEN WHEN/WHERE _____

HOW OFTEN DO YOU BRUSH YOUR TEETH _____ HOW OFTEN DO YOU FLOSS YOUR TEETH _____

IS YOUR DRINKING WATER FLUORIDATED _____

	YES	NO		YES	NO
DO YOUR GUMS BLEED WHILE BRUSHING OR FLOSSING	☐	☐	DO YOU BITE YOUR LIPS OR CHEEKS FREQUENTLY	☐	☐
ARE YOUR TEETH SENSITIVE TO HOT OR COLD LIQUIDS/FOODS	☐	☐	HAVE YOU NOTICED ANY LOOSENING OF YOUR TEETH	☐	☐
ARE YOUR TEETH SENSITIVE TO SWEET OR SOUR LIQUIDS/FOODS	☐	☐	DOES FOOD TEND TO BECOME CAUGHT BETWEEN YOUR TEETH	☐	☐
DO YOU FEEL PAIN TO ANY OF YOUR TEETH	☐	☐	HAVE YOU EVER HAD PERIODONTAL TREATMENT (GUMS)	☐	☐
DO YOU HAVE ANY SORES OR LUMPS IN OR NEAR YOUR MOUTH	☐	☐	EVER WORN A BITE PLATE OR OTHER APPLIANCE	☐	☐
HAVE YOU HAD ANY HEAD, NECK OR JAW INJURIES	☐	☐	HAVE YOU EVER HAD ANY DIFFICULT EXTRACTIONS IN THE PAST	☐	☐
HAVE YOU EVER EXPERIENCED ANY OF THE FOLLOWING PROBLEMS IN YOUR JAW?			HAVE YOU EVER HAD ANY PROLONGED BLEEDING FOLLOWING EXTRACTIONS	☐	☐
CLICKING	☐	☐	DO YOU WEAR DENTURES OR PARTIALS	☐	☐
PAIN (JOINT, EAR, SIDE OF FACE)	☐	☐	IF YES, DATE OF PLACEMENT _____		
DIFFICULTY IN OPENING OR CLOSING	☐	☐	HAVE YOU EVER RECEIVED ORAL HYGIENE		
DIFFICULTY IN CHEWING	☐	☐	INSTRUCTIONS REGARDING THE CARE OF		
DO YOU HAVE FREQUENT HEADACHES	☐	☐	YOUR TEETH AND GUMS	☐	☐
DO YOU CLENCH OR GRIND YOUR TEETH	☐	☐			

IF YOU COULD CHANGE ANYTHING ABOUT YOUR SMILE, WHAT WOULD YOU CHANGE? _____

AUTHORIZATION AND RELEASE

I CERTIFY THAT I HAVE READ AND UNDERSTAND THE ABOVE INFORMATION TO THE BEST OF MY KNOWLEDGE. THE ABOVE QUESTIONS HAVE BEEN ACCURATELY ANSWERED. I UNDERSTAND THAT PROVIDING INCORRECT INFORMATION CAN BE DANGEROUS TO MY HEALTH. I AUTHORIZE THE DENTIST TO RELEASE ANY INFORMATION INCLUDING THE DIAGNOSIS AND THE RECORDS OF ANY TREATMENT OR EXAMINATION RENDERED TO ME OR MY CHILD DURING THE PERIOD OF SUCH DENTAL CARE TO THIRD PARTY PAYORS AND/OR HEALTH PRACTITIONERS. I AUTHORIZE AND REQUEST MY INSURANCE COMPANY TO PAY DIRECTLY TO THE DENTIST OR DENTAL GROUP INSURANCE BENEFITS OTHERWISE PAYABLE TO ME. I UNDERSTAND THAT MY DENTAL INSURANCE CARRIER MAY PAY LESS THAN THE ACTUAL BILL FOR SERVICES. I AGREE TO BE RESPONSIBLE FOR PAYMENT OF ALL SERVICES RENDERED ON MY BEHALF OR MY DEPENDENTS.

X _____ DATE _____
SIGNATURE OF PATIENT OR PARENT/GUARDIAN IF MINOR

DOCTOR'S COMMENTS _____

SIGNATURE _____ DATE _____

PATIENT'S NUMBER _____

Dentrix Dental Practice
727 E Utah Valley Drive, # 500
American Fork UT 84003

(801)555-9300

What is the reason for your dental visit today?
_____

When was your last visit to the dentist (if to a different office)?
_____

What was done on your last dental visit (if to a different office)?
_____

Prior Dentist's name, address, & phone number:
_____

How frequently do you brush your teeth?
○ 3 (+) a day ○ Twice a day ○ Once a day ○ Weekly ○ Seldom

How frequently do you floss your teeth?
○ 1 (+) a day ○ 2 - 6 weekly ○ 1 - 6 monthly ○ Seldom ○ Never

Please mark any of the following to indicate Yes in response to the question:
☐ Do your gums bleed when you brush or floss?
☐ Do your teeth experience sensitivity to cold or hot temperatures?
☐ Are any of your teeth currently causing you pain?
☐ Do you grind your teeth (either consciously or during sleep)?
☐ Are any of your teeth loose, or are you concerned about any teeth loosening?
☐ Do you currently have any dental implants, dentures, or partials?

If any of the previous questions are marked, please explain:
_____

3

Examples of Registration Forms. Print form courtesy Patterson Office Supplies, Champaign, IL. Dentrix screen shot courtesy Henry Schein Practice Solutions, American Fork, UT.

PATIENT'S NAME: _____   DATE: _____

TIME: _____ (A.M.) (P.M.)

I HEREBY AUTHORIZE DR._____ AND HIS/HER ASSOCIATES AT _____
_____ TO PERFORM UPON ME OR THE NAMED PATIENT THE FOLLOWING
PROCEDURE(S): _____
_____ (EXPLAIN IN PLAIN ENGLISH).

DR. _____ HAS FULLY EXPLAINED TO ME THE PURPOSE OF THE PROCEDURE(S) AND HAS ALSO
INFORMED ME OF EXPECTED BENEFITS AND COMPLICATIONS (FROM KNOWN AND UNKNOWN CAUSES), ATTENDANT
DISCOMFORTS AND RISKS THAT MAY ARISE, AS WELL AS POSSIBLE ALTERNATIVES TO THE PROPOSED TREATMENT, INCLUDING
NO TREATMENT. THE ATTENDANT RISKS OF NO TREATMENT HAVE ALSO BEEN DISCUSSED. I HAVE BEEN GIVEN AN
OPPORTUNITY TO ASK QUESTIONS, AND ALL MY QUESTIONS HAVE BEEN ANSWERED FULLY AND SATISFACTORILY. I
ACKNOWLEDGE THAT NO GUARANTEES OR ASSURANCES HAVE BEEN MADE TO ME CONCERNING THE RESULTS INTENDED
FROM THE PROCEDURE(S).

I UNDERSTAND THAT DURING THE COURSE OF THE PROCEDURE(S), UNFORESEEN CONDITIONS MAY ARISE WHICH
NECESSITATE PROCEDURES DIFFERENT FROM THOSE CONTEMPLATED. I, THEREFORE, CONSENT TO THE PERFORMANCE OF
ADDITIONAL PROCEDURE(S) WHICH THE ABOVE-NAMED DENTIST OR HIS/HER ASSOCIATES MAY CONSIDER NECESSARY.

I ALSO UNDERSTAND THE FINANCIAL OBLIGATION ATTACHED TO THIS PROCEDURE AND AGREE TO COMPLY AS LISTED BELOW:
AMOUNT DUE _____ TO BE PAID IN _____ MONTHLY PAYMENTS OF $_____ STARTING _____.
BALANCE TO BE PAID IN FULL BY _____.

I UNDERSTAND THAT I AM RESPONSIBLE FOR ALL FEES REGARDLESS OF INSURANCE COVERAGE. I ALSO UNDERSTAND THAT AS
TREATMENT PROGRESSES THE ABOVE FEES MAY HAVE TO BE ADJUSTED, BUT THAT I WILL BE INFORMED OF THESE
ADJUSTMENTS AND HOW THEY WILL AFFECT MY PAYMENT PLAN. IN THE EVENT THAT MY PAYMENTS ARE NOT RECEIVED WITHIN
30 DAYS OF THEIR DUE DATE, I AGREE TO PAY ALL COSTS OF COLLECTIONS, INCLUDING, BUT NOT LIMITED TO, REASONABLE
ATTORNEY'S FEES.

I CONFIRM THAT I HAVE READ AND FULLY UNDERSTAND THE ABOVE AND THAT ALL BLANK SPACES HAVE BEEN COMPLETED
PRIOR TO MY SIGNING.

I HEREBY CONSENT TO THE PROPOSED DENTAL TREATMENT.

_____   _____
SIGNATURE OF PATIENT OR PARENT/GUARDIAN IF MINOR   DATE

_____   _____
INTERPRETER (IF USED)   DATE

_____   _____
SIGNATURE OF WITNESS   DATE

DENTIST CERTIFICATION:
I HEREBY CERTIFY THAT I HAVE EXPLAINED THE NATURE, PURPOSE, BENEFITS, RISKS OF, AND ALTERNATIVES (INCLUDING NO
TREATMENT AND ATTENDANT RISKS), TO THE PROPOSED PROCEDURE(S). I HAVE OFFERED ANSWERS TO ANY QUESTIONS AND
HAVE FULLY ANSWERED ALL SUCH QUESTIONS. I BELIEVE THAT THE PATIENT/PARENT/GUARDIAN FULLY UNDERSTANDS WHAT I
HAVE EXPLAINED AND ANSWERED.

DENTIST'S SIGNATURE _____

PRINT NAME _____   DATE _____

Item 881-8748/27006 Patterson Office Supplies 800-637-1140

PATIENT NUMBER

CONSENT TO DENTAL TREATMENT

Consent Form

Consent for Treatment

I, the undersigned patient, hereby authorize the undersigned provider to perform the procedure(s) or course(s) of treatment listed below. I understand my dental condition and have discussed several treatment options with the undersigned provider. I have been given a printed copy of the procedure or treatment details and any post-op instructions.

I understand the risks inherent in the treatment(s). I have discussed these risks with the dentist. The dentist has addressed all questions and concerns I have presented. I understand the expected results of the procedure(s) or course(s) of treatment. I understand that these results cannot be guaranteed and may not be achieved. I am aware of my right to waive treatment of any kind and I am aware of the possible consequences of non-treatment.

I have disclosed my health history information, including allergies, reactions to medicine, diseases, and past procedures. I understand that withholding this information may affect the outcome of the procedure(s) or course(s) of treatment.

I authorize the undersigned provider and any other qualified assistants or medical professionals to perform the procedure(s) or treatment(s)

Additional Notes...

Patient/Representative signature   Practice signature

                                Clear   Clear

Name: Brent L. Crosby Mr.   Name: Dennis Smith, D.D.S.
Date: 3/10/2011   Date: 3/10/2011
Relationship to patient: Self

                                         Print...   Save   Close

Examples of Consent to Dental Treatment Forms. Print form courtesy Patterson Office Supplies, Champaign, IL. Dentrix screen shot courtesy Henry Schein Practice Solutions, American Fork, UT.

Examples of Clinical Examination Forms. Print form courtesy Patterson Office Supplies, Champaign, IL. Dentrix screen shot courtesy Henry Schein Practice Solutions, American Fork, UT.

Examples of Treatment Plan Forms. Print form courtesy Patterson Office Supplies, Champaign, IL. Dentrix screen shot courtesy Henry Schein Practice Solutions, American Fork, UT.

PATIENT'S NAME _____ DATE OF BIRTH _____

DATE	TOOTH/ SURFACE	ANESTHETIC GIVEN	TREATMENT	DR.	ASST./HYG.

PATIENT NUMBER PAGE

PROGRESS NOTES

Progress Notes

Date	Tooth	Surface	Code	Provider	Description	N	R	D	M	Status	Amount
08/02/2010			P1111	DDS1	Prophylaxis - Adult	♪				C	85.00
08/02/2010	30		P2727	DDS1	Porcelain/HNM Crown					TP	995.00
08/02/2010	30		E6060	DDS1	Endosteal Implant Placement					TP	1,875.00
08/02/2010	30		R7171	DDS1	Routine Extraction					TP	155.00
01/27/2011	13	DLB	A2121	DDS1	Amalgam 3 Surface	♪		▽		C	195.00
02/03/2011			P0101	JJJD	Periodic Evaluation	♪		▽		CON	
02/03/2011			L0101	JJJD	Limited Evaluation			▽		C	70.00
02/07/2011	10	M,	A2323	JJJD	Anterior Resin Composite 1s	♪				CON	

Examples of Progress Notes Forms. Print form courtesy Patterson Office Supplies, Champaign, IL. Dentrix screen shot courtesy Henry Schein Practice Solutions, American Fork, UT.

COMPETENCY 26-1: REGISTERING A NEW PATIENT

Performance Objective

By following a routine procedure that meets stated protocols, the student will use the appropriate forms to gather patient registration and medical history information.

Evaluation and Grading Criteria

3   Student competently met the stated criteria without assistance.
2   Student required assistance in order to meet the stated criteria.
1   Student showed uncertainty when performing the stated criteria.
0   Student was not prepared and needs to repeat the step.
N/A   No evaluation of this step.

Instructor shall define grades for each point range earned on completion of each performance-evaluated task.

Performance Standards

The minimum number of satisfactory performances required before final evaluation is _____.

Instructor shall identify by * those steps considered critical. If step is missed or minimum competency is not met, the evaluated procedure fails and must be repeated.

PERFORMANCE CRITERIA	*	SELF	PEER	INSTRUCTOR	COMMENTS
1. Explained the need for the form to be completed.					
2. Provided the patient with a black pen and a form on a clipboard.					
3. Offered assistance to the patient in completing the form.					
4. Reviewed the completed forms to determine whether there were questions that were not answered.					
5. Reviewed the completed form for necessary information.					
6. Maintained an environment that was private and confidential when reviewing forms.					
7. Asked questions if the information on the form required clarification.					
8. Verified the patient's signature and date on the form.					

ADDITIONAL COMMENTS

Total number of points earned _____

Grade _____ Instructor's initials _____

COMPETENCY 26-2: OBTAINING A MEDICAL-DENTAL HEALTH HISTORY

Performance Objective

By following a routine procedure that meets stated protocols, the student will obtain a completed medical and dental history.

Evaluation and Grading Criteria

3 Student competently met the stated criteria without assistance.
2 Student required assistance in order to meet the stated criteria.
1 Student showed uncertainty when performing the stated criteria.
0 Student was not prepared and needs to repeat the step.
N/A No evaluation of this step.
Instructor shall define grades for each point range earned on completion of each performance-evaluated task.

Performance Standards

The minimum number of satisfactory performances required before final evaluation is _____.

Instructor shall identify by * those steps considered critical. If step is missed or minimum competency is not met, the evaluated procedure fails and must be repeated.

PERFORMANCE CRITERIA	*	SELF	PEER	INSTRUCTOR	COMMENTS
1. Explained the need for the form to be completed.					
2. Provided the patient with a black pen and a form on a clipboard.					
3. Offered assistance to the patient in completing the form.					
4. Reviewed the completed form for necessary information.					
5. Asked questions about information that required clarification.					
6. Verified the patient's signature and date on the form.					
7. Completed all additional forms requiring patient's medical-dental history					
ADDITIONAL COMMENTS					

Total number of points earned _____

Grade _____ Instructor's initials _____

COMPETENCY 26-3: ENTERING TREATMENT IN A PATIENT RECORD

Performance Objective
By following a routine procedure that meets stated protocols, the student will record dental treatment and services accurately, completely, and legibly.

Evaluation and Grading Criteria
<u>3</u>   Student competently met the stated criteria without assistance.
<u>2</u>   Student required assistance in order to meet the stated criteria.
<u>1</u>   Student showed uncertainty when performing the stated criteria.
<u>0</u>   Student was not prepared and needs to repeat the step.
<u>N/A</u>   No evaluation of this step.
Instructor shall define grades for each point range earned on completion of each performance-evaluated task.

Performance Standards
The minimum number of satisfactory performances required before final evaluation is _____.

Instructor shall identify by * those steps considered critical. If step is missed or minimum competency is not met, the evaluated procedure fails and must be repeated.

PERFORMANCE CRITERIA	*	SELF	PEER	INSTRUCTOR	COMMENTS
1. Completed all entries in black ink.					
2. Date entered.					
3. Progress notes were completed in detail: Tooth number and surface, type of dental procedure, anesthetic used, and type of dental materials used.					
4. Noted how the patient tolerated procedure.					
5. Noted what procedure is scheduled for next appointment.					
6. Signature/initials entered by dentist and dental assistant.					

ADDITIONAL COMMENTS

Total number of points earned _____

Grade _____ Instructor's initials _____

COMPETENCY 26-4: CORRECTING A CHART ENTRY

Performance Objective

By following a routine procedure that meets stated protocols, the student will correct an error on a patient's record.

Evaluation and Grading Criteria

3   Student competently met the stated criteria without assistance.
2   Student required assistance in order to meet the stated criteria.
1   Student showed uncertainty when performing the stated criteria.
0   Student was not prepared and needs to repeat the step.
N/A   No evaluation of this step.
Instructor shall define grades for each point range earned on completion of each performance-evaluated task.

Performance Standards

The minimum number of satisfactory performances required before final evaluation is _____.

Instructor shall identify by * those steps considered critical. If step is missed or minimum competency is not met, the evaluated procedure fails and must be repeated.

PERFORMANCE CRITERIA	*	SELF	PEER	INSTRUCTOR	COMMENTS
1. Drew a single line through the incorrect entry.					
2. Initialed and dated the change.					
3. Wrote the correct entry on the next available line.					
4. Initialed and dated the new entry.					
ADDITIONAL COMMENTS					

Total number of points earned _____

Grade _____ Instructor's initials _____

27 Vital Signs

SHORT-ANSWER QUESTIONS

1. List the four vital signs used to detect a person's baseline health status.

2. Describe how a person's metabolism could affect their vital signs.

3. Discuss three types of thermometers discussed in the chapter and the strengths and weaknesses of each.

4. List the common pulse sites used for taking a pulse.

5. Describe the characteristics of a pulse that you would look for when taking a patient's pulse.

6. Describe the characteristics of respiration and how they affect a patient's breathing.

7. Discuss the best way to obtain an accurate reading of a patient's respiration count.

8. Explain the importance of taking a patient's blood pressure.

9. Differentiate the Korotkoff sounds heard when a person's blood pressure is taken.

10. What does a pulse oximeter measure in the blood?

FILL-IN-THE-BLANK STATEMENTS

Select the best term from the list below and complete the following statements.

- antecubital space
- arrhythmia
- diastolic
- electrocardiogram
- metabolism
- pulse
- radial
- respiration
- rhythm
- sphygmomanometer
- stethoscope
- temperature
- thermometer
- tympanic
- volume

1. _____ is the term used to describe the blood pressure reading when the heart chambers are relaxed and dilated.

2. The _____ is a procedure that measures the electrical activity of the heartbeat and can be used in the detection and diagnosis of heart abnormalities.

3. _____ refers to the physical and chemical processes that occur within a living cell or organism that are necessary for the maintenance of life.

4. An irregularity in the force or rhythm of the heartbeat is termed _____.

5. _____ relates to the specific fold in the arm.

6. The _____ is a rhythmic throbbing of arteries produced by regular contraction of the heart.

7. The _____ artery is located at the base of the thumb on the wrist side.

8. _____ is the act or process of inhaling and exhaling (breathing).

9. The instrument used for measuring blood pressure is the _____.

10. The instrument that is used for listening to sounds produced within the body is the _____.

11. _____ is the degree of hotness or coldness of a body or an environment.

12. The instrument used for measuring a person's temperature is the _____.

13. _____ is a sequence or pattern.

14. _____ relates to or resembles a drum.

15. The quantity or amount of a substance is its _____.

MULTIPLE-CHOICE QUESTIONS

Complete each question by circling the best answer.

1. The four vital signs used to detect a patient's baseline health are _____.
   a. speech, temperature, gait, and electrocardiogram
   b. height, weight, age, and race
   c. cholesterol, blood pressure, vision, and blood sugar
   d. respiration, temperature, pulse, and blood pressure

2. A thermometer is used for _____.
   a. detecting a patient's pulse
   b. taking a patient's temperature
   c. reading a patient's blood pressure
   d. counting a patient's respiration

3. What location on the body produces the highest temperature reading?
   a. Oral
   b. Ancillary
   c. Rectal
   d. Ear

4. Where would the tympanic thermometer be placed for a temperature reading?
   a. Orally
   b. Under the arm
   c. Rectally
   d. In the ear

5. Which artery has a pulse?
   a. Carotid
   b. Radial
   c. Brachial
   d. All of the above

6. Which artery would you normally palpate when taking a patient's pulse?
   a. Carotid
   b. Radial
   c. Brachial
   d. Any of the above

7. A normal pulse rate for an adult is _____.
   a. 25 to 65 beats per minute
   b. 40 to 80 beats per minute
   c. 60 to 100 beats per minute
   d. 75 to 115 beats per minute

8. Respiration is the process of _____.
   a. speaking
   b. breathing
   c. feeling
   d. moving

9. What breathing pattern is characteristic of a very rapid rate of breathing?
   a. Bradypnea
   b. Normal pattern
   c. Tachypnea
   d. Sighing

10. The normal respiration rate for an adult is _____.
    a. 5 to 10 breaths per minute
    b. 10 to 20 breaths per minute
    c. 18 to 30 breaths per minute
    d. 20 to 40 breaths per minute

11. What is the diastolic reading of a blood pressure?
    a. The first sound heard after pressure is released from the cuff
    b. The pulse rate taken at the brachial artery
    c. The silence between the first and last sounds after pressure is released from the cuff
    d. The last sound heard after pressure is released from the cuff

12. What instruments are used to take a patient's blood pressure?
    a. A patient record and a watch with a second hand
    b. A sphygmomanometer and a stethoscope
    c. A pen and paper to record the reading
    d. A thermometer and an electrocardiogram

13. The term for the small groove or fold on the inner arm is the _____.
    a. antecubital space
    b. brachial fold
    c. radial bend
    d. femur

14. Who discovered the series of sounds that can be heard during the taking of a blood pressure reading?
    a. G.V. Black
    b. W.B. Saunders
    c. Nicolai Korotkoff
    d. C. Edmund Kells

15. The normal blood pressure reading of an adult is _____.
    a. <90/<60
    b. <100/<75
    c. <120/<80
    d. <150/<100

CASE STUDY

Mary Robins, a 53-year-old patient, is scheduled for a routine dental prophylaxis. You escort her back to the treatment area, review her health history update, and take her vital signs. The readings that were obtained today are temperature 99° F, pulse 75, respiration 20, and blood pressure 150/100.

1. What type of procedure is dental prophylaxis? Which dental professional would most likely be treating Mrs. Robins today?

2. As the clinical assistant in the office, what could be your role for seeing this patient today?

3. How would Mrs. Robins be positioned for taking vital signs?

4. Mrs. Robins states that she should not have her blood pressure taken on her left arm because she has had a mastectomy. She indicates that her lymph nodes were also removed on that side and the doctor told her not to have her blood pressure taken on that side. Why would a doctor say this? You may need to refer to the Internet for the reason why.

5. Besides the rate of respiration, what additional characteristics of the patient's respiration should you note in her patient record?

6. Are there any readings that are not within normal range? If so, which ones?

7. What is your next step when a patient's vital sign reading is abnormal?

MULTIMEDIA PROCEDURES RECOMMENDED REVIEW

ɘvolve
learning system

■ Taking a Patient's Blood Pressure

COMPETENCY 27-1: TAKING AN ORAL TEMPERATURE READING WITH A DIGITAL THERMOMETER

Performance Objective

By following a routine procedure that meets stated protocols, the student will obtain and record an oral temperature.

Evaluation and Grading Criteria

3   Student competently met the stated criteria without assistance.
2   Student required assistance in order to meet the stated criteria.
1   Student showed uncertainty when performing the stated criteria.
0   Student was not prepared and needs to repeat the step.
N/A   No evaluation of this step.
Instructor shall define grades for each point range earned on completion of each performance-evaluated task.

Performance Standards

The minimum number of satisfactory performances required before final evaluation is _____.

Instructor shall identify by * those steps considered critical. If step is missed or minimum competency is not met, the evaluated procedure fails and must be repeated.

PERFORMANCE CRITERIA	*	SELF	PEER	INSTRUCTOR	COMMENTS
1. Obtained the equipment and supplies required for taking an oral temperature.					
2. Personal protective equipment placed according to procedure.					
3. Placed a sheath over the probe of the digital thermometer.					
4. Turned the thermometer on, and after display indicates "ready" gently places it under the patient's tongue.					
5. Instructs patient to close their lips over the thermometer and not talk or move during reading.					
6. Left the thermometer in place for the appropriate time, then removed it from the patient's mouth.					
7. Reviewed the temperature reading, and recorded it in the patient record.					
8. Turned the thermometer off, removed and disposed of the sheath, and disinfected the thermometer as recommended.					
9. Procedure documented in patient record.					
ADDITIONAL COMMENTS					

Total number of points earned

Grade _____ Instructor's initials _____

COMPETENCY 27-2: TAKING A PATIENT'S PULSE

Performance Objective

By following a routine procedure that meets stated protocols, the student will take and record a patient's pulse.

Evaluation and Grading Criteria

<u>3</u>   Student competently met the stated criteria without assistance.
<u>2</u>   Student required assistance in order to meet the stated criteria.
<u>1</u>   Student showed uncertainty when performing the stated criteria.
<u>0</u>   Student was not prepared and needs to repeat the step.
<u>N/A</u> No evaluation of this step.
Instructor shall define grades for each point range earned on completion of each performance-evaluated task.

Performance Standards

The minimum number of satisfactory performances required before final evaluation is _____.

Instructor shall identify by * those steps considered critical. If step is missed or minimum competency is not met, the evaluated procedure fails and must be repeated.

PERFORMANCE CRITERIA	*	SELF	PEER	INSTRUCTOR	COMMENTS
1. Obtained the equipment and supplies required for taking a pulse.					
2. Personal protective equipment placed according to procedure.					
3. Seated the patient in an upright position.					
4. Placed the tips of index and middle fingers on the patient's radial artery.					
5. Felt for the patient's pulse before counting.					
6. Counted the pulse for 30 seconds and multiplied by 2 for a 1-minute reading.					
7. Procedure documented in patient record.					
ADDITIONAL COMMENTS					

Total number of points earned _____

Grade _____ Instructor's initials _____

COMPETENCY 27-3: TAKING A PATIENT'S RESPIRATION

Performance Objective

By following a routine procedure that meets stated protocols, the student will obtain and record a patient's respiration.

Evaluation and Grading Criteria

<u>3</u>   Student competently met the stated criteria without assistance.

<u>2</u>   Student required assistance in order to meet the stated criteria.

<u>1</u>   Student showed uncertainty when performing the stated criteria.

<u>0</u>   Student was not prepared and needs to repeat the step.

<u>N/A</u> No evaluation of this step.

Instructor shall define grades for each point range earned on completion of each performance-evaluated task.

Performance Standards

The minimum number of satisfactory performances required before final evaluation is _____.

Instructor shall identify by * those steps considered critical. If step is missed or minimum competency is not met, the evaluated procedure fails and must be repeated.

PERFORMANCE CRITERIA	*	SELF	PEER	INSTRUCTOR	COMMENTS
1. Obtained the equipment and supplies required for taking a respiration.					
2. Personal protective equipment placed according to procedure.					
3. Patient remains seated, and maintains position as in taking the pulse.					
4. Counted the rise and fall of the patient's chest for 30 seconds.					
5. Multiplied the count by 2 for a 1-minute reading.					
6. Procedure documented in patient record.					
ADDITIONAL COMMENTS					

Total number of points earned _____

Grade _____ Instructor's initials _____

COMPETENCY 27-4: TAKING A PATIENT'S BLOOD PRESSURE

Performance Objective

By following a routine procedure that meets stated protocols, the student will obtain and record a patient's blood pressure.

Evaluation and Grading Criteria

 3   Student competently met the stated criteria without assistance.
 2   Student required assistance in order to meet the stated criteria.
 1   Student showed uncertainty when performing the stated criteria.
 0   Student was not prepared and needs to repeat the step.
 N/A   No evaluation of this step.
Instructor shall define grades for each point range earned on completion of each performance-evaluated task.

Performance Standards

The minimum number of satisfactory performances required before final evaluation is _____.

Instructor shall identify by * those steps considered critical. If step is missed or minimum competency is not met, the evaluated procedure fails and must be repeated.

PERFORMANCE CRITERIA	*	SELF	PEER	INSTRUCTOR	COMMENTS
1. Obtained the equipment and supplies required for taking a blood pressure.					
2. Personal protective equipment placed according to procedure.					
3. Had patient seated with the arm extended at heart level and supported.					
4. Rolled up the patient's sleeve if possible.					
5. Palpated the patient's brachial artery to feel for a pulse.					
6. Counted the patient's brachial pulse for 30 seconds.					
7. Multiplied the count by 2 for a 1-minute reading.					
8. Added 40 mm Hg to get inflation level.					
9. Readied the cuff by expelling any air.					
10. Placed the cuff around the patient's arm 1 inch above antecubital space, with arrow over the brachial artery.					
11. Tightened the cuff and closed it using the Velcro tabs.					
12. Placed earpieces of stethoscope properly.					

Continued

13. Placed stethoscope disk over site of brachial artery.				
14. Grasped rubber bulb, locked valve, and inflated cuff to noted reading.				
15. Slowly released the valve and listened for sounds.				
16. Slowly continued to release air from the cuff until the last sound was heard.				
17. Procedure documented in patient record.				
18. Disinfected the diaphragm and ear pieces of the stethoscope.				

ADDITIONAL COMMENTS

Total number of points earned

Grade _____ Instructor's initials _____

COMPETENCY 27-5: TAKING A PATIENT'S PULSE OXIMETRY (EXPANDED FUNCTION)

Performance Objective

By following a routine procedure that meets stated protocols, the student will obtain and record a patient's oximetry level.

Evaluation and Grading Criteria

3 Student competently met the stated criteria without assistance.
2 Student required assistance in order to meet the stated criteria.
1 Student showed uncertainty when performing the stated criteria.
0 Student was not prepared and needs to repeat the step.
N/A No evaluation of this step.
Instructor shall define grades for each point range earned on completion of each performance-evaluated task.

Performance Standards

The minimum number of satisfactory performances required before final evaluation is _____.

Instructor shall identify by * those steps considered critical. If step is missed or minimum competency is not met, the evaluated procedure fails and must be repeated.

PERFORMANCE CRITERIA	*	SELF	PEER	INSTRUCTOR	COMMENTS
1. Obtained the equipment and supplies required for performing oximetry.					
2. Personal protective equipment placed according to procedure.					
3. Seated the patient with his or her arm extended on the chair arm.					
4. Turned the pulse oximeter machine on and waited for it to go through its calibration and check tests.					
5. Ensured that the finger was cleaned and any nail polish removed. Selected the correct size probe and positioned the probe on the finger, avoiding excess force.					
6. Allowed several seconds for the pulse oximeter to detect the pulse and calculate the oxygen saturation.					
7. Procedure documented in patient record.					
ADDITIONAL COMMENTS					

Total number of points earned

Grade _____   Instructor's initials _____

COMPETENCY 27-6: TAKING A PATIENT'S ECG (EXPANDED FUNCTION)

Performance Objective

By following a routine procedure that meets stated protocols, the student will obtain and record a patient's electrocardiographic reading.

Evaluation and Grading Criteria

3   Student competently met the stated criteria without assistance.
2   Student required assistance in order to meet the stated criteria.
1   Student showed uncertainty when performing the stated criteria.
0   Student was not prepared and needs to repeat the step.
N/A   No evaluation of this step.
Instructor shall define grades for each point range earned on completion of each performance-evaluated task.

Performance Standards

The minimum number of satisfactory performances required before final evaluation is _____.

Instructor shall identify by * those steps considered critical. If step is missed or minimum competency is not met, the evaluated procedure fails and must be repeated.

PERFORMANCE CRITERIA	*	SELF	PEER	INSTRUCTOR	COMMENTS
1. Obtained the equipment and supplies required for taking an ECG.					
2. Personal protective equipment placed according to procedure.					
3. Explains procedure to the patient, and answers any questions.					
4. Instructs the patient to lay down.					
5. Labeled all forms and tracing paper with the patient's name, the date, the time, and any medication the patient was receiving intravenously or orally.					
6. At each location wiped the patient's chest with an alcohol wipe, and placed the electrodes at the six positions on the patient's chest.					
7. Connected the lead wires to the correct electrodes, making sure the lead wires were not crossed.					
8. At the surgeon's request, proceeds by pressing the auto button. (The machine automatically begins the tracing.)					

Continued

9. Continued the tracings until the completion of the procedure.					
10. Removed the lead wires and electrodes from the patient's chest.					
12. Turns off the electrocardiograph, properly disinfected it, and placed it in its storage area.					
13. Procedure documented in patient record.					

ADDITIONAL COMMENTS

Total number of points earned _____

Grade _____ Instructor's initials _____

28 Oral Diagnosis and Treatment Planning

SHORT-ANSWER QUESTIONS

1. List and describe the examination and diagnostic techniques used for patient assessment.

2. Discuss the role of the assistant in the clinical examination of a patient.

3. List the six classifications of Black's classification of cavities.

4. Differentiate between an anatomic and a geometric diagram for charting.

5. Differentiate between red and black for color-coding a charted diagram.

6. Describe the pocket depth and probing index of the gingival tissues, and explain how they should be recorded.

7. Describe the need for a soft tissue examination.

8. Discuss the importance of a treatment plan.

FILL-IN-THE-BLANK STATEMENTS

Select the best term from the list below and complete the following statements.

- detection
- extraoral
- furcation
- intraoral
- mobility
- morphology
- mucogingival
- palpation
- probing
- recession
- restoration
- symmetric

1. _____ is the process of bringing a tooth back to its functional permanent unit.

2. _____ is the process of discovering decay.

3. To divide into branches or separate as with roots on a tooth is termed _____.

4. _____ is to have movement.

183

5. _____ is the branch of biology that deals with the form and structure of organisms without attention to function.

6. To touch or feel for abnormalities within soft tissue is _____.

7. _____ is the term that is used to mean outside the oral cavity.

8. The periodontal probe is used for _____ and for measuring the periodontal pocket.

9. _____ is to recede or wear away from its normal location.

10. _____ is below the gingival tissue surrounding a tooth.

11. An object is considered to be _____ if it is balanced on both sides.

12. _____ is the term that means within the oral cavity.

MULTIPLE-CHOICE QUESTIONS

Complete each question by circling the best answer.

1. The four reasons why a patient would seek dental care are _____.
   a. proximity to home, reasonable price, nice decor, good dentist
   b. as a new patient, for an emergency, for a consultation, as a returning patient
   c. sterile techniques, knowledgeable staff, appropriate attire, clean environment
   d. takes insurance, has flexible hours, performs specialty procedures, no waiting

2. What technique(s) could be used to diagnose decay within a tooth?
   a. Visual
   b. Instrumentation
   c. Radiographic
   d. All of the above

3. Which material is not used to restore a tooth?
   a. Silver
   b. Gold
   c. Brass
   d. Porcelain

4. What charting symbol indicates a tooth that is not visible in the mouth?
   a. Circle around the tooth
   b. Outline with diagonal lines
   c. X through the tooth
   d. a and c

5. Intraoral imaging is similar to _____.
   a. use of a video camera
   b. use of a laser
   c. radiography
   d. photocopying

6. Which of G.V. Black's classifications of cavities would involve the premolars and molars?
   a. Class I
   b. Class II
   c. Class III
   d. a and b

7. Which classifications of cavities would involve the incisors?
   a. Class I
   b. Class III
   c. Class IV
   d. All of the above

8. How would an MOD amalgam be charted for tooth number 4?
   a. The gingival one third on the facial surface would be outlined in blue and colored in.
   b. The mesial, occlusal, and distal surfaces would be outlined in blue and colored in.
   c. The occlusal surface would be outlined in blue, with an A placed in the center.
   d. The mesial and distal surfaces of the tooth would be outlined in red, and the occlusal portion would be colored in blue.

9. What dental professional can legally perform periodontal probing and a bleeding index for a patient?
   a. Dentist
   b. Assistant
   c. Hygienist
   d. a and c

10. Which classification of dental mobility is most severe?
    a. Class I
    b. Class II
    c. Class III
    d. Class IV

11. The cervical lymph nodes are examined for
    _____.
    a. bruising
    b. swelling
    c. tenderness
    d. b and c

12. When two halves of the face are not identical mirror
    images, the face is said to be _____.
    a. symmetrical
    b. disproportionate
    c. distorted
    d. asymmetrical

13. To avoid triggering the gag reflex during a soft tissue
    examination, the mouth mirror can be_____.
    a. warmed before placing it in the mouth
    b. moved from left to right in the back of the
       tongue
    c. placed firmly on the back of the tongue
    d. a and b

14. To examine the tongue, a _____ is used
    to gently pull it forward.
    a. pair of cotton pliers
    b. gauze square
    c. tongue retractor
    d. suture material

15. The abbreviation PFM stands for _____.
    a. patient fainted momentarily
    b. porcelain filling on mesial
    c. porcelain fused to metal
    d. protrusive forward movement

Ɵvolve
learning system

MULTIMEDIA PROCEDURES RECOMMENDED REVIEW

■ Extraoral and Intraoral Photography

CHARTING IDENTIFICATION

List the condition depicted by each charting symbol. Please note that areas in gray would normally appear in red within a
dental chart; these are areas in which treatment has yet to be completed. The areas in black indicate treatment that has been
completed.

CHARTING SYMBOL	CONDITION

Chapter **28** **Oral Diagnosis and Treatment Planning**

CHARTING SYMBOL	CONDITION

CHARTING SYMBOL	CONDITION

CHARTING SYMBOL	CONDITION

CHARTING SYMBOL	CONDITION

CHARTING SYMBOL	CONDITION

CHARTING EXERCISE

Chart the following findings on the diagram:

#1	impacted
#2	DO amalgam
#3	MOD amalgam
#4	porcelain crown
#5-7	three-unit gold bridge
#8	root canal with porcelain crown
#9	root canal with porcelain crown
#10	class V facial composite
#11	class V facial decay
#12	MO decay
#13	abscess
#14	class I lingual pit amalgam with sealant placed on occlusal surface

#15	sealant on occlusal surface
#16-17	impacted
#18-21	four-unit gold bridge with #18 having a root canal
#24	mesial composite
#25	distal composite
#26	fractured mesial/incisal edge
#28	MO composite
#29	missing
#30	MOD amalgam with recurrent decay
#31	occlusal amalgam with recurrent decay
#32	impacted

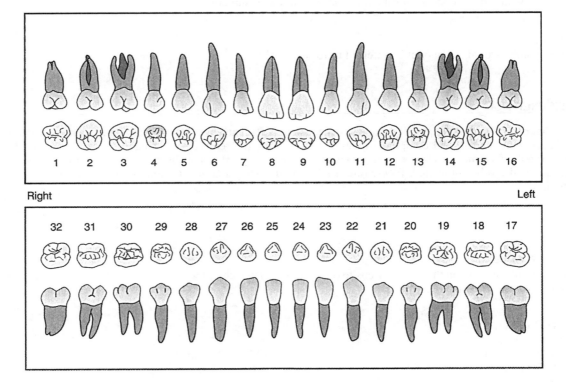

Right   Left

From your charting, answer the following questions:

1. Which teeth are missing that are replaced by a bridge?

2. Which teeth have Class II restorations?

3. Is there an area within the mouth in which drifting could take place? If so, where would this occur?

4. Why do you think the dentist chose to place composite resin material in tooth #28?

5. What teeth would be of concern for the oral and maxillofacial surgeon?

6. What specialist would the patient be referred to for tooth #13?

DENTRIX EXERCISE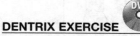

An important component of the practice management system is Patient Chart, which makes it easy to enter electronically all existing, recommended, and completed treatment or conditions. Dentrix uses standard, easy-to-recognize textbook charting symbols. Treatment is color-coded, making it easy to see at a glance whether a procedure is completed, existing, a condition, or still to be completed. Please refer to the Dentrix *User's Guide*, Chapter 4, to review how to chart within the system.

Exercise: Charting

Please refer to information on the Evolve website on **Charting.** Then chart the following conditions and completed treatment for the patient listed below:

Gregory H Brooks

#1	Missing	#14	MOD amalgam
#2	MO amalgam	#15	MO amalgam
#3	MOD amalgam	#16	Missing
#4	PFM crown	#17	Missing
#5	DO amalgam	#18	MO amalgam
#8	Missing	#19	Root canal treatment with gold crown
#11	Amalgam restoration	#20	MO amalgam
#12	MOD amalgam	#30	Missing with three-unit gold bridge
#13	MOD amalgam	#32	Missing

COMPETENCY 28-1: EXTRAORAL AND INTRAORAL PHOTOGRAPHY (EXPANDED FUNCTION)

Performance Objective

By following a routine procedure that meets stated protocols, when provided with a camera, the student will demonstrate the proper technique for taking extraoral and intraoral photographs.

Evaluation and Grading Criteria

 3   Student competently met the stated criteria without assistance.
 2   Student required assistance in order to meet the stated criteria.
 1   Student showed uncertainty when performing the stated criteria.
 0   Student was not prepared and needs to repeat the step.
 N/A No evaluation of this step.

Instructor shall define grades for each point range earned on completion of each performance-evaluated task.

Performance Standards

The minimum number of satisfactory performances required before final evaluation is _____.

Instructor shall identify by * those steps considered critical. If step is missed or minimum competency is not met, the evaluated procedure fails and must be repeated.

PERFORMANCE CRITERIA	*	SELF	PEER	INSTRUCTOR	COMMENTS
1. Obtained the equipment and supplies required for the procedure.					
2. Calibrated the camera system for intraoral and extraoral photographs. For intraoral photography, camera was set to landscape mode; and for extraoral photography, camera was set to portrait mode.					
3. Seated the patient in the dental chair in an upright position with a neutral color background.					
4. For extraoral photographs, t positioned himself or herself 5 to 6 feet from the patient.					
5. For intraoral photographs, the mouth was visible and partially dried.					
6. The retractors were positioned symmetrically and then pulled out and away from the mouth.					
7. If a mouth mirror or reflection mirror was used, it was free of fog and kept clean.					
8. Kept fingertips, mirror edges, and retractors out of the picture.					

Continued

9. Photographs of the teeth were correct and in alignment.				
10. Cleaned and disinfected all supplies and returned to case.				
11. Procedure documented in patient record.				
ADDITIONAL COMMENTS				

Total number of points earned _____

Grade _____ Instructor's initials _____

COMPETENCY 28-2: THE SOFT TISSUE EXAMINATION (EXPANDED FUNCTION)

Performance Objective

By following a routine procedure that meets stated protocols, the student will demonstrate the proper technique for performing a soft tissue examination.

Evaluation and Grading Criteria

_3_   Student competently met the stated criteria without assistance.
_2_   Student required assistance in order to meet the stated criteria.
_1_   Student showed uncertainty when performing the stated criteria.
_0_   Student was not prepared and needs to repeat the step.
_N/A_   No evaluation of this step.
Instructor shall define grades for each point range earned on completion of each performance-evaluated task.

Performance Standards

The minimum number of satisfactory performances required before final evaluation is _____.

Instructor shall identify by * those steps considered critical. If step is missed or minimum competency is not met, the evaluated procedure fails and must be repeated.

PERFORMANCE CRITERIA	*	SELF	PEER	INSTRUCTOR	COMMENTS
1. Obtained the equipment and supplies required for the procedure.					
2. Escorted the patient to the treatment area, observing patient's general appearance, speech, and behavior.					
3. Personal protective equipment placed according to procedure.					
4. Seated the patient in the dental chair in an upright position.					
5. Explained the procedure to the patient.					
Extraoral Features					
6. Examined the patient's face, neck, and ears for asymmetry or abnormal swelling.					
7. Looked for abnormal tissue changes, skin abrasions, and discolorations.					
8. Evaluated the texture, color, and continuity of the vermilion border, commissures of the lips, philtrum, and smile line.					
9. Procedure documented in patient record.					

Continued

Cervical Lymph Nodes					
10. Positioned self in front and to the side of patient.					
11. Examined the right side of the neck using fingers and thumb of the right hand to follow the chain of lymph nodes starting in front of the ear and continuing to the collarbone.					
12. Examined the left side of the neck in the same manner.					
13. Procedure documented in patient record.					
Temporomandibular Joint					
14. Evaluated TMJ movement in centric, lateral, protrusive, and retrusive movements. Asked the patient to open and close mouth normally and to move jaw from side to side.					
15. Listened for noise in the TMJ as the patient opened and closed the mouth.					
16. Procedure documented in patient record.					
Indications of Oral Habits					
17. Looked for oral habits of thumb sucking, tongue-thrust swallow, mouth breathing, and tobacco use.					
18. Looked for signs of oral habits such as bruxism, grinding, and clenching.					
Interior of the Lips					
19. Examined the mucosa and the labial frenum of the patient's upper lip.					
20. Examined the mucosa and the labial frenum of the patient's lower lip.					
21. Palpated tissues to detect lumps or abnormalities.					
Oral Mucosa and Tongue					
22. Palpated the tissue of the buccal mucosa.					
23. Examined the tissue covering the hard palate.					
24. Examined the buccal mucosa and the opening of Stensen's duct.					

25. Evaluated the patient's tongue by pulling it forward and from side to side, noting color, papillae, and abnormalities.					
26. Instructed patient to open, stick their tongue out and say "Ahh" and examined the uvula and the base of the tongue.					
Floor of the Mouth					
27. Palpated the soft tissues of the face above and below the mandible.					
28. Palpated the interior of the floor of the mouth.					
29. Observed the quantity and consistency of the flow of the saliva.					
30. Procedure documented in patient record.					

ADDITIONAL COMMENTS

Total number of points earned _____

Grade_____ Instructor's initials_____

COMPETENCY 28-3: CHARTING OF TEETH

Performance Objective
By following a routine procedure that meets stated protocols, when provided with a patient chart and colored pencils, the student will demonstrate the proper technique for recording the dentist's findings as dictated during an examination.

Evaluation and Grading Criteria
3   Student competently met the stated criteria without assistance.
2   Student required assistance in order to meet the stated criteria.
1   Student showed uncertainty when performing the stated criteria.
0   Student was not prepared and needs to repeat the step.
N/A   No evaluation of this step.
Instructor shall define grades for each point range earned on completion of each performance-evaluated task.

Performance Standards
The minimum number of satisfactory performances required before final evaluation is _____.

Instructor shall identify by * those steps considered critical. If step is missed or minimum competency is not met, the evaluated procedure fails and must be repeated.

PERFORMANCE CRITERIA	*	SELF	PEER	INSTRUCTOR	COMMENTS
1. Obtained the equipment and supplies required for the procedure.					
2. Personal protective equipment placed according to procedure.					
3. Seated the patient in the dental chair in a supine position and draped with a patient napkin.					
4. Had colored pencils, eraser, and clinical examination form readily available.					
5. Recorded specific notations the operator called out for each tooth.					
6. Throughout the procedure, used the air syringe to dry the mouth mirror.					
7. Adjusted the operating light as necessary.					
8. Procedure documented in patient record.					
9. Accurately read back the operator's findings.					
ADDITIONAL COMMENTS					

Total number of points earned _____

Grade _____ Instructor's initials _____

COMPETENCY 28-4: PERIODONTAL SCREENING: EXAMINATION OF THE GINGIVAL TISSUES

Performance Objective
By following a routine procedure that meets stated protocols, the student will assist the dentist or the dental hygienist in the examination and charting of gingival tissues.

Evaluation and Grading Criteria
3   Student competently met the stated criteria without assistance.
2   Student required assistance in order to meet the stated criteria.
1   Student showed uncertainty when performing the stated criteria.
0   Student was not prepared and needs to repeat the step.
N/A   No evaluation of this step.
Instructor shall define grades for each point range earned on completion of each performance-evaluated task.

Performance Standards
The minimum number of satisfactory performances required before final evaluation is _____.

Instructor shall identify by * those steps considered critical. If step is missed or minimum competency is not met, the evaluated procedure fails and must be repeated.

PERFORMANCE CRITERIA	*	SELF	PEER	INSTRUCTOR	COMMENTS
1. Obtained the equipment and supplies required for the procedure.					
2. Personal protective equipment placed according to procedure.					
3. Seated the patient in the dental chair in a supine position and draped with a patient napkin.					
4. Provided air from the air-water syringe on the mirror during the examination.					
5. Transferred instruments as needed.					
6. Recorded depths of the sulcus greater than 3 mm on the examination form.					
7. Charted bleeding.					
8. Noted sensitivity, calculus, mobility, saliva changes, and furcation involvement.					
9. Procedure documented in patient record.					
10. Accurately read back the operator's findings.					

ADDITIONAL COMMENTS

Total number of points earned _____

Grade _____ Instructor's initials _____

29 The Special Needs and Medically Compromised Patient

SHORT-ANSWER QUESTIONS

1. Give the three categories of how an individual can be defined through his or her aging process. Explain how they differ with regard to dental care?

2. List the five most common oral health conditions that affect the older patient.

3. What additional information is important to obtain from a medically compromised patient besides the medical-dental history?

4. You are scheduling a patient with early onset Alzheimer's. Describe what clinical considerations should be taken into consideration for this patient

5. You will be transferring a patient from a wheelchair to the patient chair. What will you need to have on hand to help in the moving process?

FILL-IN-THE-BLANK STATEMENTS

Select the best term from the list below and complete the following statements.

- aging
- Alzheimer's
- anemia
- angina
- arthritis
- asthma
- atrophy
- bacteremia
- bronchitis
- diabetes
- epilepsy
- hemophilia
- hyperplasia
- hyperthyroidism
- hypothyroidism
- leukemia
- myocardial infarction
- seizure
- stroke
- xerostomia

1. A person with a deficiency in the oxygen-carrying component of blood is said to have _____.

2. Wasting away or deterioration is termed _____.

3. A(n) _____ is a sudden attack, spasm, or convulsion that occurs in specific disorders.

4. The presence of bacteria in the blood is termed _____.

5. _____ is the loss of saliva production that causes a dry mouth.

6. _____ is severe pain in the chest that results from an insufficient supply of blood to the heart.

7. _____ is a neurologic disorder with sudden recurring seizures of motor, sensory, or psychological malfunction.

8. _____ refers to becoming mature or older.

9. _____ is a disorder in which progressive mental deterioration occurs in middle to old age.

10. A blood coagulation disorder in which the blood fails to clot normally is _____.

11. _____ is an abnormal increase in the number of cells in an organ or tissue.

12. _____ is a disorder in which inflammation of the mucous membrane of the bronchial tubes occurs.

13. A condition that results from excessive activity of the thyroid gland is _____.

14. A disease of the bone marrow in which an abnormal development of white blood cells occurs is _____.

15. _____ is also known as a *heart attack*.

16. Inflammation, pain, and swelling of the joints are symptoms of _____.

17. _____ is a chronic respiratory disease that is often associated with allergies and is characterized by sudden recurring attacks of labored breathing, chest constriction, and coughing.

18. _____ is a condition that results from severe thyroid insufficiency.

19. A sudden loss of brain function caused by a blockage or rupture of a blood vessel to the brain is a _____.

20. _____ is a metabolic disorder that is characterized by high blood glucose and insufficient insulin.

MULTIPLE-CHOICE QUESTIONS

Complete each question by circling the best answer.

1. The fastest-growing segment of the population is _____.
   a. infants
   b. young adults
   c. middle-aged adults
   d. older adults

2. How would you describe a frail older adult?
   a. Better educated
   b. Beginning to have multiple health problems
   c. Having fewer natural teeth
   d. a and c

3. Xerostomia is a condition of _____.
   a. excessive saliva
   b. eye infection
   c. loss of hearing
   d. dry mouth

4. What oral health condition(s) affects the aging population?
   a. Periodontal disease
   b. Root caries
   c. Bone resorption
   d. All of the above

5. Dementia is a condition of _____.
   a. bone loss
   b. deterioration of mental capacity
   c. aging
   d. body senses

6. What common oral adverse effect results from taking Dilantin?
   a. Hyperplasia
   b. Allergies
   c. Endocarditis
   d. Anxiety

7. Another term that is used to describe a cerebrovascular accident is _____.
   a. angina
   b. stroke
   c. seizure
   d. Alzheimer's

8. An example of a neurologic disorder is _____.
   a. emphysema
   b. multiple sclerosis
   c. Parkinson's disease
   d. b and c

9. The leading cause of death in the United States is _____.
   a. emphysema
   b. Alzheimer's disease
   c. heart disease
   d. drug abuse

10. What anesthetic agent should be of concern for the dentist when treating patients with heart disease?
    a. Nitrous oxide/oxygen
    b. Epinephrine
    c. Carbocaine
    d. Novocain

11. Another term for hypertension is _____.
    a. high blood pressure
    b. seizure
    c. depression
    d. anemia

12. What organ in the body is affected by pulmonary disorders?
    a. Heart
    b. Brain
    c. Lungs
    d. Kidneys

13. The abbreviation COPD stands for _____.
    a. common older population disorders
    b. category of pulmonary diseases
    c. cardiovascular patients in dentistry
    d. chronic obstructive pulmonary disease

14. What body system would be affected if a patient has an overactive thyroid gland?
    a. Digestive
    b. Endocrine
    c. Pulmonary
    d. Neurologic

15. A Type I diabetic patient is classified as _____.
    a. chronic
    b. adult
    c. insulin dependent
    d. non–insulin dependent

16. What is the psychological condition in which patients experience alternating, prolonged episodes of extreme elation followed by depression?
    a. Bulimia
    b. Angina
    c. Bipolar disorder
    d. Schizophrenia

17. Which developmental disorder typically shows signs before a child is 3 years old?
    a. Autism
    b. Epilepsy
    c. Arthritis
    d. Angina

18. Which category best describes a modification of care by the dental team with a patient requiring scheduling changes or shorter appointments?
    a. Category I
    b. Category II
    c. Category III
    d. Category IV

Chapter **29** The Special Needs and Medically Compromised Patient

Josh Allen is a 37-year-old patient of the practice who has been diagnosed with multiple sclerosis. His condition has deteriorated such that he now uses a wheelchair. He has called the office to schedule an appointment to have two teeth restored.

1. How would you categorize this patient with regard to how treatment is to proceed?

2. Do you think a certain time of day would be better for the dental team to see Josh? If so, what would be the best time for his appointment?

3. As you are reviewing the health history update, Josh indicates that he has recently been diagnosed with trigeminal neuralgia. What is this and how will it affect his dental care?

4. Are there any specific drugs that Josh may be taking that should be noted before the time of treatment? If so, what would they be?

5. Your dental treatment area is not designed to treat patients in a wheelchair. Where should Josh be seen by the dentist?

6. Describe specific techniques that help when one is moving a patient from a wheelchair to the dental chair.

7. Describe specific ergonomic techniques that will protect you from injuring yourself while moving a patient from a wheelchair to the dental chair.

8. Should Josh be positioned in an upright or supine position, based on his disease?

MULTIMEDIA PROCEDURES RECOMMENDED REVIEW ⊖volve
learning system

■ Medical Emergencies Animations (7 videos)

COMPETENCY 29-1: TRANSFERRING A PATIENT FROM A WHEELCHAIR

Performance Objective

By following a routine procedure that meets stated protocols, the student will demonstrate proper technique for transferring a patient from a wheelchair.

Evaluation and Grading Criteria

 3   Student competently met the stated criteria without assistance.
 2   Student required assistance in order to meet the stated criteria.
 1   Student showed uncertainty when performing the stated criteria.
 0   Student was not prepared and needs to repeat the step.
N/A   No evaluation of this step.
Instructor shall define grades for each point range earned on completion of each performance-evaluated task.

Performance Standards

The minimum number of satisfactory performances required before final evaluation is _____.

Instructor shall identify by * those steps considered critical. If step is missed or minimum competency is not met, the evaluated procedure fails and must be repeated.

PERFORMANCE CRITERIA	*	SELF	PEER	INSTRUCTOR	COMMENTS
1. Cleared all items from the pathway of the wheelchair.					
2. Determined whether it was best to enter the treatment room forward or backward.					
3. Moved the wheelchair as close to the dental chair as possible.					
4. Locked the wheelchair.					
5. Brought the patient to the edge of the wheelchair.					
6. Positioned the gait belt around the waist, with the clip in front.					
7. Placed your fingers between the gait belt and the patient, using an underhand motion to grasp the gait belt.					
8. Assisted the patient to stand slowly.					
9. Pivoted the patient so that the back side was closest to the dental chair.					
10. Lowered the patient into the dental chair.					
11. Swung the patient's legs over and onto the dental chair.					
ADDITIONAL COMMENTS					

Total number of points earned _____

Grade _____ Instructor's initials _____

Chapter **29** The Special Needs and Medically Compromised Patient

30 Principles of Pharmacology

1. Differentiate among a drug's chemical, generic, and trade names.

2. Describe the stages a drug goes through once it enters the body.

3. List each part of a prescription.

4. Describe the various methods of administering a medication.

5. Define the DEA and explain why drugs are categorized in five Schedules of the Controlled Substance Act.

6. Describe the negative effects of drug use.

7. Describe why drug reference materials would be located in a dental office.

8. Describe the classification of prescription drugs and their effects.

9. Describe why a drug would be prescribed for a patient in the dental office.

FILL-IN-THE-BLANK STATEMENTS

Select the best term from the list below and complete the following statements.

absorption
antibiotic prophylaxis
distribution
dosage
dose
drug
excretion
generic

patent
pharmacology
prescription
signature
subscription
superscription
systemic

1. _____ is the action by which a drug leaves the body.

2. The action by which the body takes in or receives a drug is _____.

3. The _____ are the patient's name, address, date, and Rx on the prescription.

4. The term _____ relates to a drug that affects a specific system of the body.

5. A specified quantity or volume of a drug or medicine is termed a(n) _____.

6. A substance that is used in the diagnosis, treatment, or prevention of a disease is a(n) _____.

7. _____ is the process or action of a drug when it is released throughout the body.

8. The _____ refers to specific instructions on a prescription about how to take a prescribed medicine.

9. _____ is the amount of drug to be administered according to time and specific body weight.

10. A drug that can be obtained without a prescription is referred to as a(n) _____ drug.

11. _____ is the science of drugs.

12. A(n) _____ is a written order to the pharmacist for a specific drug.

13. A patient may be prescribed a(n) _____ for the prevention of infective endocarditis.

14. The _____ are the directions provided to the pharmacist for mixing a specific medication.

15. A(n) _____ name of a drug will not have a brand name or a trademark.

MULTIPLE-CHOICE QUESTIONS

Complete each question by circling the best answer.

1. Where do drugs come from?
   a. Plants
   b. Animals
   c. Laboratories
   d. All of the above

2. What type of drug name is Advil?
   a. Generic name
   b. Brand name
   c. Chemical name
   d. Company name

3. The slowest route of absorption for a drug is
   _____.
   a. intramuscular
   b. rectal
   c. oral
   d. intravenous

4. Who is responsible for regulating the sale of medicines?
   a. Pharmaceutical company
   b. U.S. Department of Public Health
   c. Centers for Disease Control and Prevention
   d. U.S. Food and Drug Administration

5. Within the dental profession, who can prescribe drugs to a patient?
   a. Oral surgeon
   b. General dentist
   c. Dental hygienist
   d. a and b

6. What part of the prescription includes the name and the quantity of the drug?
   a. Subscription
   b. Inscription
   c. Superscription
   d. Description

7. If a medication were placed sublingually, where would it be placed?
   a. Ancillary
   b. Rectally
   c. Under the tongue
   d. Topically

8. By which route is a subcutaneous injection given?
   a. Muscular
   b. Intravenous
   c. Nerve
   d. Under the skin

9. What Schedule of drug is Tylenol with codeine?
   a. I
   b. II
   c. III
   d. IV

10. Which of the following is the term used to describe the body's negative reaction to a drug?
    a. Adverse effect
    b. Response
    c. Symptom
    d. Sign

11. An analgesic would be prescribed for

    _____.
    a. treatment of hives
    b. reduction of fever
    c. pain relief
    d. b and c

12. Which would be an example of an antibiotic?
    a. Aspirin
    b. Codeine
    c. Erythromycin
    d. Meperidine

13. A drug that is prescribed to slow the clotting of blood

    is _____.
    a. epinephrine
    b. Valium
    c. Coumadin
    d. Monistat

14. _____ may be taken when a patient has a cold.
    a. Dilantin
    b. Prozac
    c. Sudafed
    d. Ventolin

15. The main reason that Ritalin is considered a Schedule

    II drug is because of _____.
    a. its hallucinogenic effects
    b. its high potential for abuse
    c. its depressant effects
    d. its high cost

Listed are different types of prescription drugs. Indicate next to the drug which body system it affects (cardiovascular, respiratory, gastrointestinal, neurologic, psychoactive, endocrine).

1. Prozac

2. Zocor

3. Tagamet

4. Dilantin

5. Bronchodilator

6. Metformin

7. Valium

8. Nitroglycerin

9. Albuterol

10. HCTZ

211

ABBREVIATION IDENTIFICATION

List the meaning of each abbreviation.

ABBREVIATION	MEANING
a.a.	
a.c.	
a.m.	
b.i.d.	
disp.	
H	
h.s.	
NPO	
p.c.	
PRN	
q.	
q.d.	
q.i.d.	
Sl	
t, tsp	
T, tbs	
t.i.d.	

CASE STUDY

John Miller is scheduled for a gingivectomy on the lower right quadrant. While setting up the treatment area, you remove the patient's radiographs and health history from the chart for the dentist to review. While assembling the documents, you notice an alert sticker indicating that Mr. Miller has a history of congenital heart disease and is allergic to penicillin.

1. What is an alert sticker?

2. Where would you find the alert sticker?

3. Is there any significance to Mr. Miller's heart disease in terms of today's procedure? If so, what is it?

4. What type of procedure is Mr. Miller having today?

5. Is this procedure considered a high-risk procedure? If so, what does that mean?

6. Why is it important to know that Mr. Miller is allergic to penicillin?

7. What classification of antibiotic could be the choice when penicillin is contraindicated?

8. According to the American Heart Association, should a prophylactic antibiotic be prescribed for Mr. Miller before the time of his appointment?

9. At the conclusion of the procedure you provide Mr. Miller with postoperative instructions, which include a prescription for Tylenol with codeine. Why would this drug be prescribed for Mr. Miller?

31 Assisting in a Medical Emergency

SHORT-ANSWER QUESTIONS

1. Define a medical emergency.

2. Give the specific role each staff member should be responsible for during a medical emergency.

3. List the basic items to be included in an emergency kit.

4. Discuss the use of a defibrillator for the purpose of an emergency.

5. What are the physical changes most often seen in a medical emergency situation?

6. What are the most common causes of a patient experiencing hypoglycemia?

FILL-IN-THE-BLANK STATEMENTS

Select the best term from the list below and complete the following statements.

acute
allergen
allergy
anaphylaxis
antibodies
antigen
aspiration
asthma
cardiopulmonary resuscitation

convulsion
erythema
gait
hyperglycemia
hyperventilating
hypoglycemia
hypotension
myocardial infarction
syncope

1. A(n) _____ is a sudden uncontrollable physical act.

2. _____ is a redness that most likely is caused by inflammation or infection.

3. _____ is an emergency method for restoring consciousness or life.

4. Rapid onset of a symptom can be termed _____.

5. A person who is highly sensitive to a certain substance has a(n) _____ to that substance.

6. A(n) _____ can trigger an allergic state.

7. _____ is the loss of consciousness caused by lack of blood going to the brain.

8. A person's _____ is his or her particular way or manner of moving by foot.

9. _____ is a chronic respiratory disease.

10. _____ is a life-threatening hypersensitivity to a substance.

11. _____ are the immunoglobulins produced by lymphoid tissue in response to a foreign substance.

12. A substance that is introduced into the body to stimulate the production of an antibody is an _____.

13. _____ is the act of inhaling or swallowing something by mouth.

14. An abnormally low level of glucose in the blood is the condition of _____.

15. _____ is a condition that is diagnosed in a patient with abnormally low blood pressure.

16. A(n) _____ can occur when an area of heart tissue undergoes necrosis as a result of obstruction of blood supply.

17. An abnormally high presence of glucose in the blood is the condition diagnosed as _____.

18. When a patient is breathing abnormally fast or deeply, he or she is said to be _____.

MULTIPLE-CHOICE QUESTIONS

Complete each question by circling the best answer.

1. The best way to prevent an emergency is to _____.
   a. have the drug kit open and ready for all procedures
   b. know your patient
   c. call the patient's physician before the appointment
   d. take vital signs before seating the patient in the dental treatment area

2. Most medical emergencies occur because a person is _____.
   a. overweight
   b. not taking his or her medication
   c. under stress
   d. not active

3. What member of the dental team is ultimately responsible for a patient's safety in the dental office?
   a. Dental assistant
   b. Dental hygienist
   c. Business assistant
   d. Dentist

4. What member of the dental team would most likely be in charge of calling emergency medical services?
   a. Dentist
   b. Business assistant
   c. Dental laboratory technician
   d. Another patient

5. Emergency phone numbers should be kept _____.
   a. next to each phone
   b. in each treatment area
   c. in the business area
   d. in the sterilization area

6. What minimum credentials must a dental assistant have to meet emergency care standards?
   a. RN license
   b. CPR and Heimlich certification
   c. EMT certification
   d. DDS

7. In emergency care, the acronym *CAB* represents _____.
   a. certified assisted breathing
   b. continue airway breathing
   c. chest compressions, airway, breathing
   d. call ambulance before

8. What is the ratio of breaths to compressions when CPR is performed on an adult?
   a. 5 compressions/1 breath
   b. 7 compressions/2 breaths
   c. 15 compressions/1 breath
   d. 30 compressions/2 breaths

9. The drug most commonly used in a medical emergency is _____.
   a. an ammonia capsule
   b. nitroglycerin
   c. epinephrine
   d. oxygen

10. In emergency care, the acronym *AED* represents _____.
    a. automated external defibrillator
    b. auxiliary examination device
    c. acute emergency drill
    d. airway that is externally directed

11. What does the AED provide to the heart?
    a. Oxygen
    b. Jolt of an electrical current
    c. Blood
    d. Heat

12. If a patient tells you how he or she is feeling, the patient is referring to a(n) _____.
    a. diagnosis
    b. sign
    c. explanation
    d. symptom

13. When a patient is not responsive to sensory stimulation, he or she is said to be _____.
    a. agitated
    b. unconscious
    c. comatose
    d. paralyzed

14. What is the medical term for fainting?
    a. Stroke
    b. Seizure
    c. Syncope
    d. Senile

15. The medical term for chest pain is _____.
    a. angioplasty
    b. angina
    c. angiogram
    d. anemia

16. The medical term for a stroke is _____.
    a. cerebrovascular accident
    b. cardiovascular accident
    c. cardiopulmonary obstruction
    d. obstructed airway

17. The medication a patient with asthma would most commonly have with him or her is _____.
    a. nitroglycerin
    b. insulin
    c. a bronchodilator
    d. an analgesic

18. What kind of allergic response could be life-threatening?
    a. Grand mal seizure
    b. Anaphylaxis
    c. Myocardial infarction
    d. Airway obstruction

19. An abnormal increase of glucose in the blood can cause _____.
    a. angina
    b. hypoglycemia
    c. seizure
    d. hyperglycemia

20. The universal sign for someone choking is _____.
    a. wheezing
    b. placement of the hands to the throat
    c. turning blue
    d. screaming

Renee Miller is a 26-year-old woman who is in her third trimester of pregnancy. Renee is scheduled to have a root canal on tooth #12. Her health history and treatment record show no indication of adverse reactions to prior treatment. Renee is seated in the dental chair, and pretreatment instructions have been provided. The procedure goes well, and you are repositioning the chair in an upright position while the dentist is discussing posttreatment steps. Renee comments that she feels faint.

1. How was the dental chair positioned for Renee during the procedure?

2. Should Renee have dental care while she is pregnant? If so, what is your reasoning?

3. What might be the cause for Renee's feeling faint?

4. What type of medical emergency may Renee be experiencing?

5. How do you respond to this medical emergency?

6. What drug would be retrieved from the emergency medical kit?

7. Is there anything that could have prevented Renee from feeling this way?

COMPETENCY 31-1: PERFORMING CARDIOPULMONARY RESUSCITATION (ONE PERSON)

Performance Objective

By following a routine procedure that meets stated protocols, the student will use an American Heart Association–approved mannequin to demonstrate the proper technique for performing CPR.

Evaluation and Grading Criteria

<u>3</u>   Student competently met the stated criteria without assistance.
<u>2</u>   Student required assistance in order to meet the stated criteria.
<u>1</u>   Student showed uncertainty when performing the stated criteria.
<u>0</u>   Student was not prepared and needs to repeat the step.
<u>N/A</u> No evaluation of this step.
Instructor shall define grades for each point range earned on completion of each performance-evaluated task.

Performance Standards

The minimum number of satisfactory performances required before final evaluation is _____.

Instructor shall identify by * those steps considered critical. If step is missed or minimum competency is not met, the evaluated procedure fails and must be repeated.

PERFORMANCE CRITERIA	*	SELF	PEER	INSTRUCTOR	COMMENTS
1. Approached victim and checked for signs of breathing, coughing, or movement.					
2. Asked, "Are you OK?"					
3. Call 911 • If alone, and patient is an adult phoned first. • If alone, and patient is a child gave 2 minutes of compressions and then phoned.					
4. Provide 30 chest compressions at a rate of 100/minute with adequate depth. • For adults and children over the age of 8, compression depth was at least 2 inches. • For children under the age of 8, compression depth was about 2 inches. • For infants, compression depth was at least 1½ inches.					
5. During compressions • Minimized interruptions in compressions. • Allowed complete recoil between compressions.					
6. Opened the victim's airway and delivered 2 breaths.					
7. Continued a 30:2 compression-to-ventilation ratio.					

Continued

8. Attached and initiated AED as soon as available.				
9. Reassessed victim.				
10. Continued CPR until medical service arrives.				
11. Procedure documented in patient record.				
ADDITIONAL COMMENTS				

Total number of points earned _____

Grade _____ Instructor's initials _____

COMPETENCY 31-2: RESPONDING TO THE PATIENT WITH AN OBSTRUCTED AIRWAY

Performance Objective

By following a routine procedure that meets stated protocols, the student will demonstrate the proper technique for the Heimlich maneuver.

Evaluation and Grading Criteria

 3   Student competently met the stated criteria without assistance.
 2   Student required assistance in order to meet the stated criteria.
 1   Student showed uncertainty when performing the stated criteria.
 0   Student was not prepared and needs to repeat the step.
N/A No evaluation of this step.

Instructor shall define grades for each point range earned on completion of each performance-evaluated task.

Performance Standards

The minimum number of satisfactory performances required before final evaluation is _____.

Instructor shall identify by * those steps considered critical. If step is missed or minimum competency is not met, the evaluated procedure fails and must be repeated.

PERFORMANCE CRITERIA	*	SELF	PEER	INSTRUCTOR	COMMENTS
1. If victim could not speak, cough, or breathe, immediately called for assistance					
2. Made a fist and placed the thumb side of the hand against the victim's abdomen just above the belly button.					
3. Grasped the fist with the other hand, and forcefully thrust both hands inward and upward					
4. Repeated thrusts until object was expelled.					
5. Verbally described the procedure if the victim is seated					
6. Procedure documented in patient record.					
ADDITIONAL COMMENTS					

Total number of points earned _____

Grade _____ Instructor's initials _____

COMPETENCY 31-3: OPERATING THE AUTOMATED EXTERNAL DEFIBRILLATOR

Performance Objective

By following a routine procedure that meets stated protocols, the student will demonstrate the proper technique for operating an automated external defibrillator for use in an emergency situation.

Evaluation and Grading Criteria

__3__   Student competently met the stated criteria without assistance.
__2__   Student required assistance in order to meet the stated criteria.
__1__   Student showed uncertainty when performing the stated criteria.
__0__   Student was not prepared and needs to repeat the step.
__N/A__   No evaluation of this step.
Instructor shall define grades for each point range earned on completion of each performance-evaluated task.

Performance Standards

The minimum number of satisfactory performances required before final evaluation is _____.

Instructor shall identify by * those steps considered critical. If step is missed or minimum competency is not met, the evaluated procedure fails and must be repeated.

PERFORMANCE CRITERIA	*	SELF	PEER	INSTRUCTOR	COMMENTS
1. Verified the absence of breathing and pulse.					
2. Began CPR.					
3. Positioned the defibrillator machine on the left side of the patient's head.					
4. Turned the power on.					
5. Attached the electrode lines to the paddles.					
6. Attached the paddles to the patient. Positioned one paddle at the left sternal border and the second on the right side above the nipple area.					
7. Stopped CPR and cleared the patient.					
8. Pressed the "analyze" button.					
9. If the machine advised shock, delivered a shock.					
10. Reanalyzed the cardiac rhythm. Completed three intervals and then reassessed.					
11. Procedure documented in patient record.					
ADDITIONAL COMMENTS					

Total number of points earned _____

Grade _____ Instructor's initials _____

COMPETENCY 31-4: PREPARING THE OXYGEN SYSTEM

Performance Objective

By following a routine procedure that meets stated protocols, the student will demonstrate the proper technique for preparing an oxygen system for an emergency.

Evaluation and Grading Criteria

3	Student competently met the stated criteria without assistance.
2	Student required assistance in order to meet the stated criteria.
1	Student showed uncertainty when performing the stated criteria.
0	Student was not prepared and needs to repeat the step.
N/A	No evaluation of this step.

Instructor shall define grades for each point range earned on completion of each performance-evaluated task.

Performance Standards

The minimum number of satisfactory performances required before final evaluation is _____.

Instructor shall identify by * those steps considered critical. If step is missed or minimum competency is not met, the evaluated procedure fails and must be repeated.

PERFORMANCE CRITERIA	*	SELF	PEER	INSTRUCTOR	COMMENTS
1. Obtained the equipment and supplies required for the procedure.					
2. Confirmed the oxygen cylinder is an adequate level of oxygen					
3. Positioned the regulator over the pin. Aligned the pin index and cylinder holes.					
4. Opened the valve with two full turns, and checked to ensure that cylinders contained oxygen.					
5. Checked pressure gauge for a minimum of 2000 pounds per square inch.					
6. Attached tubing.					
7. Positioned the mask comfortably over the patient's face.					
8. Monitored the patient.					
9. Procedure documented in patient record.					
ADDITIONAL COMMENTS					

Total number of points earned _____

Grade _____ Instructor's initials _____

COMPETENCY 31-5: RESPONDING TO THE UNCONSCIOUS PATIENT

Performance Objective

By following a routine procedure that meets stated protocols, the student will physically and verbally respond to an unconscious patient.

Evaluation and Grading Criteria

<u>3</u>   Student competently met the stated criteria without assistance.
<u>2</u>   Student required assistance in order to meet the stated criteria.
<u>1</u>   Student showed uncertainty when performing the stated criteria.
<u>0</u>   Student was not prepared and needs to repeat the step.
<u>N/A</u>   No evaluation of this step.
Instructor shall define grades for each point range earned on completion of each performance-evaluated task.

Performance Standards

The minimum number of satisfactory performances required before final evaluation is _____.

Instructor shall identify by * those steps considered critical. If step is missed or minimum competency is not met, the evaluated procedure fails and must be repeated.

PERFORMANCE CRITERIA	*	SELF	PEER	INSTRUCTOR	COMMENTS
1. Placed the patient in subsupine position with head lower than feet.					
2. Called for assistance.					
3. Loosened any binding clothing.					
4. Had an ammonia inhalant ready to administer under the patient's nose.					
5. Had oxygen ready for use.					
6. Monitored and recorded vital signs.					
7. Procedure documented in patient record.					
ADDITIONAL COMMENTS					

Total number of points earned _____

Grade _____ Instructor's initials _____

COMPETENCY 31-6: RESPONDING TO THE PATIENT WITH CHEST PAIN

Performance Objective

By following a routine procedure that meets stated protocols, the student will act out and verbally respond to a patient with chest pain.

Evaluation and Grading Criteria

_3_   Student competently met the stated criteria without assistance.
_2_   Student required assistance in order to meet the stated criteria.
_1_   Student showed uncertainty when performing the stated criteria.
_0_   Student was not prepared and needs to repeat the step.
_N/A_   No evaluation of this step.
Instructor shall define grades for each point range earned on completion of each performance-evaluated task.

Performance Standards

The minimum number of satisfactory performances required before final evaluation is _____.

Instructor shall identify by * those steps considered critical. If step is missed or minimum competency is not met, the evaluated procedure fails and must be repeated.

PERFORMANCE CRITERIA	*	SELF	PEER	INSTRUCTOR	COMMENTS
1. Called for medical assistance.					
2. Positioned the patient in an upright position.					
3. Obtained nitroglycerin from the patient or emergency kit.					
4. Administers oxygen as directed by the dentist					
5. Monitored and recorded vital signs.					
6. Procedure documented in patient record.					
ADDITIONAL COMMENTS					

Total number of points earned _____

Grade _____ Instructor's initials _____

COMPETENCY 31-7: RESPONDING TO THE PATIENT WHO IS EXPERIENCING A CEREBROVASCULAR ACCIDENT (STROKE)

Performance Objective

By following a routine procedure that meets stated protocols, the student will act out and verbally respond to a patient who is experiencing a stroke (CVA).

Evaluation and Grading Criteria

3   Student competently met the stated criteria without assistance.
2   Student required assistance in order to meet the stated criteria.
1   Student showed uncertainty when performing the stated criteria.
0   Student was not prepared and needs to repeat the step.
N/A   No evaluation of this step.
Instructor shall define grades for each point range earned on completion of each performance-evaluated task.

Performance Standards

The minimum number of satisfactory performances required before final evaluation is _____.

Instructor shall identify by * those steps considered critical. If step is missed or minimum competency is not met, the evaluated procedure fails and must be repeated.

PERFORMANCE CRITERIA	*	SELF	PEER	INSTRUCTOR	COMMENTS
1. Called for medical assistance.					
2. Initiated basic life support if patient became unconscious.					
3. Monitored and recorded vital signs.					
4. Administers oxygen as directed by the dentist.					
5. Procedure documented in patient record.					
ADDITIONAL COMMENTS					

Total number of points earned _____

Grade _____ Instructor's initials _____

COMPETENCY 31-8: RESPONDING TO THE PATIENT WITH A BREATHING PROBLEM

Performance Objective

By following a routine procedure that meets stated protocols, the student will physically and verbally respond to a patient with a breathing problem.

Evaluation and Grading Criteria

 3   Student competently met the stated criteria without assistance.
 2   Student required assistance in order to meet the stated criteria.
 1   Student showed uncertainty when performing the stated criteria.
 0   Student was not prepared and needs to repeat the step.
 N/A   No evaluation of this step.

Instructor shall define grades for each point range earned on completion of each performance-evaluated task.

Performance Standards

The minimum number of satisfactory performances required before final evaluation is _____.

Instructor shall identify by * those steps considered critical. If step is missed or minimum competency is not met, the evaluated procedure fails and must be repeated.

PERFORMANCE CRITERIA	*	SELF	PEER	INSTRUCTOR	COMMENTS
1. Called for medical assistance.					
2. Positioned the patient in a comfortable position.					
3. Used a quiet voice to calm and reassure the patient.					
4. If asthma induced, had the patient self-medicate with inhaler.					
5. If hyperventilating, instructed the patient to breathe into their cupped hands.					
6. Administers oxygen as directed by the dentist.					
7. Monitored and recorded vital signs.					
8. Procedure documented in patient record.					
ADDITIONAL COMMENTS					

Total number of points earned _____

Grade _____ Instructor's initials _____

COMPETENCY 31-9: RESPONDING TO THE PATIENT WHO IS EXPERIENCING AN ALLERGIC REACTION

Performance Objective

By following a routine procedure that meets stated protocols, the student will physically and verbally respond to a patient who is experiencing an allergic reaction.

Evaluation and Grading Criteria

__3__   Student competently met the stated criteria without assistance.
__2__   Student required assistance in order to meet the stated criteria.
__1__   Student showed uncertainty when performing the stated criteria.
__0__   Student was not prepared and needs to repeat the step.
__N/A__   No evaluation of this step.
Instructor shall define grades for each point range earned on completion of each performance-evaluated task.

Performance Standards

The minimum number of satisfactory performances required before final evaluation is _____.

Instructor shall identify by * those steps considered critical. If step is missed or minimum competency is not met, the evaluated procedure fails and must be repeated.

PERFORMANCE CRITERIA	*	SELF	PEER	INSTRUCTOR	COMMENTS
Localized Rash					
1. Identified area of rash.					
2. Monitored and recorded vital signs.					
3. Readied an antihistamine or epinephrine for administration if needed.					
4. Initiated basic life support if needed.					
5. Referred the patient for medical consultation.					
6. Procedure documented in patient record.					
Anaphylaxis					
1. Called for emergency assistance.					
2. Placed the patient in supine position.					
3. If patient became unconsious, started basic life support (CPR).					
4. Prepared epi pen for administration.					

Continued

5. Administered oxygen.					
6. Monitored and recorded vital signs.					
7. Procedure documented in patient record.					
ADDITIONAL COMMENTS					

Total number of points earned _____

Grade _____ Instructor's initials _____

COMPETENCY 31-10: RESPONDING TO THE PATIENT WHO IS EXPERIENCING A CONVULSIVE SEIZURE

Performance Objective

By following a routine procedure that meets stated protocols, the student will physically and verbally respond to a patient who is experiencing a convulsive seizure.

Evaluation and Grading Criteria

_3_   Student competently met the stated criteria without assistance.
_2_   Student required assistance in order to meet the stated criteria.
_1_   Student showed uncertainty when performing the stated criteria.
_0_   Student was not prepared and needs to repeat the step.
_N/A_ No evaluation of this step.
Instructor shall define grades for each point range earned on completion of each performance-evaluated task.

Performance Standards

The minimum number of satisfactory performances required before final evaluation is _____.

Instructor shall identify by * those steps considered critical. If step is missed or minimum competency is not met, the evaluated procedure fails and must be repeated.

PERFORMANCE CRITERIA	*	SELF	PEER	INSTRUCTOR	COMMENTS
Grand Mal Seizure					
1. Called for medical assistance.					
2. If the patient is in the dental chair, quickly removed all materials from the mouth and placed the patient in a supine position.					
3. Prevented self-injury of the patient during the seizure.					
4. Readied the anticonvulsant from the drug kit if needed.					
5. Initiated basic life support if needed.					
6. Monitored and recorded vital signs.					
7. Procedure documented in patient record.					
Petit Mal Seizure					
1. Protected patient from self-injury.					
2. Monitored and recorded vital signs.					

Continued

3. Referred patient for medical consultation.					
4. Procedure documented in patient record.					
ADDITIONAL COMMENTS					

Total number of points earned _____

Grade _____ Instructor's initials _____

COMPETENCY 31-11: RESPONDING TO THE PATIENT WHO IS EXPERIENCING A DIABETIC EMERGENCY

Performance Objective

By following a routine procedure that meets stated protocols, the student will physically and verbally respond to a patient who is experiencing a diabetic emergency.

Evaluation and Grading Criteria

 3   Student competently met the stated criteria without assistance.
 2   Student required assistance in order to meet the stated criteria.
 1   Student showed uncertainty when performing the stated criteria.
 0   Student was not prepared and needs to repeat the step.
 N/A   No evaluation of this step.

Instructor shall define grades for each point range earned on completion of each performance-evaluated task.

Performance Standards

The minimum number of satisfactory performances required before final evaluation is _____.

Instructor shall identify by * those steps considered critical. If step is missed or minimum competency is not met, the evaluated procedure fails and must be repeated.

PERFORMANCE CRITERIA	*	SELF	PEER	INSTRUCTOR	COMMENTS
1. Called for medical assistance.					
2. If the patient was conscious, inquired about when they last ate, or when insulin was last taken.					
3. Retrieved patient's insulin if hyperglycemic, or provided concentrated carbohydrate if hypoglycemic.					
4. If the patient was unconscious, provided basic life support.					
5. Monitored and recorded vital signs.					
6. Procedure documented in patient record.					
ADDITIONAL COMMENTS					

Total number of points earned _____

Grade _____ Instructor's initials _____

32 The Dental Office

SHORT-ANSWER QUESTIONS

1. Describe how the dental office environment should be maintained as a professional office.

2. Discuss the important qualities of a reception area.

3. Describe the goals to achieve when designing a dental treatment area.

4. List the main clinical equipment required for the treatment area.

5. Discuss the basic function of the dental unit.

FILL-IN-THE-BLANK STATEMENTS

Select the best term from the list below and complete the following statements.

air/water syringe	**HVE**
amalgamator	**rheostat**
compressor	**saliva ejector**
condensation	**subsupine**
consultation	**supine**
curing light	**triturate**
dental operatory	**upright**
dental unit	

1. Of the two types of suction systems, _____ is the less powerful type of suction system.

2. In the _____ position, commonly used in emergency situations, the patient's head is below the heart.

3. To mechanically mix something is to _____.

4. The _____ provides the necessary electrical and air to the handpiece.

5. The _____ provides compressed air to the air-water syringe and dental handpieces.

6. A(n) _____ is a means of delivering air and water to the oral cavity.

7. A(n) _____ is a type of meeting held to discuss a diagnosis or treatment.

8. A _____ is a wandlike attachment used to harden or cure light sensitive dental materials.

9. _____ is the process by which a liquid is removed from vapor.

10. A patient who is sitting in the _____ position is in a vertical position.

11. A system used to remove fluid and debris from the oral cavity is _____.

12. A room designed for the treatment of dentistry is referred to as the _____.

13. A foot-controlled device that is used to operate the dental handpiece is a _____.

14. A _____ is an electrical machine used to mechanically mix dental materials

15. When a patient is in the _____ position, the head, chest, and knees are at the same level.

MULTIPLE-CHOICE QUESTIONS

Complete each question by circling the best answer.

1. What is an ideal temperature for the reception area of a dental practice?
   a. 68° F
   b. 72° F
   c. 75° F
   d. 78° F

2. What type of flooring would be most suitable for the clinical area?
   a. Carpet
   b. Wood
   c. Vinyl
   d. Tile

3. What items are important to have in the reception area?
   a. Seating
   b. Lighting
   c. Reading material
   d. All of the above

4. Where would the money transactions take place in the dental office?
   a. In the operatory
   b. In the laboratory
   c. In the administrative area
   d. In the sterilization area

5. Another term for operatory is _____.
   a. rheostat
   b. treatment area
   c. radiography
   d. laboratory

6. The dental chair is situated in the position for most dental procedures.
   a. Upright
   b. Subsupine
   c. Supine
   d. Flat

7. Which two items would be found on the dental assistant's stool that are not found on the operator's stool?
   a. Light switch and up-and-down button
   b. Back cushion and wheeled coasters
   c. Headrest and armrests
   d. Footrest and abdominal bar

8. What foot-controlled device is used to operate the dental handpiece?
   a. Dental unit
   b. Amalgamator
   c. Rheostat
   d. Central air compressor

9. What does the acronym HVE stand for?
   a. High-volume evacuator
   b. Hose vacuum evacuator
   c. High-velocity evacuator
   d. Handle volume evacuator

10. Where do you place dental materials to be triturated?
    a. In the dental unit
    b. In the amalgamator
    c. In the rheostat
    d. In the central air compressor

CASE STUDY

You are responsible for showing a new staff member around the office. Nancy has been in dentistry for 26 years and is quite familiar with her role as a professional dental assistant. She has conveyed to you that she really likes the design and setup of the dental office and is excited about adding her personal touches toward making the office more functional.

1. What would be your role in showing Nancy the office and the design and setup?

2. The office has four dental treatment areas and three full-time dental assistants. Describe how each assistant could create an environment in which he or she feels comfortable.

3. What types of items can be placed in the dental operatory to make it more personal and to show a team atmosphere?

4. How do you feel about a new employee wanting to make changes so quickly?

5. Nancy has requested that the temperature be turned up in the clinical area because she is "cold natured" and does not want to have to wear multiple layers of clothing to stay warm. How should the office manager handle this concern? Why is the temperature set differently throughout the office?

COMPETENCY 32-1: PERFORMING THE MORNING ROUTINE (OPENING THE OFFICE)

Performance Objective

By following a routine procedure that meets stated protocols, the student will open and prepare the dental office for patients.

Evaluation and Grading Criteria

  3   Student competently met the stated criteria without assistance.

  2   Student required assistance in order to meet the stated criteria.

  1   Student showed uncertainty when performing the stated criteria.

  0   Student was not prepared and needs to repeat the step.

N/A   No evaluation of this step.

Instructor shall define grades for each point range earned on completion of each performance-evaluated task.

Performance Standards

The minimum number of satisfactory performances required before final evaluation is _____.

Instructor shall identify by * those steps considered critical. If step is missed or minimum competency is not met, the evaluated procedure fails and must be repeated.

PERFORMANCE CRITERIA	*	SELF	PEER	INSTRUCTOR	COMMENT
1. Arrived 30 minutes before the first scheduled patient.					
2. Personal protective equipment placed according to procedure.					
3. Turned on the master switches for the central air compressor and vacuum units.					
4. Turned on the master switches for the dental and radiographic units.					
5. Determined that the dental treatment area was ready for patient care.					
6. Checked appointment schedule.					
7. Set up the treatment room for the first patient.					
ADDITIONAL COMMENTS					

Total number of points earned _____

Grade _____ Instructor's initials _____

COMPETENCY 32-2: PERFORMING THE EVENING ROUTINE (CLOSING THE OFFICE)

Performance Objective

By following a routine procedure that meets stated protocols, the student will close the dental office at the end of the day.

Evaluation and Grading Criteria

 3 Student competently met the stated criteria without assistance.
 2 Student required assistance in order to meet the stated criteria.
 1 Student showed uncertainty when performing the stated criteria.
 0 Student was not prepared and needs to repeat the step.
 N/A No evaluation of this step.

Instructor shall define grades for each point range earned on completion of each performance-evaluated task.

Performance Standards

The minimum number of satisfactory performances required before final evaluation is _____.

Instructor shall identify by * those steps considered critical. If step is missed or minimum competency is not met, the evaluated procedure fails and must be repeated.

PERFORMANCE CRITERIA	*	SELF	PEER	INSTRUCTOR	COMMENT
1. Completed the treatment room exposure control cleanup and preparation protocols.					
2. Personal protective equipment placed according to procedure.					
3. Turned off all equipment.					
4. Restocked treatment rooms.					
5. Posted appointment schedules for the next day.					
6. Checked appointment schedules to ensure that instruments, patient records, and laboratory work were ready for the next day.					
7. Ensured that all contaminated instruments had been processed and sterilized.					
8. Ensured that treatment rooms were ready for use.					
9. Placed any soiled PPE in the appropriate container.					
ADDITIONAL COMMENTS					

Total number of points earned _____

Grade _____ Instructor's initials _____

33 Delivering Dental Care

1. Describe how you would prepare the dental operatory for a patient's arrival.

2. What specific items would be set out for patient treatment?

3. Describe how the operator is positioned for treatment.

4. Describe how the assistant is positioned for treatment.

5. Explain the single-handed instrument transfer technique.

6. Describe the three grasps used by the operator or assistant when carrying out an expanded function.

7. Identify five areas in which the dental assistant must become proficient in when carrying out an expanded function.

FILL-IN-THE-BLANK STATEMENTS

Select the best term from the list below and complete the following statements.

classification of motions
delegate
direct supervision
expanded function
four-handed dentistry
fulcrum

grasp
indirect supervision
indirect vision
operating zones

1. The dentist provides _____ when he or she is physically in the same treatment area overseeing the expanded-function procedure.

2. By using the clock concept, the dental team is following the four _____ of positioning to practice four-handed dentistry.

3. _____ is the method of viewing something through the use of a mirror.

4. The five categories that describe the extent of movement by the clinical assistant when assisting are called the

    _____.

5. _____ is a dental procedure that is delegated to the dental assistant by the dentist.

6. A(n) _____ is a finger rest that is used while one is working intraorally with a dental instrument or handpiece.

7. The process by which a skilled dental assistant and dentist work together as a team to perform clinical tasks is _____.

8. A(n) _____ is the manner in which a specific instrument or handpiece is held.

9. The dentist provides _____ when he or she is present in the immediate area to oversee the dental assistant's expanded function.

10. To _____ is when the dentist assigns or entrusts a specific procedure to the dental assistant.

MULTIPLE-CHOICE QUESTIONS

Complete each question by circling the best answer.

1. What can increase productivity in a dental office?
   a. Patient comfort
   b. Minimization of stress and fatigue
   c. Delegation of expanded functions
   d. All of the above

2. When using the clock concept for a right-handed operator, where is the static zone located?
   a. Twelve o'clock to two o'clock
   b. Two o'clock to four o'clock
   c. Four o'clock to seven o'clock
   d. Seven o'clock to twelve o'clock

3. According to the clock concept, instruments are to be exchanged during a procedure in the _____.
   a. static zone
   b. assistant's zone
   c. transfer zone
   d. operator's zone

4. Besides the assistant, what else could be located in the assistant's zone?
   a. Mobile dental unit
   b. Patient light
   c. Assistant's stool
   d. a and c

5. In relation to the seated operator, how is the assistant positioned?
   a. At the same height
   b. 4 to 6 inches higher than the operator
   c. Level with the patient's head
   d. 4 to 6 inches lower than the operator

6. How should the operator maintain his or her posture when treating a patient?
   a. Upright
   b. Elbows at the side
   c. Feet flat on the ground
   d. All of the above

7. The chairside assistant should use _____ hand(s) in the transfer of single instruments.
   a. both
   b. one
   c. varying
   d. b or c

8. What hand is used primarily to transfer instruments to a right-handed dentist?
   a. Left
   b. Right
   c. Either

9. Depending on the operator's position, indirect vision could be used for which of the following tooth surface(s)?
   a. Lingual area of tooth #7
   b. Facial area of tooth #25
   c. Occlusal area of tooth #3
   d. All of the above

10. Another term for finger rest is _____.
    a. rheostat
    b. intraoral
    c. fulcrum
    d. tactile

11. Depending on the instrument, the assistant can use the _____ of his or her left hand when retrieving a used instrument from a right-handed dentist.
    a. last two fingers
    b. middle and index fingers
    c. palm
    d. a and c

12. How should the working end of an instrument be positioned for transfer when working on tooth #13?
    a. Downward toward the mandibular
    b. Upward toward the maxillary
    c. It does not matter; the dentist will position the instrument
    d. Facing to the right

13. The exchange of surgical instruments is best executed with the use of a _____ transfer.
    a. single-handed
    b. two-handed
    c. pen-grasp
    d. reverse palm-thumb

14. During instrument transfer, the handles of the instruments are held parallel to avoid _____.
    a. injuring the patient
    b. injuring the dental team
    c. tangling
    d. All of the above

15. During a procedure, you transfer instruments using your left hand and hold the _____ in your right hand.
    a. next instrument to transfer
    b. air-water syringe
    c. HVE
    d. anesthetic syringe

TOPIC FOR DISCUSSION

Dr. Williams is a general dentist who has been practicing dentistry for 35 years. She views her dental assistants and dental hygienists as an important part of the practice and recognizes everyone as a contributor toward provision of patient care. Dr. Williams advocates advanced functions and believes that dental assistants should be allowed to practice procedures that they are legally permitted to perform.

1. How can you find out what procedures are legal for you to practice in your state?

2. As you begin your clinical training, describe specific skills that you could practice to help you become more proficient in expanded functions.

3. What preparation could you use to maintain a high level of competency when performing advanced functions?

4. If a new clinical procedure became an advanced function in your state, how would you acquire the knowledge and skill to practice the procedure?

5. Are there any procedures that you believe dental assistants could perform but are not legal for them to perform in your state?

LABELING EXERCISE

Label the operating zones for a right-handed operator.

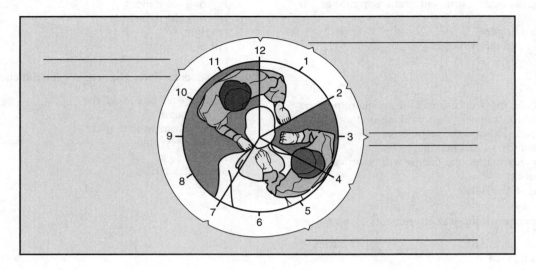

MULTIMEDIA PROCEDURES RECOMMENDED REVIEW

■ Transferring Instruments (Single-Handed)

COMPETENCY 33-1: ADMITTING AND SEATING OF THE PATIENT

Performance Objective
By following a routine procedure that meets stated protocols, the student will admit, seat, and prepare the patient for treatment.

Evaluation and Grading Criteria
 3 Student competently met the stated criteria without assistance.
 2 Student required assistance in order to meet the stated criteria.
 1 Student showed uncertainty when performing the stated criteria.
 0 Student was not prepared and needs to repeat the step.
 N/A No evaluation of this step.
Instructor shall define grades for each point range earned on completion of each performance-evaluated task.

Performance Standards
The minimum number of satisfactory performances required before final evaluation is _____.

Instructor shall identify by * those steps considered critical. If step is missed or minimum competency is not met, the evaluated procedure fails and must be repeated.

PERFORMANCE CRITERIA	*	SELF	PEER	INSTRUCTOR	COMMENT
1. Ensured that the treatment room is properly cleaned and prepared, with the chair properly positioned and the patient's path clear.					
2. Performed instrument setup and placed materials.					
3. Identified and greeted the patient appropriately.					
4. Escorted the patient to the treatment area.					
5. Placed the patient's personal items in a safe place within the treatment room.					
6. Properly seated the patient.					
7. Placed the patient's napkin around the neck.					
8. Properly positioned the dental chair for the procedure.					
9. Adjusted the operating light and then turned it on.					

Continued

Chapter **33** **Delivering Dental Care**

10. Initiates conversation with the patient about any questions about the procedure.				
11. Maintained patient comfort throughout these preparations.				

ADDITIONAL COMMENTS

Total number of points earned _____

Grade _____ Instructor's initials _____

COMPETENCIES 33-2 AND 33-3: TRANSFERRING INSTRUMENTS WITH SINGLE-HANDED AND TWO-HANDED TECHNIQUES

Performance Objective

By following a routine procedure that meets stated protocols, the student will perform single-handed and specialized instrument transfer in a safe and efficient manner.

Evaluation and Grading Criteria

 3   Student competently met the stated criteria without assistance.
 2   Student required assistance in order to meet the stated criteria.
 1   Student showed uncertainty when performing the stated criteria.
 0   Student was not prepared and needs to repeat the step.
 N/A   No evaluation of this step.
Instructor shall define grades for each point range earned on completion of each performance-evaluated task.

Performance Standards

The minimum number of satisfactory performances required before final evaluation is _____.

Instructor shall identify by * those steps considered critical. If step is missed or minimum competency is not met, the evaluated procedure fails and must be repeated.

PERFORMANCE CRITERIA	*	SELF	PEER	INSTRUCTOR	COMMENT
Single-Handed Transfer and Exchange					
1. Personal protective equipment placed according to procedure.					
2. Retrieved the instrument from the instrument tray using their left hand grasping the instrument with the thumb, index and middle finger, opposite the working end.					
3. Held the instrument in the transfer zone, in a ready position 8 to 10 inches away from the dentist.					
4. Anticipated the dentist's transfer signal, and positioned the new instrument parallel to the instrument in the dentist's hand.					
5. Retrieved the used instrument using the last two fingers, tucking it into their palm.					
6. Delivered the new instrument to the dentist.					
7. Maintained safety throughout the transfer.					
Nonlocking Cotton Pliers Transfer					
1. Personal protective equipment placed according to procedure.					
2. Retrieved the cotton pliers grasping a cotton pellet securely by pinching the beaks together.					

Continued

3. Carries the instrument to the transfer zone reading is transfer.				
4. Delivered the pliers so the dentist can grasp it correctly and hold the beaks together.				
5. Retrieved the pliers without dropping the cotton pellet.				
Forceps Transfer				
1. Personal protective equipment placed according to procedure.				
2. Used the right hand to retrieve the forceps from the tray. Carries the forcep to the transfer zone in the position of use.				
3. Used the left hand to retrieve the used instrument from the dentist.				
4. Delivered the new instrument to the dentist in a palm grasp in the appropriate position of use.				
5. Returned the used instrument to its proper position on the tray.				
Handpiece Exchange				
1. Personal protective equipment placed according to procedure.				
2. Used the left hand to retrieve the handpiece, holding it for delivery in the position of use in the transfer zone.				
3. Used the right hand to take the used instrument from the dentist.				
4. Delivered the handpiece to the dentist in the appropriate position.				
5. When exchanging two handpieces, did not tangle the cords.				
Air-Water Syringe Transfer				
1. Personal protective equipment placed according to procedure.				
2. Held the nozzle of the air-water syringe in the delivery position holding the tip in-between the fingers.				
3. Retrieved the instrument the dentist was using, and then delivered the syringe.				

Scissors Transfer					
1. Personal protective equipment placed according to procedure.					
2. Retrieved the scissors from the tray, holding them near the working end with the beaks slightly open.					
3. Positioned the handle of the scissors over the dentist's fingers.					
4. Retrieved the used instrument with the right hand.					
ADDITIONAL COMMENTS					

Total number of points earned _____

Grade _____ Instructor's initials _____

COMPETENCY 33-4: USING THE DENTAL MIRROR INTRAORALLY

Performance Objective

By following a routine procedure that meets stated protocols, the student will demonstrate the proper technique for using the dental mirror intraorally.

Evaluation and Grading Criteria

 3 Student competently met the stated criteria without assistance.
 2 Student required assistance in order to meet the stated criteria.
 1 Student showed uncertainty when performing the stated criteria.
 0 Student was not prepared and needs to repeat the step.
 N/A No evaluation of this step.

Instructor shall define grades for each point range earned on completion of each performance-evaluated task.

Performance Standards

The minimum number of satisfactory performances required before final evaluation is _____.

Instructor shall identify by * those steps considered critical. If step is missed or minimum competency is not met, the evaluated procedure fails and must be repeated.

PERFORMANCE CRITERIA	*	SELF	PEER	INSTRUCTOR	COMMENT
1. Personal protective equipment placed according to procedure.					
2. Positioned the patient in a supine position.					
3. Positioned self as the operator.					
4. Turned on patient light and illuminated oral cavity.					
5. Asked the patient to position the head with mandibular incisors vertical to the floor.					
6. Grasped the dental mirror in the left hand using a pen grasp.					
7. Positioned the dental mirror for indirect vision of the lingual surfaces of the maxillary anteriors.					
8. Positioned the dental mirror for light illumination on the lingual aspects of the mandibular anteriors.					
9. Positioned the dental mirror for retraction.					
10. Maintained patient comfort throughout these steps.					
ADDITIONAL COMMENTS					

Total number of points earned _____

Grade _____ Instructor's initials _____

COMPETENCY 33-5: USING AN INSTRUMENT INTRAORALLY (EXPANDED FUNCTION)

Performance Objective
By following a routine procedure that meets stated protocols, the student will demonstrate the proper technique for using an instrument intraorally.

Evaluation and Grading Criteria
 3 Student competently met the stated criteria without assistance.
 2 Student required assistance in order to meet the stated criteria.
 1 Student showed uncertainty when performing the stated criteria.
 0 Student was not prepared and needs to repeat the step.
 N/A No evaluation of this step.
Instructor shall define grades for each point range earned on completion of each performance-evaluated task.

Performance Standards
The minimum number of satisfactory performances required before final evaluation is _____.

Instructor shall identify by * those steps considered critical. If step is missed or minimum competency is not met, the evaluated procedure fails and must be repeated.

PERFORMANCE CRITERIA	*	SELF	PEER	INSTRUCTOR	COMMENT
1. Personal protective equipment placed according to procedure.					
2. Seated and positioned the patient in the supine position.					
3. Positioned self as the operator.					
4. Instructed the patient to open the mouth.					
5. Adjusted the dental light to illuminate the oral cavity.					
6. Retrieved the dental mirror in the left hand and the explorer in the right hand, using a pen grasp for both instruments.					
7. With the tip of the instrument, followed around each tooth beginning with #1 and continuing through #32.					
8. With the mirror and explorer, examined all surfaces using visualization and touch.					
9. Using a fulcrum and indirect vision, adapted the instruments to all areas of the mouth.					

Continued

10. Identified specific dental landmarks through the dentition.				
11. Maintained patient comfort throughout these steps.				
ADDITIONAL COMMENTS				

Total number of points earned _____

Grade _____ Instructor's initials _____

34 Dental Hand Instruments

SHORT-ANSWER QUESTIONS

1. Describe the three parts of a dental hand instrument.

2. Describe why an instrument formula was designed by G.V. Black.

3. List the commonly used examination instruments and their uses.

4. List the types of hand cutting instruments commonly set out for a restorative procedure.

5. List the types of restorative instruments and their uses.

6. Describe additional accessory instruments used in restorative dentistry.

7. List the reasons for using preset trays and tubs in dentistry.

8. Discuss the theory of placing instruments in a specific sequence.

FILL-IN-THE-BLANK STATEMENTS

Select the best term from the list below and complete the following statements.

beveled	point
blade	serrated
handle	shank
nib	tactile
plane	working end

1. _____ means to have a sense of touch or feeling.

2. The _____ is the portion of a dental instrument that is used on the tooth surface or for mixing dental materials.

3. The portion of a dental instrument that the operator grasps is the _____.

263

4. The working end of an instrument that is angled or slanted is referred to as being _____.

5. A flat edge of the working end of an instrument that is sharp enough to cut is a _____.

6. The working end of an explorer has a _____.

7. A(n) _____ is a(n) instrument that has notchlike projections that extend from a flat surface.

8. A flat or level surface is a _____.

9. The _____ is the portion of a dental instrument that attaches the handle to the working end.

10. A _____ can be designed with a sharp or tapered working end.

MULTIPLE-CHOICE QUESTIONS

Complete each question by circling the best answer.

1. What dental instruments are more commonly referred to by a number than by their name?
   a. Mirrors
   b. Restorative instruments
   c. Pliers
   d. Excavators

2. What part of the instrument is located between the handle and the working end?
   a. Nib
   b. Shank
   c. Blade
   d. Plane

3. Instruments of what classification are used to manually remove decay?
   a. Examination
   b. Hand cutting
   c. Restorative
   d. Accessory

4. Besides indirect vision, the mouth mirror is used for

   _____.
   a. moisture control
   b. anesthesia
   c. retraction
   d. placement of restorations

5. The main characteristic of the working end of an

   explorer is _____.
   a. dull
   b. flat
   c. serrated
   d. pointed

6. What instrument is part of the basic setup?
   a. Spoon excavator
   b. Cotton pliers
   c. Condenser
   d. Carver

7. What instrument is used to measure the sulcus of a tooth?
   a. Spoon excavator
   b. Cotton pliers
   c. Explorer
   d. Periodontal probe

8. What instrument is similar to the spoon excavator in appearance and use?
   a. Explorer
   b. Black spoon
   c. Discoid-cleoid
   d. Gingival margin trimmer

9. What instrument is used to carve the interproximal portion of the amalgam restoration?
   a. Black spoon
   b. Discoid-cleoid
   c. Explorer
   d. Hollenback

10. What instrument is used to pack amalgam in the tooth preparation?
    a. Cotton pliers
    b. Amalgam knife
    c. Condenser
    d. Burnisher

11. What kind of instrument is a discoid-cleoid?
    a. Carver
    b. Examination
    c. Hand cutting
    d. Packing

12. What type of scissors would commonly be seen on a restorative tray setup?
    a. Tissue
    b. Suture
    c. Crown and bridge
    d. Surgical

13. Howe pliers are also referred to as _____.
    a. cotton pliers
    b. 110 pliers
    c. articulating pliers
    d. chisel pliers

14. Newly triturated amalgam is placed in the _____ before it is packed in the amalgam carrier.
    a. syringe
    b. cotton pliers
    c. spoon excavator
    d. amalgam well

15. On which tooth surface would the Hollenback carver be used to carve amalgam?
    a. Occlusal
    b. Facial
    c. Distal
    d. Lingual

ACTIVITY

You are assisting with a class II amalgam procedure on tooth #29. In order of use, list the instruments you would place in the setup, beginning from the left and working toward the right of the tray. Next to each instrument, describe its use for the procedure.

COMPETENCIES 34-1 THROUGH 34-4: IDENTIFYING DENTAL INSTRUMENTS FOR A RESTORATIVE PROCEDURE

Performance Objective

By following a routine procedure that meets stated protocols, the student will retrieve and organize the appropriate examination, hand cutting, restorative, and accessory instruments and supplies for a specified restorative procedure.

Evaluation and Grading Criteria

3   Student competently met the stated criteria without assistance.
2   Student required assistance in order to meet the stated criteria.
1   Student showed uncertainty when performing the stated criteria.
0   Student was not prepared and needs to repeat the step.
N/A   No evaluation of this step.
Instructor shall define grades for each point range earned on completion of each performance-evaluated task.

Performance Standards

The minimum number of satisfactory performances required before final evaluation is _____.

Instructor shall identify by * those steps considered critical. If step is missed or minimum competency is not met, the evaluated procedure fails and must be repeated.

PERFORMANCE CRITERIA	*	SELF	PEER	INSTRUCTOR	COMMENT
1. Reviewed the patient record and determined the type of procedure and setup.					
2. Selected correct instruments for the procedure.					
3. Placed instruments in the appropriate order of use on the tray.					
4. Stated verbally or recorded the use for each instrument and item placed on the tray setup.					
ADDITIONAL COMMENTS					

Total number of points earned _____

Grade _____ Instructor's initials _____

35 Dental Handpieces and Accessories

SHORT-ANSWER QUESTIONS

1. Discuss the historical importance of the dental handpiece.

2. Describe the use of the low-speed handpiece in dentistry.

3. What three attachments can be used on the low-speed handpiece?

4. Describe the high-speed handpiece and its use.

5. Give a brief description of other types of handpieces used in dentistry.

6. Describe rotary instruments and explain how they are used.

7. List the parts of a bur.

8. Describe the composition, shape, and uses of carbide and diamond burs.

FILL-IN-THE-BLANK STATEMENTS

Select the best term from the list below and complete the following statements.

- console
- fiberoptic
- flutes
- friction grip
- laser
- latch-type
- mandrel
- rotary
- shank
- torque
- tungsten carbide
- ultrasonic

1. A(n) _____ bur is designed with no retention grooves in the shank end.

2. The _____ handpiece uses a beam of light to cauterize soft tissue or to vaporize decayed tooth structure.

3. A(n) _____ instrument is a part or device that rotates around an axis.

4. The _____ or grooves in the cutting portion of a bur resemble pleats.

5. A(n) _____ is a freestanding cabinet that is used to hold something.

6. A(n) _____ bur is rigid and stronger than steel and remains sharper for longer periods.

7. The narrow portion of the bur that fits into the handpiece is called a(n) _____.

8. The _____ bur has a shank with a small groove at the end that mechanically locks into a contra-angle attachment.

9. The high-speed handpiece has a(n) _____ lighting system to provide light on the tooth during use.

10. A(n) _____ handpiece provides mechanical energy that creates water and sound vibrations.

11. The twisting or turning of the internal components of a handpiece is referred to as _____.

12. Sandpaper discs are mounted on a _____.

MULTIPLE-CHOICE QUESTIONS

Complete each question by circling the best answer.

1. How did the first handpiece operate?
   a. Operated with a hand pedal
   b. Operated with electricity
   c. Driven by a belt
   d. Powered by water

2. What is the most versatile handpiece in dentistry?
   a. Low-speed
   b. High-speed
   c. Laboratory
   d. Air abrasion

3. How fast does the low-speed handpiece rotate?
   a. 10,000 rpm
   b. 20,000 rpm
   c. 30,000 rpm
   d. 40,000 rpm

4. What attachment on the low-speed handpiece is used to hold a latch-type bur?
   a. Prophy angle
   b. Contra-angle
   c. Straight
   d. Mandrel

5. How fast does the high-speed handpiece rotate?
   a. 250,000 rpm
   b. 450,000 rpm
   c. 650,000 rpm
   d. 950,000 rpm

6. During cavity preparation, how does the high-speed handpiece keep the tooth at a proper temperature and free of debris?
   a. Air
   b. Suction system
   c. Water coolant
   d. Application of a dental material

7. A bur is held in place in the high-speed handpiece with a _____.
   a. friction grip
   b. locking key
   c. latch-type lock
   d. twist and lock

8. On the high-speed handpiece, the _____ helps illuminate the working field.
   a. water
   b. air
   c. fiberoptic light
   d. suction

9. What type of handpiece resembles a sandblaster?
   a. Laser
   b. Low-speed
   c. Air abrasion
   d. High-speed

10. A _____ shank fits into the contra-angle attachment.
    a. friction grip
    b. mandrel
    c. long
    d. latch-type

11. Restorative burs are commonly manufactured from what material?
    a. Stainless steel
    b. Tungsten carbide
    c. Gold
    d. Nickel

12. What design of bur is a 33½?
    a. Round
    b. Tapered
    c. Inverted cone
    d. Pear

13. _____ is an advantage when a diamond bur is used.
    a. Cutting ability
    b. Fineness
    c. Polishing ability
    d. Nonabrasive ability

14. What type of restorative material would a finishing bur commonly be used for?
    a. Amalgam
    b. Stainless steel
    c. Gold
    d. Composite resin

15. What is used to hold a disc in the low-speed handpiece?
    a. Contra-angle attachment
    b. Bur
    c. Mandrel
    d. Prophy angle

CASE STUDY

You are setting up the treatment area for a patient who will be receiving a class II composite resin on tooth #5. Your tray setup includes a high-speed handpiece, low-speed motor, contra-angle attachment, #169 friction grip bur, #4 round latch-type bur, mandrel, sandpaper disks, and rubber points.

1. Which hose on the dental unit do you attach to the high-speed handpiece?

2. Which handpiece do you attach to the contra-angle attachment?

3. In which handpiece do you insert the #169 bur?

4. In which handpiece do you insert the #4 round bur?

5. At what step in the procedure would the operator use the #4 bur?

6. At what step in the procedure would the operator use the #169 bur?

7. What handpiece would the mandrel be attached to?

8. When would the disks and points be used during the procedure?

9. At the completion of the procedure, how are the dental handpieces and rotary instruments removed from the dental unit and prepared for the next procedure?

MULTIMEDIA PROCEDURES RECOMMENDED REVIEW

- Identifying and Attaching Handpieces

COMPETENCIES 35-1 AND 35-2: IDENTIFYING AND ATTACHING HANDPIECES AND ROTARY INSTRUMENTS

Performance Objective
By following a routine procedure that meets stated protocols, given instructions for which size or type to select, the student will place and remove burs in a high-speed and a low-speed handpiece.

Evaluation and Grading Criteria
3	Student competently met the stated criteria without assistance.
2	Student required assistance in order to meet the stated criteria.
1	Student showed uncertainty when performing the stated criteria.
0	Student was not prepared and needs to repeat the step.
N/A	No evaluation of this step.

Note: The student is provided with an appropriate assortment of burs and handpieces with which to work.
Instructor shall define grades for each point range earned on completion of each performance-evaluated task.

Performance Standards
The minimum number of satisfactory performances required before final evaluation is _____.

Instructor shall identify by * those steps considered critical. If step is missed or minimum competency is not met, the evaluated procedure fails and must be repeated.

PERFORMANCE CRITERIA	*	SELF	PEER	INSTRUCTOR	COMMENT
1. Attached the high-speed handpiece to the correct receptor on the dental unit.					
2. Attached the low-speed handpiece to the correct receptor on the dental unit.					
3. Attached the straight attachment, contra-angle attachment, and prophylaxis angle to the low-speed handpiece.					
4. Identified varying shapes of burs for the low-speed and the high-speed handpieces.					
5. Selected the specified size and type of bur for the high-speed handpiece.					
6. Placed burs in the handpiece in accordance with the manufacturer's instructions.					
7. Removed burs from the handpiece in accordance with the manufacturer's instructions.					
8. Selected the specified size and type of bur for the low-speed handpiece.					

Continued

Chapter **35** Dental Handpieces and Accessories

9. Placed the bur in the handpiece in accordance with the manufacturer's instructions.					
10. Removed the bur from the handpiece in accordance with the manufacturer's instructions.					

ADDITIONAL COMMENTS

Total number of points earned _____

Grade _____ Instructor's initials _____

36 Moisture Control

SHORT-ANSWER QUESTIONS

1. List the isolation techniques used to decrease moisture during a dental procedure.

2. Define the two types of oral evacuation systems used in dentistry.

3. Describe the grasp and positioning of the high-volume oral evacuator (HVE) tip.

4. Define the use of the air-water syringe.

5. Describe the dental dam, and explain its role in moisture control.

6. List the equipment and supplies used in dental dam application.

7. Describe a special situation in the preparation and placement of the dental dam.

FILL-IN-THE-BLANK STATEMENTS

Select the best term from the list below and complete the following statements.

aspirate   jaw
beveled   malaligned
bow   septum
exposed   stylus
inverted   universal

1. The _____ is the rounded part of the dental dam clamp that is visible in the mouth after the dam material has been placed.

2. The end of the HVE tip is _____ so that it can be positioned parallel to the site for better suction.

3. The dental dam is _____ around each tooth to create a seal to prevent the leakage of saliva.

4. The _____ is the part of the dental dam clamp that is stabilized around the anchor tooth.

5. The rubber dam punch has a _____, which is a sharp pointed tool used for cutting.

6. An instrument or item that is adaptable or adjustable to the maxillary or mandibular right or left is said to be

_____.

7. When something is not straight or in line, it is _____.

8. A(n) _____ is the piece of the dental dam between each punched hole.

9. When a tooth is visible in the dental dam, it becomes _____.

10. _____ means to inhale or swallow something.

MULTIPLE-CHOICE QUESTIONS

Complete each question by circling the best answer.

1. What are the two types of evacuators used in dental procedures?
   a. Cotton rolls and saliva ejector
   b. High-volume suction and saliva ejector
   c. Dental dam and high-volume suction
   d. Air-water syringe and saliva ejector

2. The main function of the saliva ejector is to

_____.
   a. remove dental materials
   b. remove blood
   c. remove saliva and water
   d. remove tooth fragments

3. Operative suction tips are made from

_____.
   a. surgical steel
   b. stainless steel
   c. plastic
   d. b and c

4. What rinsing technique is regularly completed throughout a procedure?
   a. Limited
   b. Full
   c. Gargle
   d. Spray

5. What method of isolation could be used for sealant placement?
   a. Dental dam
   b. Cotton roll
   c. Cheek retractors
   d. a and b

6. Which would provide a moisture-free isolation for the restoration of a class IV composite resin?
   a. Dental dam
   b. Cotton roll
   c. Gauze squares
   d. Saliva ejector

7. Why is it important to wet a cotton roll before removing it from the mouth?
   a. The cotton roll may interfere with the setting of the dental materials.
   b. The cotton roll may stick to the teeth.
   c. The cotton roll may pull on the lining mucosa.
   d. The cotton roll may be sucked up in the suction tip.

8. Teeth that are visible after the dam material is placed

are referred to as being _____.
   a. open
   b. exposed
   c. revealed
   d. inverted

9. What piece of equipment stabilizes and stretches the dam away from the face?
   a. Dental dam frame
   b. Dental dam clamp
   c. Ligature tie
   d. Dental dam forceps

10. If you are unable to slide the dam material inter-proximally, what can be placed on the underside of the dam to help in the application?
    a. Water
    b. Petroleum jelly
    c. Water-soluble lubricant
    d. Powder

11. What hole size would you punch in the dental dam for the anchor tooth?
    a. 2
    b. 3
    c. 4
    d. 5

276

Chapter 36 **Moisture Control**

32 31 30 29 28

12. What cavity classification would indicate the use of an anterior dental dam clamp?
    a. Class I on tooth #4
    b. Class II on tooth #18
    c. Class V on tooth #7
    d. Class VI on tooth #28

13. The assistant uses the _____ grasp when holding the HVE.
    a. pen
    b. thumb-to-nose
    c. reverse-palm
    d. a or b

14. The dentist is preparing a Class V on the buccal surface of tooth #5, the HVE tip would be placed on the.
    a. Mesial lingual surface of the tooth
    b. Mesial facial surface of the tooth
    c. Distal facial surface of the tooth
    d. Distal lingual surface of the tooth

15. The rationale for inverting the dental dam is to _____.
    a. prevent saliva leakage
    b. remove excess material
    c. stabilize the restoration
    d. All of the above

16. The working end of the HVE tip should be positioned _____ the occlusal surface of the tooth being prepared.
    a. even with
    b. slightly beyond
    c. gingivally with
    d. directly on

17. The _____ is used to place holes in the dental dam to expose the teeth for isolation.
    a. dental dam clamp
    b. dental dam punch
    c. dental dam frame
    d. dental dam forceps

18. What should be positioned on the dental dam clamp before it is positioned on the tooth in a patient's mouth?
    a. Dental dam material
    b. Cotton roll
    c. Compound wax
    d. Dental floss

19. What equipment is used to perform a limited rinse?
    a. Dry-angle
    b. Air-water syringe
    c. HVE
    d. b and c

20. With the high-speed handpiece positioned on the occlusal surface of tooth #4, where would the HVE be positioned?
    a. Lingual surface of tooth #3
    b. Occlusal surface of tooth #5
    c. Buccal surface of tooth #15
    d. Lower right buccal vestibule

CASE STUDY

Candy Allen is scheduled to have a Class III composite resin placed on the mesial surface of tooth #8. Candy has several restorations placed and is comfortable with the dental treatment she will be receiving today. Throughout the procedure, it will be your responsibility to maintain moisture control.

1. After administration of anesthesia, what type of moisture control would be used to rinse the taste from her mouth?

2. The dentist has indicated for you to place the dental dam. At what point in the procedure will you place the dental dam?

3. What teeth are to be isolated? What size hole will be punched for each tooth?

4. When placing the dam, you find that the contacts are very tight, which is making it difficult to slide the dam interproximally. What surfaces of the teeth are involved in the contact area? How can you adapt the dam to fit interproximally?

5. How will the dental dam be held away from the working area?

6. At what stage of the procedure will you remove the dental dam?

7. When the dam is removed, you see that a piece of the dam has been torn away and is missing. What do you do to retrieve this missing piece?

ACTIVITY

(Requires stamped dental dam)
Tooth #29 will be receiving a class II amalgam restoration today. The dentist would like the dam to be isolated from one tooth distal of tooth #29 to the opposite canine. Place an X on each tooth to be punched. Beside each X, indicate the size of hole to be punched.

MULTIMEDIA PROCEDURES RECOMMENDED REVIEW ⊖volve
learning system

- Positioning the high-volume evacuator during a procedure
- Preparing, placing, and removing the dental dam

COMPETENCY 36-1: POSITIONING THE HIGH-VOLUME EVACUATOR DURING A PROCEDURE

Performance Objective

By following a routine procedure that meets stated protocols, the student will maintain moisture control, access, and visibility during patient care by appropriately positioning the high-volume oral evacuator (HVE).

Evaluation and Grading Criteria

 3   Student competently met the stated criteria without assistance.
 2   Student required assistance in order to meet the stated criteria.
 1   Student showed uncertainty when performing the stated criteria.
 0   Student was not prepared and needs to repeat the step.
 N/A   No evaluation of this step.

Instructor shall define grades for each point range earned on completion of each performance-evaluated task.

Performance Standards

The minimum number of satisfactory performances required before final evaluation is _____.

Instructor shall identify by * those steps considered critical. If step is missed or minimum competency is not met, the evaluated procedure fails and must be repeated.

PERFORMANCE CRITERIA	*	SELF	PEER	INSTRUCTOR	COMMENTS
1. Personal protective equipment placed according to procedure.					
2. HVE tip and air water syringe tip placed and readied for procedure.					
3. Assumed the correct seated position to accommodate a left-handed or a right-handed dentist.					
4. Used the proper grasp when holding the HVE.					
5. Grasped the air-water syringe in the left hand during HVE placement.					
6. Positioned the HVE correctly for the maxillary left posterior treatment.					
7. Positioned the HVE correctly for the maxillary right posterior treatment.					
8. Positioned the HVE correctly for the mandibular left posterior treatment.					
9. Positioned the HVE correctly for the mandibular right posterior treatment.					
10. Positioned the HVE correctly for the anterior treatment with lingual access.					

Continued

11. Positioned the HVE correctly for the anterior treatment with facial access.				
12. Maintained patient comfort and followed appropriate infection control measures throughout the procedure.				

ADDITIONAL COMMENT

Total number of points earned _____

Grade _____ Instructor's initials _____

COMPETENCY 36-2: PERFORMING A MOUTH RINSE

Performance Objective

By following a routine procedure that meets stated protocols, the student will perform a limited-area rinse and a complete mouth rinse using the high-volume oral evacuator (HVE) and air-water syringe.

Evaluation and Grading Criteria

__3__ Student competently met the stated criteria without assistance.
__2__ Student required assistance in order to meet the stated criteria.
__1__ Student showed uncertainty when performing the stated criteria.
__0__ Student was not prepared and needs to repeat the step.
__N/A__ No evaluation of this step.
Instructor shall define grades for each point range earned on completion of each performance-evaluated task.

Performance Standards

The minimum number of satisfactory performances required before final evaluation is _____.

Instructor shall identify by * those steps considered critical. If step is missed or minimum competency is not met, the evaluated procedure fails and must be repeated.

PERFORMANCE CRITERIA	*	SELF	PEER	INSTRUCTOR	COMMENTS
Limited-Area Rinse					
1. Personal protective equipment placed according to procedure.					
2. Grasped the air-water syringe with the left hand.					
3. Grasped the HVE in the right hand using the proper grasp.					
4. Positioned the HVE in the area being worked on, and rinsed and suctioned the area.					
5. Maintained patient comfort and followed appropriate infection control measures throughout the procedure.					
Complete Mouth Rinse					
6. Held the air-water syringe in the left hand.					
7. Held the HVE in the right hand using a proper grasp.					
8. Instructed patient to turn towards you.					

Continued

9. Positioned the HVE in the vestibule of the mouth and, starting at one area, rinsed the mouth thoroughly, suctioning the accumulated water and debris.				
10. Maintained patient comfort and followed appropriate infection control measures throughout the procedure.				

ADDITIONAL COMMENT

Total number of points earned _____

Grade _____ Instructor's initials _____

Performance Objective

By following a routine procedure that meets stated protocols, the student will place and properly remove cotton roll isolation for each area of the mouth.

Evaluation and Grading Criteria

 3   Student competently met the stated criteria without assistance.
 2   Student required assistance in order to meet the stated criteria.
 1   Student showed uncertainty when performing the stated criteria.
 0   Student was not prepared and needs to repeat the step.
 N/A   No evaluation of this step.

Instructor shall define grades for each point range earned on completion of each performance-evaluated task.

Performance Standards

The minimum number of satisfactory performances required before final evaluation is _____.

Instructor shall identify by * those steps considered critical. If step is missed or minimum competency is not met, the evaluated procedure fails and must be repeated.

PERFORMANCE CRITERIA	*	SELF	PEER	INSTRUCTOR	COMMENTS
Maxillary Placement					
1. Personal protective equipment placed according to procedure.					
2. Positioned the patient with head turned toward assistant and chin raised.					
3. Used cotton pliers to transfer cotton rolls to the mouth.					
4. Positioned the cotton rolls securely in the mucobuccal fold.					
5. Positioned the cotton rolls close to the working field.					
Mandibular Placement					
6. Positioned the patient with head turned toward assistant and chin lowered.					
7. Used cotton pliers to transfer cotton rolls to the mouth.					
8. Positioned the cotton rolls securely in the mucobuccal fold.					
9. Positioned the second cotton roll in the floor of the mouth between the working field and the tongue.					

Continued

10. Positioned cotton rolls close to the working field.				
Cotton Roll Removal				
11. If cotton rolls were dry, moistened them with water from the air-water syringe.				
12. Removed cotton rolls with cotton pliers.				
13. Performed a limited rinse.				
14. Maintained patient comfort and followed appropriate infection control measures throughout the procedure.				
ADDITIONAL COMMENT				

Total number of points earned _____

Grade _____ Instructor's initials _____

COMPETENCY 36-4: PREPARING, PLACING, AND REMOVING OF THE DENTAL DAM (EXPANDED FUNCTION)

Performance Objective
By following a routine procedure that meets stated protocols, the student will prepare, place, stabilize, and remove the dental dam.

Evaluation and Grading Criteria
<u>3</u>   Student competently met the stated criteria without assistance.
<u>2</u>   Student required assistance in order to meet the stated criteria.
<u>1</u>   Student showed uncertainty when performing the stated criteria.
<u>0</u>   Student was not prepared and needs to repeat the step.
<u>N/A</u> No evaluation of this step.
Instructor shall define grades for each point range earned on completion of each performance-evaluated task.

Performance Standards

The minimum number of satisfactory performances required before final evaluation is _____.

Instructor shall identify by * those steps considered critical. If step is missed or minimum competency is not met, the evaluated procedure fails and must be repeated.

PERFORMANCE CRITERIA	*	SELF	PEER	INSTRUCTOR	COMMENTS
1. Personal protective equipment placed according to procedure.					
2. Selected instrument setup for the procedure.					
3. Used a mouth mirror and explorer to examine the site to be isolated.					
4. Flossed all contacts involved in placement of dental dam.					
5. Correctly punched the dam for the teeth to be isolated.					
6. Selected the correct size of clamp and tied a ligature to it.					
7. Placed prepared clamp in the dental dam forceps in the position of use.					
8. Prepared the dental dam material and clamp for placement.					
9. Seated the clamp so that it is secure around the anchor tooth.					
10. Slid the dam over the clamp, making sure to pull the ligature through the keyhole of the dam.					
11. Positioned the dental dam frame correctly, making sure to fasten all notches to the dam.					

Continued

12. Slid the dam through all contacts, using floss to push the dam interproximally.				
13. Inverted the dental dam using floss, air, or a blunted instrument.				
14. Ensured that the dam was ligated and stabilized for the procedure.				
15. When removing the dental dam, the stabilization ligature is removed.				
16. Cut the dental dam septum with scissors.				
17. Removed the dental dam clamp, dental dam frame, and dental dam.				
18. Examined the dental dam for tears or missing pieces.				
19. Used the air-water syringe and HVE tip to rinse the patient's mouth.				
20. Gently wiped debris from the area around the patient's mouth.				
21. Maintained patient comfort and followed appropriate infection control measures throughout the procedure.				

ADDITIONAL COMMENT

Total number of points earned _____

Grade _____ Instructor's initials _____

37 Anesthesia and Pain Control

SHORT-ANSWER QUESTIONS

1. Discuss the importance of pain control in dentistry.

2. Describe the chemical makeup and application of topical anesthetic agents.

3. Discuss the chemical makeup and application of local anesthetic agents.

4. Describe nitrous oxide/oxygen (N_2O/O_2) sedation and explain its use in dentistry.

5. Discuss the importance of reducing the exposure of N_2O/O_2 for the dental team.

6. Discuss intravenous sedation and its use in dentistry.

7. Discuss general anesthesia and its use in dentistry.

FILL-IN-THE-BLANK STATEMENTS

Select the best term from the list below and complete the following statements.

analgesia   **lumen**
anesthesia   **oximetry**
anesthetic   **permeate**
duration   **porous**
gauge   **tidal volume**
induction   **titration**
innervation   **vasoconstrictor**

1. A drug that produces a temporary loss of feeling or sensation is a(n) _____.

2. The measurement of the oxygen concentration in the blood is its _____.

3. The time from induction of an anesthetic to its complete reversal is its_____

4. The_____ is the standard dimension or measurement of the thickness of an injection needle.

5. The_____ is a measurement of the amount of air inhaled and exhaled with each breath during N_2O/O_2 sedation.

6. _____is a temporary loss of feeling or sensation.

7. A(n) _____ is a type of drug used to prolong anesthetic action and constrict blood vessels.

8. To spread or flow throughout is to _____.

9. _____ is determining the exact amount of drug used to achieve a desired level of sedation.

10. Something that is _____ will have openings to allow gas or fluid to pass through.

11. _____ is the supply or distribution of nerves to an organ or a specific body part.

12. The _____ is the hollow center of the injection needle.

13. The time from injection to the point at which anesthesia takes effect is the _____.

14. _____ is a stage in which the perception of pain is dulled without unconsciousness.

MULTIPLE-CHOICE QUESTIONS

Complete each question by circling the best answer.

1. Topical anesthetics are used in dentistry for _____.
   a. sedating the patient
   b. numbing localized nerves
   c. numbing surface tissue
   d. inhalation sedation

2. The most frequently selected form of pain control used in dentistry is _____.
   a. prescribed drugs
   b. local anesthesia
   c. N_2O/O_2 sedation
   d. intravenous sedation

3. Local anesthetics are injected near _____ to create a numbing effect.
   a. an artery
   b. a vein
   c. a nerve
   d. the pulp

4. What drug is added to a local anesthetic solution to prolong its physiological effect?
   a. Alcohol
   b. Ammonia
   c. Nitrous oxide
   d. Epinephrine

5. What type of injection technique will the dentist most frequently use on maxillary teeth?
   a. Block
   b. Infiltration
   c. Intraosseous
   d. Intravenous

6. What needle sizes are most commonly used in dentistry?
   a. ½-inch and ¾-inch needles
   b. 1-inch and 2-inch needles
   c. 1½-inch and $1\frac{5}{8}$-inch needles
   d. 1-inch and $1\frac{5}{8}$-inch needles

7. Is it common for a patient with an acute infection in a tooth to feel the numbing sensation of local anesthesia?
   a. No
   b. Only when the anesthesia has a vasoconstrictor
   c. Yes
   d. Only with a block injection

8. What type of condition is paresthesia?
   a. A localized toxic reaction
   b. An injection into a blood vessel
   c. Numbness that lasts longer than normal
   d. An infected area

9. The first dentist to offer N_2O for his patients was

   _____.
   a. G.V. Black
   b. Horace Wells
   c. C. Edmund Kells
   d. Pierre Fauchard

10. How could the dental team be at risk for exposure to N_2O/O_2 in a dental office?
    a. Gases leaking or escaping from the nasal mask
    b. Patients exhaling gases
    c. Gases leaking from the hoses
    d. All of the above

11. What will the patient receive at the beginning and end of an N_2O/O_2 sedation procedure?
    a. Local anesthesia
    b. Oxygen
    c. Gauze to bite down on
    d. Topical fluoride

12. What level or stage of anesthesia has a patient reached if he or she is relaxed and fully conscious?
    a. Analgesia
    b. Excitement
    c. General anesthesia
    d. Respiratory failure

13. What level of consciousness should a patient reach during general anesthesia?
    a. Stage I
    b. Stage II
    c. Stage III
    d. Stage IV

14. In what environment would general anesthesia be most safely administered to a dental patient?
    a. Dental office
    b. Outpatient clinic
    c. Hospital
    d. a and b

15. The tank or cylinder of _____ is always color-coded green.
    a. topical anesthetic
    b. vasoconstrictor
    c. nitrous oxide
    d. oxygen

16. Anesthetic cartridges should be _____.
    a. refrigerated before use
    b. enclosed in their packaging before use
    c. sterilized before use
    d. soaked in disinfectant before use

17. _____ anesthesia is achieved by injecting the anesthetic into the inferior alveolar nerve.
    a. IV sedation
    b. General
    c. Block
    d. Infiltration

18. A _____ needle is commonly used for infiltration injections.
    a. 1-inch
    b. ⅝-inch
    c. 2-inch
    d. 2⅝-inch

19. The most commonly used form of topical anesthetic for controlling a gag reflex would be _____.
    a. ointment
    b. liquid
    c. spray
    d. a patch

20. A used or contaminated needle should be discarded in the _____.
    a. medical waste
    b. sharps container
    c. sterilization center
    d. general garbage

CASE STUDY

Meredith Smith is coming in to begin treatment for a new bridge on teeth #3, #4, and #5. She is apprehensive about the procedure. Ms. Smith has discussed the option of receiving N_2O analgesia during the procedure and seems reassured that this will help alleviate her worries.

1. What methods or types of anesthesia will most likely be provided to Ms. Smith throughout the procedure today?

2. Could any contraindications prevent Ms. Smith from receiving any of the anesthesia methods you have mentioned? If so, give examples.

3. Where would you find these contraindications?

4. In what order would Ms. Smith receive the methods of anesthesia?

5. What specific supplies and equipment would be placed out for the pain control procedures?

6. At the completion of the procedure, what postoperative instructions will you provide to Meredith regarding her numbness?

7. How would you write up in the patient's chart the anesthetics used today?

MULTIMEDIA PROCEDURES RECOMMENDED REVIEW

- Applying a topical anesthetic
- Assembling the local anesthetic syringe

COMPETENCY 37-1: APPLYING A TOPICAL ANESTHETIC

Performance Objective

By following a routine procedure that meets stated protocols, the student will select the necessary setup, identify the injection site, and apply topical anesthetic.

Evaluation and Grading Criteria

_3_ Student competently met the stated criteria without assistance.
_2_ Student required assistance in order to meet the stated criteria.
_1_ Student showed uncertainty when performing the stated criteria.
_0_ Student was not prepared and needs to repeat the step.
_N/A_ No evaluation of this step.
Instructor shall define grades for each point range earned on completion of each performance-evaluated task.

Performance Standards

The minimum number of satisfactory performances required before final evaluation is _____.

Instructor shall identify by * those steps considered critical. If step is missed or minimum competency is not met, the evaluated procedure fails and must be repeated.

PERFORMANCE CRITERIA	*	SELF	PEER	INSTRUCTOR	COMMENT
1. Personal protective equipment placed according to procedure.					
2. Gathered the appropriate setup.					
3. Used a sterile cotton-tipped applicator to remove a small amount of topical anesthetic ointment from the container; replaced the cover immediately.					
4. Explained the procedure to the patient.					
5. Determined the injection site.					
6. Wiped the injection site dry using a sterile 2- × 2-inch gauze pad.					
7. Applied topical anesthetic ointment to the injection site only.					
8. Left the topical anesthetic ointment in contact with the oral tissues for 2 to 5 minutes.					
9. Removed the cotton-tipped applicator just before the injection was made by the dentist.					

Continued

10. Maintained patient comfort and followed appropriate infection control measures throughout the procedure.					
11. Procedure documented in patient record.					
ADDITIONAL COMMENTS					

Total number of points earned _____

Grade _____ Instructor's initials _____

COMPETENCIES 37-2 AND 37-3: ASSISTING IN THE ASSEMBLY AND ADMINISTRATION OF LOCAL ANESTHESIA

Performance Objective

By following a routine procedure that meets stated protocols, the student will select the necessary setup, prepare an aspirating-type syringe for local anesthetic injection, and assist in administration.

Evaluation and Grading Criteria

  3   Student competently met the stated criteria without assistance.
  2   Student required assistance in order to meet the stated criteria.
  1   Student showed uncertainty when performing the stated criteria.
  0   Student was not prepared and needs to repeat the step.
 N/A   No evaluation of this step.
Instructor shall define grades for each point range earned on completion of each performance-evaluated task.

Performance Standards

The minimum number of satisfactory performances required before final evaluation is _____.

Instructor shall identify by * those steps considered critical. If step is missed or minimum competency is not met, the evaluated procedure fails and must be repeated.

PERFORMANCE CRITERIA	*	SELF	PEER	INSTRUCTOR	COMMENT
1. Personal protective equipment placed according to procedure.					
2. Gathered the necessary instruments and supplies.					
3. Inspected the syringe, needle, and anesthetic cartridge, and prepared the syringe out of the patient's sight.					
4. Double-checked the anesthetic cartridge to confirm that the anesthetic was the type the dentist had indicated.					
5. Retracted the piston using the thumb ring, and inserted the anesthetic cartridge with the rubber stopper end first.					
6. Released the piston and gently engaged the harpoon.					
7. Gently pulled back on the thumb ring to make certain the harpoon was securely in place.					
8. Removed the plastic cap from the syringe end of the needle, and screwed the needle onto the syringe.					
9. Loosened the colored plastic cap from the injection end of the needle.					
10. Transferred the syringe below the patient's chin or behind the patient's head as instructed.					

Continued

Chapter **37 Anesthesia and Pain Control**

11. Took appropriate safety precaution measures while transferring the syringe.					
12. When disassembling the syringe, retracted the piston of the syringe by pulling back on the thumb ring.					
13. While still retracting the piston, removed the anesthetic cartridge from the syringe.					
14. Unscrewed and removed the needle from the syringe.					
15. Disposed of the needle in an appropriate sharps container.					
16. Disposed of the used cartridge in the appropriate waste container.					
17. Followed appropriate infection control measures throughout the procedure.					
18. Procedure documented in patient record.					

ADDITIONAL COMMENTS

Total number of points earned _____

Grade _____ Instructor's initials _____

COMPETENCY 37-4: ASSISTING IN THE ADMINISTRATION AND MONITORING OF NITROUS OXIDE/OXYGEN SEDATION (EXPANDED FUNCTION)

Performance Objective

By following a routine procedure that meets stated protocols, the student will assist with the administration of nitrous oxide analgesia by monitoring the patient's reactions and recording appropriate information in the patient's record.

Evaluation and Grading Criteria

 3 Student competently met the stated criteria without assistance.
 2 Student required assistance in order to meet the stated criteria.
 1 Student showed uncertainty when performing the stated criteria.
 0 Student was not prepared and needs to repeat the step.
N/A No evaluation of this step.

Instructor shall define grades for each point range earned on completion of each performance-evaluated task.

Performance Standards

The minimum number of satisfactory performances required before final evaluation is _____.

Instructor shall identify by * those steps considered critical. If step is missed or minimum competency is not met, the evaluated procedure fails and must be repeated.

PERFORMANCE CRITERIA	*	SELF	PEER	INSTRUCTOR	COMMENT
1. Personal protective equipment placed according to procedure.					
2. Checked the nitrous oxide and oxygen tanks for adequate supply.					
3. Gathered appropriate supplies and placed a sterile mask of the appropriate size on the tubing.					
4. Updated the patient's health history, then took and recorded the patient's blood pressure and pulse.					
5. Instructed the patient with the procedure of nitrous oxide analgesia, and what to expect.					
6. Placed the patient in a supine position.					
7. Assisted the patient with placement of the mask.					
8. Made necessary adjustments to the mask and tubing to ensure proper fit.					
9. At the dentist's direction, adjusted the flow of oxygen to the established tidal volume.					
10. At the dentist's direction, adjusted the flow of nitrous oxide and oxygen.					

Continued

11. Noted on the patient's chart the times and volumes of gas needed to achieve baseline.				
12. Monitored the patient's status throughout the procedure.				
13. At the dentist's direction, turned off the flow of nitrous oxide and increased the flow of oxygen.				
14. After oxygenation was complete, removed the nosepiece, and then slowly returned the patient to the upright position.				
15. Recorded in the patient's record the concentrations of gases administered and any the patient reaction to the analgesia.				
16. Maintained patient comfort and followed appropriate infection control measures throughout the procedure.				

ADDITIONAL COMMENTS

Total number of points earned _____

Grade _____ Instructor's initials _____

38 Foundations of Radiography, Radiographic Equipment, and Radiation Safety

SHORT-ANSWER QUESTIONS

1. Describe the uses of dental imaging.

2. Describe the discovery of x-radiation.

3. Describe the process of ionization.

4. Describe the properties of x-radiation.

5. Describe in detail how x-rays are produced.

6. Label the parts of the dental x-ray tubehead and the dental x-ray tube.

7. Describe the effect of kilovoltage on the quality of the x-ray beam.

8. Describe how milliamperage affects the quality of the x-ray beam.

9. Define the range of kilovoltage and milliamperage required for dental radiography.

10. Discuss the effects of radiation exposure on the human body.

11. Discuss the risks versus benefits of dental images.

12. List the critical organs that are sensitive to radiation.

13. Discuss the ALARA concept.

14. Describe the methods of protecting the patient from excess radiation.

15. Describe the methods of protecting the operator from excess radiation.

FILL-IN-THE-BLANK STATEMENTS

Select the best term from the list below and complete the following statements.

ALARA	**kilovoltage peak**
anode	**latent period**
cathode	**matter**
contrast	**milliampere**
density	**penumbra**
dental radiography	**photon**
digital imaging	**primary beam**
dose	**radiation**
electrons	**radiograph**
energy	**radiology**
genetic effects	**somatic effects**
image	**tungsten target**
image receptor	**x-radiation**
ion	**x-ray**
ionizing radiation	

1. _____ is the emission of energy in the form of waves through space or a material.

2. _____ is a high-energy ionizing electromagnetic radiation.

3. A form of ionizing radiation is the _____.

4. _____ is the science or study of radiation as used in medicine.

5. A(n) _____ is an image produced on photosensitive film by exposing the film to x-rays and then processing it.

6. The making of radiographs of the teeth and adjacent structures through exposure to x-rays is _____.

7. _____ is radiation that produces ionization.

8. The positive electrode in the x-ray tube is the _____.

9. The negative electrode in the x-ray tube is the _____.

10. The _____ is the most penetrating beam produced at the target of the anode.

11. An electrically charged particle is a(n) _____.

12. The _____ is the x-ray tube peak voltage used during an x-ray exposure.

13. A(n) _____ is 1/1000 of an ampere, a unit of measurement used to describe the intensity of an electric current.

14. Tiny negatively charged particles found in the atom are _____.

15. The _____ is a focal spot in the anode.

16. _____ is the difference in degrees of blackness on a radiograph.

17. _____ is the overall darkness or blackness of a radiograph.

18. The amount of energy absorbed by tissues is its _____.

19. _____ are effects of radiation that are passed on to future generations through genetic cells.

20. Effects of radiation that cause illness that is responsible for poor health are _____.

21. The period of time between exposure to ionizing radiation and the appearance of symptoms is the _____.

22. _____ is a concept of radiation protection that states that all exposures should be kept "as low as reasonably achievable."

23. A(n) _____ is a minute bundle of pure energy that has no weight or mass.

24. Anything that occupies space and has form or shape is _____.

25. _____ is a filmless method of capturing an image and displaying it by using an image sensor, an electronic signal, and a computer to process and store the image.

26. The blurred or indistinct area that surrounds an image is _____.

27. A film-based or digitally produced recording of an anatomic structure is a(n) _____.

28. A(n) _____ is a recording medium for images such as a film or sensor.

29. The ability to do work takes _____.

LABELING EXERCISE

1. Label the components of the dental x-ray tubehead.

    a. X-ray tube
    b. Metal housing of x-ray tubehead
    c. Insulating oil
    d. Unleaded glass window of x-ray tube
    e. Lead collimator
    f. Positioning indicating device
    g. Aluminum discs
    h. Tubehead seal
    i. Filament circuit
    j. Cathode (−)
    k. Anode (+)

MULTIPLE-CHOICE QUESTIONS

Complete each question by circling the best answer.

1. Who discovered x-rays?
    a. G.V. Black
    b. W.C. Roentgen
    c. Pierre Fauchard
    d. Horace Wells

2. Who was the first person to make practical use of radiographs in dentistry?
    a. C. Edmund Kells
    b. G.V. Black
    c. W.C. Roentgen
    d. Horace Wells

3. _____ is the process by which electrons are removed from electrically stable atoms.
    a. Physics
    b. Radiation
    c. Ionization
    d. Roentgen

4. The primary components of a dental x-ray machine are the _____.
    a. tubehead
    b. PID
    c. extension arm
    d. All of the above

5. The name of the negative electrode inside the x-ray tube is the _____.
   a. cathode
   b. nucleus
   c. anode
   d. photon

6. The name of the positive electrode inside the x-ray tube is the _____.
   a. cathode
   b. nucleus
   c. anode
   d. neutron

7. What is located on the x-ray machine control panel?
   a. Filter
   b. Collimator
   c. Milliamperage (mA) selector
   d. Tubehead

8. During the production of x-rays, how much energy is lost as heat?
   a. 5%
   b. 25%
   c. 50%
   d. 99%

9. What are the types of radiation?
   a. Primary
   b. Secondary
   c. Scatter
   d. All of the above
   e. a and b

10. A structure that appears dark on a processed radiograph is termed _____.
    a. radiopaque
    b. radiolucent
    c. contrast
    d. density

11. A structure that appears light on a processed radiograph is termed _____.
    a. radiopaque
    b. density
    c. contrast
    d. radiolucent

12. What exposure factor controls contrast?
    a. mA
    b. kVp
    c. Time
    d. Distance

13. Density is the _____.
    a. overall lightness of a processed radiograph
    b. structure that appears light on a processed radiograph
    c. overall darkness of a processed radiograph
    d. structure that appears dark on a processed radiograph

14. The name of the process for the harmful effects of x-rays is _____.
    a. radiation
    b. ionization
    c. ultraviolet rays
    d. infrared rays

15. The period of time between x-ray exposure and the appearance of symptoms is the _____.
    a. exposure time
    b. primary radiation
    c. development
    d. latent period

16. Radiation that is passed on to future generations is the _____.
    a. cumulative effect
    b. somatic effect
    c. genetic effect
    d. exposure effect

17. _____ is a system that is used to measure radiation.
    a. The traditional or standard system
    b. The metric system
    c. Systeme Internationale
    d. a and c

18. The maximum permissible dose of radiation for occupationally exposed persons is _____.
    a. 5.0 rems/year
    b. 15 rems/year
    c. 50 rems/year
    d. 0.05 rems/year

19. The purpose of the collimator is to _____.
    a. filter the primary beam
    b. reduce the exposure of the primary beam
    c. restrict the size of the primary beam
    d. both b and c

20. The purpose of the aluminum filter is to

_____.
   a. reduce the exposure of the primary beam
   b. remove the low-energy, long-wavelength rays
   c. restrict the size of the primary beam
   d. remove the high-energy, short-wavelength rays

21. Which patients should wear a lead apron and thyroid collar?
   a. Patients with a pacemaker
   b. Patients with lung cancer
   c. Children
   d. All patients

22. What is the purpose of personnel monitoring?
   a. To record the amount of radiation a patient receives
   b. To record the amount of radiation the operator receives
   c. To record the amount of radiation that is produced
   d. To check for radiation leakage

23. What is the purpose of equipment monitoring?
   a. To record the amount of radiation a patient receives
   b. To determine the amount of radiation produced during exposure of a radiograph
   c. To record the amount of radiation that reaches a body
   d. To check for radiation leakage

24. What states that "all exposure to radiation should be kept to a minimum" or "as low as reasonably achievable"?
   a. Right to Know Law
   b. ALARA concept
   c. Patient's Bill of Rights
   d. Dental Assistant Creed

25. What is the purpose of using a position indicator device (PID)?
   a. To increase the contrast on the radiograph
   b. To direct the x-ray beam
   c. To increase the density on the radiograph
   d. All of the above

26. What is the primary type of radiation produced in the dental x-ray tubehead?
   a. Roentgen radiation
   b. Bavarian radiation
   c. Tungsten radiation
   d. Bremsstrahlung radiation

TOPICS FOR DISCUSSION

Your next patient is a 37-year-old woman who is new to the practice. She is scheduled today for a series of radiographs, but she appears apprehensive and is asking you a lot of questions. How would you respond to her questions?

1. "I don't know why the dentist wants x-rays; my teeth look fine."

2. "Why are you putting that heavy thing on my lap?"

3. "Why do you leave the room?"

4. "How do you know how many pictures you are going to take?"

5. "Are dental x-rays really safe?"

Access the *Interactive Dental Office* on *Evolve* and click on the patient case file for Margaret Brown.
- Review Margaret's record.
- Answer the following question.

1. Would it be better if the dental assistant held the film in the proper position for the child? It was only for one film.

39 Digital Imaging, Dental Film, and Processing Radiographs

SHORT-ANSWER QUESTIONS

1. Identify the types of dental image receptor holding devices.

2. Describe the composition of a dental x-ray film.

3. Describe the care and maintenance of the processing solutions, equipment, and equipment accessories used in manual and automatic film processing.

4. List and identify the component parts of an automatic film processor.

5. Describe the film-processing problems that result from time and temperature errors.

6. Describe the film-processing problems that result from chemical contamination errors.

7. Describe the film-processing problems that result from film-handling errors.

8. Describe the film-processing problems that result from lighting errors.

9. State the types and indications for the three types of dental images.

10. Identify the five basic sizes of intraoral dental x-ray film.

11. Explain the purpose of an intensifying screen.

12. Describe the process for duplicating radiographs.

13. Discuss the requirements necessary for the darkroom.

14. Describe the differences between direct and indirect digital imaging.

15. Describe the advantages and disadvantages of digital radiography.

16. Describe the equipment necessary for digital radiography.

FILL-IN-THE-BLANK STATEMENTS

Select the best term from the list below and complete the following statements.

beam alignment devices
bitewing radiograph
charge-coupled device (CCD)
digital image
duplicating film
emulsion
extraoral film
film cassette
film-holding devices

film speed
intraoral film
label side
manual processing
occlusal radiograph
periapical radiograph
processing errors
teledentistry
tube side

1. A(n) _____ is an electronic signal captured by sensors and displayed on computer monitors.

2. A coating on the x-ray film that contains energy-sensitive crystals is the _____.

3. The _____ is the solid white side of the film that faces the x-ray tube.

4. The _____ is the colored side of the film that faces the tongue.

5. _____ is a method of film processing that uses film racks and processing tanks.

6. _____ is the process of using electronic transfer of images and other information for consultation and/or insurance purposes in dentistry.

7. _____ are used to hold the film in position in the patient's mouth.

8. _____ are used to indicate the position indicator device (PID) position in relation to the tooth and film.

9. _____ is film that is used for placement in the patient's mouth.

10. Film designed for use in cassettes is _____.

11. Film designed for use in film-duplicating machines is _____.

12. A radiograph that shows the crown, root tip, and surrounding structures is a(n) _____.

13. A(n) _____ shows the crowns of both arches on one film.

14. A radiograph that shows large areas of the maxilla or mandible is the _____.

15. The holder for extraoral films during exposure is a(n) _____.

16. The _____ is determined by the sensitivity of the emulsion on the film to radiation.

17. _____ is a solid-state image sensor used in intraoral digital imaging.

18. _____ are faults that occur on the radiograph during processing.

MULTIPLE-CHOICE QUESTIONS

Complete each question by circling the best answer.

1. How does a film holder protect the patient from unnecessary radiation?
   a. It filters the scatter radiation.
   b. It keeps the patient's hands and fingers from being exposed to x-radiation.
   c. It speeds up the process.
   d. It shows the correct teeth.

2. Describe a basic type of image receptor.
   a. Hemostat device
   b. Resembles a clothespin
   c. Square with adhesive on the back
   d. Bite-block with a backing plate and a slot for film-sensor retention

3. Name a component of an intraoral film.
   a. Film emulsion
   b. Aluminum foil
   c. Plastic
   d. Alginate

4. The image on the film before it is processed is the

   _____.
   a. density
   b. latent image
   c. contrast
   d. mirror image

5. Which side of the film faces toward the tube?
   a. Envelope-looking side
   b. Silver side
   c. Plain side

6. What size film is used for posterior periapical radiographs?
   a. 0
   b. 1
   c. 2
   d. 3

7. What size film is used for occlusal radiographs?
   a. 2
   b. 3
   c. 4
   d. 5

8. Describe the types of extraoral film cassettes.
   a. Flexible
   b. Rigid
   c. Expandable
   d. a and b

9. What converts x-ray energy into visible light?
   a. Aluminum foil
   b. Cardboard
   c. Intensifying screen
   d. Collimator

10. When would you need to duplicate a radiograph?
    a. To get a second opinion
    b. To send to an insurance company
    c. To refer a patient to a specialist
    d. b and c

11. How should x-ray film be stored?
    a. Away from light
    b. In heat
    c. In a moist environment
    d. Submersed in chemicals

12. Where is the expiration date on a package of x-ray film?
    a. On each film
    b. Outside the box
    c. On the package insert
    d. On the bar code

13. What is the second step involved in manually processing dental radiographs?
    a. Developing
    b. Fixing
    c. Rinsing
    d. Washing

14. Indirect digital imaging involves the use of:
    a. Digital sensor
    b. Phosphor storage plate (PSP)
    c. Intraoral film
    d. Extraoral film

15. How often should processing solution be replenished?
    a. Daily
    b. Weekly
    c. Bimonthly
    d. Monthly

16. What low-intensity light is composed of long wave-lengths in the red-orange spectrum?
    a. X-rays
    b. Safelight
    c. Intensifying screen
    d. Filter

17. What is the minimum distance between a safelight and the working area?
    a. 1 foot
    b. 2 feet
    c. 3 feet
    d. 4 feet

18. What is the optimum temperature for the water in the manual processing tanks?
    a. 65° F
    b. 68° F
    c. 72° F
    d. 75° F

19. What is the major advantage of automatic film processing?
    a. The quality of the radiograph is better.
    b. It saves time.
    c. There are fewer chemicals.
    d. It is safer.

20. Are manual processing solutions and automatic processing solutions interchangeable?
    a. Yes
    b. No

ACTIVITY

You are scheduled to take radiographs of the following patients. Listed are the areas of the mouth on which you will be taking films. For each area, give the size of film that you will need to set up for the procedure.

Patient One: 28 years old

Maxillary right molar: _____

Maxillary left molar: _____

Maxillary central: _____

Mandibular right molar: _____

Mandibular left molar: _____

Mandibular central: _____

Right bitewing: _____

Left bitewing: _____

Patient Two: 8 years old

Maxillary right molar: _____

Maxillary left molar: _____

Maxillary central: _____

Mandibular right molar: _____

Mandibular left molar: _____

Mandibular central: _____

Right bitewing: _____

Left bitewing: _____

Patient Three: 4 years old

Maxillary occlusal: _____

Mandibular occlusal: _____

Ⓔvolve
learning system

MULTIMEDIA PROCEDURES RECOMMENDED REVIEW

■ Automatic processing of dental radiographs
■ Duplicating radiographs
■ Manual processing of radiographs
■ Digital imaging (4 videos)

⊖volve
learning system

Access the *Interactive Dental Office* on *Evolve* and click on the patient case file for Miguel Ricardo.
- Review Mr. Ricardo's record.
- Mount his radiographs.
- Answer the following questions.

1. Is the dark area below the roots of the mandibular molars a processing error?

2. What size film was used for the bitewings?

Access the *Interactive Dental Office* on *Evolve* and click on the patient case file for Mrs. Harriet Ross.
- Review Mrs. Ross' record.
- Mount her radiographs.
- Answer the following questions.

3. Why were only 13 films taken?

4. Are there any processing errors on her FMX?

Access the *Interactive Dental Office* on *Evolve* and click on the patient case file for Mr. Lee Wong.
- Review Mr. Wong's record.
- Mount his radiographs.
- Answer the following questions.

5. Is the dark area around the roots caused by a processing error?

6. Did a processing error cause the round circle at the bottom on the right side of the film?

COMPETENCY 39-1: DUPLICATING DENTAL RADIOGRAPHS

Performance Objective

By following a routine procedure that meets stated protocols, the student will demonstrate the proper technique for duplicating dental radiographs.

Evaluation and Grading Criteria

<u>3</u>   Student competently met the stated criteria without assistance.
<u>2</u>   Student required assistance in order to meet the stated criteria.
<u>1</u>   Student showed uncertainty when performing the stated criteria.
<u>0</u>   Student was not prepared and needs to repeat the step.
<u>N/A</u> No evaluation of this step.
Instructor shall define grades for each point range earned on completion of each performance-evaluated task.

Performance Standards

The minimum number of satisfactory performances required before final evaluation is _____.

Instructor shall identify by * those steps considered critical. If step is missed or minimum competency is not met, the evaluated procedure fails and must be repeated.

PERFORMANCE CRITERIA	*	SELF	PEER	INSTRUCTOR	COMMENT
1. Turned on the safelight, and turned off the white light.					
2. Placed the radiographs on the duplicator machine glass.					
3. Placed the duplicating film on top of the radiographs with the emulsion side against the radiographs.					
4. Turned on the light in the duplicating machine for the manufacturer's recommended time.					
5. Removed the duplicating film from the machine and processed it normally, using manual or automatic techniques.					
6. Procedure documented in patient record.					
ADDITIONAL COMMENTS					

Total number of points earned _____

Grade _____ Instructor's initials _____

COMPETENCY 39-2: PROCESSING DENTAL FILMS MANUALLY

Performance Objective

By following a routine procedure that meets stated protocols, the student will demonstrate the proper technique for processing films manually.

Evaluation and Grading Criteria

__3__   Student competently met the stated criteria without assistance.
__2__   Student required assistance in order to meet the stated criteria.
__1__   Student showed uncertainty when performing the stated criteria.
__0__   Student was not prepared and needs to repeat the step.
__N/A__   No evaluation of this step.

Instructor shall define grades for each point range earned on completion of each performance-evaluated task.

Performance Standards

The minimum number of satisfactory performances required before final evaluation is _____.

Instructor shall identify by * those steps considered critical. If step is missed or minimum competency is not met, the evaluated procedure fails and must be repeated.

PERFORMANCE CRITERIA	*	SELF	PEER	INSTRUCTOR	COMMENT
1. Followed all infection control steps.					
2. Stirred the solutions, and checked solution levels and temperature. The temperature was 65° F to 70° F.					
3. Labeled the film rack with the patient's name and the date of exposure.					
4. Turned on the safelight, then turned off the white light.					
5. Washed and dried hands and put on gloves.					
6. Opened the film packets and allowed the films to drop onto the clean paper towel. Used care not to touch the films.					
7. Removed contaminated gloves, and washed and dried hands.					
8. Attached each film to the film rack so that films were parallel and not touching.					
9. Agitated the rack slightly while inserting it into the solution.					

Continued

10. Started the timer. The timer was set according to the manufacturer's instructions on the basis of the temperature of the solutions.				
11. Removed the rack of films after the timer went off, and rinsed it in running water in the center tank for 20 to 30 seconds.				
12. Determined the fixation time and set the timer. Immersed the rack of films in the fixer tank.				
13. Returned the rack of films to the center tank with circulating water for a minimum of 20 minutes.				
14. Removed the rack of films from the water and allowed it to dry.				
15. When the rack of films was completely dry, removed the films from the rack and mounted them in an appropriately labeled mount.				

ADDITIONAL COMMENTS

Total number of points earned _____

Grade _____ Instructor's initials _____

COMPETENCY 39-3: PROCESSING DENTAL FILMS IN AN AUTOMATIC FILM PROCESSOR

Performance Objective

By following a routine procedure that meets stated protocols, the student will demonstrate the proper technique for processing dental radiographs in an automatic film processor.

Evaluation and Grading Criteria

3   Student competently met the stated criteria without assistance.
2   Student required assistance in order to meet the stated criteria.
1   Student showed uncertainty when performing the stated criteria.
0   Student was not prepared and needs to repeat the step.
N/A No evaluation of this step.

Instructor shall define grades for each point range earned on completion of each performance-evaluated task.

Performance Standards

The minimum number of satisfactory performances required before final evaluation is _____.

Instructor shall identify by * those steps considered critical. If step is missed or minimum competency is not met, the evaluated procedure fails and must be repeated.

PERFORMANCE CRITERIA	*	SELF	PEER	INSTRUCTOR	COMMENT
1. Before the machine was operational, turned it on and allowed the chemicals to warm up (according to manufacturer's recommendations for proper temperature).					
2. Followed infection control steps.					
3. Opened the lid on the daylight loader and placed a paper towel over the bottom, then placed two disposable cups on the paper towel.					
4. Put on gloves and slid gloved hands through the sleeves of the daylight loader.					
5. Opened film packet, then removed the black paper and lead foil. Placed the films in the processor.					
6. Fed the films slowly into the machine and kept them straight. Allowed at least 10 seconds between inserting each film into the processor. Alternated slots within the processor when possible.					

Continued

7. After the last film was inserted into the machine, removed gloves and dropped them into the center of the paper towel. Wrapped the paper towel over the contaminated film packets and gloves, touching only the corners and underside of the paper towel. Placed the paper towel into the second cup.				
8. Removed the cup that contains the lead foil and took it to the recycling container.				
9. Removed the processed radiographs from the film recovery slot on the outside of the automatic processor and allowed 4-6 minutes for the automated process to be completed.				

ADDITIONAL COMMENTS

Total number of points earned _____

Grade _____ Instructor's initials _____

40 Legal Issues, Quality Assurance, and Infection Prevention

SHORT-ANSWER QUESTIONS

1. Describe what must be included for informed consent with regard to dental imaging.

2. Define the types of laws that affect the practice of dental radiography.

3. Describe what is included in the Consumer-Patient Radiation Health and Safety Act.

4. Identify the individual who "owns" the dental images.

5. Describe the purpose of a quality assurance program.

6. Describe the components of a quality assurance program.

7. Describe quality control tests for processing solutions.

8. Explain the use of a stepwedge.

9. Explain the purpose of a "reference radiograph."

10. Explain the infection control requirements for preparing an x-ray operatory.

11. Describe the infection control protocol for making exposures using phosphor storage plates (PSPs).

12. Describe the infection control protocol for making exposures using digital sensors.

13. Describe the infection control protocol for making exposures using conventional dental x-ray film.

FILL-IN-THE-BLANK STATEMENTS

Select the best term from the list below and complete the following statements.

disclosure
informed consent
liable

quality assurance
quality control tests
stepwedge

1. _____ is the process of informing the patient about dental imaging procedures.

2. _____ is permission granted by a patient after he or she has been informed about the particulars of the procedure.

3. _____ means that a person is accountable, or legally responsible.

4. _____ ensures that high-quality diagnostic radiographs are produced.

5. Specific tests that are used to ensure quality in dental x-ray equipment, supplies, and film processing are _____.

6. A(n) _____ is used to demonstrate film densities and contrasts.

MULTIPLE-CHOICE QUESTIONS

Complete each question by circling the best answer.

1. What federal act requires persons who take radiographs to be trained and certified?
   a. Hazard Communication Standard
   b. Blood-Borne Pathogen Standard
   c. Consumer-Patient Radiation Health and Safety Act
   d. Bill of Rights Act

2. What type of agreement is most desirable before radiographs of a patient are taken?
   a. Verbal consent
   b. Dentist's signature
   c. Written consent
   d. Medical approval

3. Under state laws, who is allowed to prescribe dental images?
   a. Radiologist
   b. Specialist
   c. Physician
   d. Dentist

4. Who legally owns a patient's dental images?
   a. The patient
   b. The radiologist
   c. The dentist
   d. The physician

5. A way to ensure that high-quality diagnostic radiographs are produced is by having _____.
   a. the best type of film
   b. quality assurance
   c. certified dental assistants
   d. Kodak approval

6. What are quality control tests?
   a. Specific tests that are used to monitor dental x-ray equipment, supplies, and film processing
   b. Specific tests that dental personnel must take and pass
   c. National board examinations for dentists
   d. Radiology certification

7. When should you check a box of film for freshness?
   a. Daily
   b. Monthly
   c. Every Monday morning
   d. Each time you open a new box

8. Should you use a film cassette that has scratches?
   a. Yes
   b. No

9. Which of the following is a critical area in a quality control program?
   a. Patient consent
   b. Film mounting
   c. Film processing
   d. Use of PPE

10. What is the purpose of the coin test?
    a. To check the x-ray machine
    b. To check the safelight
    c. To check the processor
    d. To check the technique

11. How often should processing solutions be replenished?
    a. Daily
    b. Weekly
    c. Monthly
    d. Twice a year

12. Why are a reference radiograph and a stepwedge used?
    a. To check the absorbed dose
    b. To check the processing technique
    c. To check the densities and contrast
    d. To check the radiolucency and radiopacity

13. How can you tell when the fixer is losing its strength?
    a. Films take longer to clear.
    b. Films appear dark.
    c. Films are black.
    d. Films appear light.

14. What is the purpose of a quality administration program?
    a. It deals with credentialing of the quality assurance program.
    b. It deals with management of the quality assurance program.
    c. It deals with who takes the x-rays in the office.
    d. It deals with being compensated more for taking x-rays.

15. Which staff members need to be aware of the quality administration program?
    a. Dentist
    b. Dental assistant
    c. Dental hygienist
    d. All of the above

16. What surfaces must be covered with a barrier?
    a. All surfaces
    b. Surfaces that are not easily cleaned and disinfected
    c. No surfaces should be covered with a barrier
    d. Only surfaces in the darkroom

17. What precautions should NOT be taken when one is handling contaminated phosphor storage plates (PSPs)?
    a. Wearing overgloves
    b. Placing the films in a paper cup
    c. Soaking the plates in a liquid sterilant
    d. Wiping saliva off the film as soon as the film is removed from the mouth

18. What is the minimum personal protective equipment the operator should wear while exposing radiographs?
    a. Mask
    b. Eyewear
    c. Gloves
    d. Hair cover

19. How do you sterilize sensors?
    a. Heat
    b. Moisture
    c. Vapor
    d. You cannot sterilize sensors.

TOPICS FOR DISCUSSION

A series of films has just been processed in the automatic processor, and something has happened to them. You take them to the view box, and all of the films are dark. Dark films can be the result of a variety of processing errors. Explain how the following factors can affect the processing of a film:

Time:

Solution strength:

Temperature:

Light leaks:

Improper fixation:

Paper left on film:

COMPETENCY 40-1: PRACTICING INFECTION CONTROL DURING FILM EXPOSURE

Performance Objective

By following a routine procedure that meets stated protocols, the student will demonstrate the proper technique for implementing appropriate infection control procedures during film exposure.

Evaluation and Grading Criteria

3	Student competently met the stated criteria without assistance.
2	Student required assistance in order to meet the stated criteria.
1	Student showed uncertainty when performing the stated criteria.
0	Student was not prepared and needs to repeat the step.
N/A	No evaluation of this step.

Instructor shall define grades for each point range earned on completion of each performance-evaluated task.

Performance Standards

The minimum number of satisfactory performances required before final evaluation is _____.

Instructor shall identify by * those steps considered critical. If step is missed or minimum competency is not met, the evaluated procedure fails and must be repeated.

PERFORMANCE CRITERIA	*	SELF	PEER	INSTRUCTOR	COMMENT
1. Washed and dried hands, and placed barriers.					
2. Set out the packaged positioning device. Film, labelled container for exposed film, paper towel, and other miscellaneous items needed.					
3. Seated the patient and placed the lead apron.					
4. Washed and dried hands, and put on gloves.					
5. Placed each exposed film into the container, being careful not to touch the external surface.					
6. Wiped the exposed packet on the paper towel.					
7. After exposures were complete, removed lead apron and dismissed patient.					
8. When finished exposing films and while still gloved, discarded the barriers and paper towel.					

Continued

9. Removed gloves and washed hands before leaving the treatment room.				
10. Carried the cup or bag of exposed films to the processing area.				

ADDITIONAL COMMENTS

Total number of points earned _____

Grade _____ Instructor's initials _____

COMPETENCY 40-2: PRACTICING INFECTION CONTROL IN THE DARKROOM

Performance Objective
By following a routine procedure that meets stated protocols, the student will demonstrate the proper technique for implementing proper infection control in the darkroom.

Evaluation and Grading Criteria
  3   Student competently met the stated criteria without assistance.
  2   Student required assistance in order to meet the stated criteria.
  1   Student showed uncertainty when performing the stated criteria.
  0   Student was not prepared and needs to repeat the step.
 N/A   No evaluation of this step.
Instructor shall define grades for each point range earned on completion of each performance-evaluated task.

Performance Standards
The minimum number of satisfactory performances required before final evaluation is _____.

Instructor shall identify by * those steps considered critical. If step is missed or minimum competency is not met, the evaluated procedure fails and must be repeated.

PERFORMANCE CRITERIA	*	SELF	PEER	INSTRUCTOR	COMMENT
1. Placed a paper towel and a clean cup on the counter near the processor.					
2. Washed hands and put on a new pair of gloves.					
3. Opened the film packets, and allowed each exposed film to drop onto the paper towel. Ensured that unwrapped films did not come into contact with gloves.					
4. Removed the lead foil from the packet and placed it into the foil container.					
5. Placed the empty film packets into the clean cup.					
6. Discarded the cup, and removed gloves with insides turned out and discarded them.					
7. Placed the films into the processor or on developing racks with bare hands.					
ADDITIONAL COMMENTS					

Total number of points earned _____

Grade _____ Instructor's initials _____

Chapter **40 Legal Issues, Quality Assurance, and Infection Prevention**

COMPETENCY 40-3: PRACTICING INFECTION CONTROL WITH USE OF A DAYLIGHT LOADER

Performance Objective

By following a routine procedure that meets stated protocols, the student will demonstrate proper infection control techniques while using the daylight loader.

Evaluation and Grading Criteria

__3__   Student competently met the stated criteria without assistance.
__2__   Student required assistance in order to meet the stated criteria.
__1__   Student showed uncertainty when performing the stated criteria.
__0__   Student was not prepared and needs to repeat the step.
__N/A__   No evaluation of this step.
Instructor shall define grades for each point range earned on completion of each performance-evaluated task.

Performance Standards

The minimum number of satisfactory performances required before final evaluation is _____.

Instructor shall identify by * those steps considered critical. If step is missed or minimum competency is not met, the evaluated procedure fails and must be repeated.

PERFORMANCE CRITERIA	*	SELF	PEER	INSTRUCTOR	COMMENT
1. Washed and dried hands, then placed a paper towel or piece of plastic as a barrier inside the bottom of the daylight loader.					
2. Placed the cup with the contaminated film, a clean pair of gloves, and a second paper cup on the barrier, and closed the top.					
3. Put clean hands through the sleeves and put on the gloves.					
4. Opened the packets and allowed the films to drop onto the clean barrier. Placed the contaminated packets into the second cup and the lead foil into the foil container.					
5. After opening the last packet, removed gloves with insides turned out, and inserted the films into the developing slots.					
6. After inserting the last film, pulled ungloved hands through sleeves.					
7. Opened the top of the loader and carefully pulled the ends of the barrier over the paper cup; used gloves and discarded them. Used care not to touch the contaminated parts of the barrier with bare hands.					
8. Washed and dried hands.					

Continued

9. Labeled a film mount, paper cup, or envelope with the patient's name and used it to collect the processed films.				
ADDITIONAL COMMENTS				

Total number of points earned _____

Grade _____ Instructor's initials _____

COMPETENCY 40-4: PRACTICING INFECTION CONTROL WITH DIGITAL SENSORS

Performance Objective

By following a routine procedure that meets stated protocols, the student will demonstrate all infection control practices using digital sensors.

Evaluation and Grading Criteria

_3_   Student competently met the stated criteria without assistance.
_2_   Student required assistance in order to meet the stated criteria.
_1_   Student showed uncertainty when performing the stated criteria.
_0_   Student was not prepared and needs to repeat the step.
N/A   No evaluation of this step.
Instructor shall define grades for each point range earned on completion of each performance-evaluated task.

Performance Standards

The minimum number of satisfactory performances required before final evaluation is_____.

Instructor shall identify by * those steps considered critical. If step is missed or minimum competency is not met, the evaluated procedure fails and must be repeated.

PERFORMANCE CRITERIA	*	SELF	PEER	INSTRUCTOR	COMMENT
1. Washed and dried hands, then placed surface barriers on equipment, computer keyboard and mouse, and work area.					
2. Set out the packaged positioning device, barriers for the sensor and cable, and a paper towel or gauze squares.					
3. Secured the barrier around the digital sensor.					
4. Seated the patient and positioned the lead apron.					
5. Washed and dried hands and donned gloves.					
6. After all exposures were complete, removed the lead apron using appropriate aseptic techniques and dismissed the patient.					
7. Put on utility gloves and removed barriers from the x-ray equipment, keyboard, and mouse, taking care not to touch the surfaces underneath.					
8. Disposed of barriers and paper towels.					
9. Placed the positioning device on a tray to be returned to the instrument processing area.					

Continued

10. Disinfected the lead apron and any surfaces that may have become contaminated during the removal of surface barriers.					
11. Washed and dried hands.					

ADDITIONAL COMMENTS

Total number of points earned _____

Grade _____ Instructor's initials _____

COMPETENCY 40-5: PRACTICING INFECTION CONTROL WITH PHOSPHOR STORAGE PLATES (PSPs)

Performance Objective
By following a routine procedure that meets stated protocols, the student will demonstrate all infection control practices when using phosphor storage plates.

Evaluation and Grading Criteria
3   Student competently met the stated criteria without assistance.
2   Student required assistance in order to meet the stated criteria.
1   Student showed uncertainty when performing the stated criteria.
0   Student was not prepared and needs to repeat the step.
N/A   No evaluation of this step.
Instructor shall define grades for each point range earned on completion of each performance-evaluated task.

Performance Standards
The minimum number of satisfactory performances required before final evaluation is _____.

Instructor shall identify by * those steps considered critical. If step is missed or minimum competency is not met, the evaluated procedure fails and must be repeated.

PERFORMANCE CRITERIA	*	SELF	PEER	INSTRUCTOR	COMMENT
Procedural Steps					
1. Turned on the computer and logged on to link the patient's images to his or her chart. Chose the image layout.					
2. Washed and dried hands.					
3. Placed surface barriers on equipment and work area.					
4. Slid the phosphor plates into barrier envelopes.					
5. Sealed barrier envelope by removing protective strip, and gently pressed to seal the edge.					
6. Set out the packaged positioning device, transfer box, paper towel, and any other miscellaneous items necessary.					
Exposures					
7. Seated the patient and positioned the lead apron.					
8. Washed and dried hands and donned gloves.					
9. Placed the PSP into the film holder for each exposure.					
10. After each exposure, wiped the excess saliva from the PSP using a paper towel or gauze.					
11. Placed each exposed PSP into the paper cup that was labeled with the patient's name.					

Continued

12. After exposures were complete, removed the lead apron and dismissed the patient.				
13. Removed barriers, taking care not to touch the surfaces underneath.				
14. Disposed of barriers and placed positioning devices on tray to be returned to the instrument processing area.				
Preparation for Scanning				
15. While gloved, removed PSP from paper cup.				
16. Carefully opened sealed envelope and allowed PSP to drop into the black transfer box.				
17. Disposed of contaminated envelopes.				
18. Removed gloves and washed hands.				
Scanning				
19. Followed the manufacturer's directions for insertion of PSPs into the scanner.				
20. When imaging was complete, logged off the system.				
21. Procedure documented in patient record.				
ADDITIONAL COMMENTS				

Total number of points earned _____

Grade _____ Instructor's initials _____

41 Intraoral Imaging

SHORT-ANSWER QUESTIONS

1. Describe the procedure for preparing a patient for dental images.

2. Name and describe the two primary types of projections used in an intraoral technique.

3. Explain the advantages and disadvantages of the paralleling and bisection of the angle technique.

4. Explain the basic principle of the paralleling technique.

5. Explain why a film or sensor holder is necessary with the paralleling technique.

6. State the five basic rules of the paralleling technique.

7. Label the parts of the Rinn XCP instruments.

8. State the recommended vertical angulation for all bitewing exposures.

9. State the basic rules for the bitewing technique.

10. Describe the appearance of opened and overlapped contact areas on a dental image.

11. State the basic rules of the bisecting technique.

12. Describe the film-sensor size used in the bisecting technique.

13. Describe correct vertical angulation.

14. Describe incorrect vertical angulation.

15. Describe the technique for exposing occlusal radiographs.

16. Describe techniques for managing the patient with a hypersensitive gag reflex.

17. Describe techniques for managing patients with physical and mental disabilities.

FILL-IN-THE-BLANK STATEMENTS

Select the best term from the list below and complete the following statements.

alveolar bone
bisection of the angle technique
bitewing
central ray
contact area
crestal bone
diagnostic quality

interproximal
intersecting
long axis of the tooth
parallel
paralleling technique
perpendicular
right angle

1. The _____ is an intraoral technique of exposing periapical images in which the teeth and the image receptor are parallel to each other.

2. The _____ is an intraoral technique of exposing periapical images in which the film and the teeth create an angle that is bisected by the beam.

3. Dental images with the proper landmarks and optimum density, contrast, definition, and detail have good

    _____.

4. _____ is the term that is used to describe a space between two adjacent surfaces.

5. A(n) _____ is the type of image used for the interproximal examination.

6. The bone that supports and encases the roots of the teeth is the _____.

7. The _____ is the coronal portion of alveolar bone found between the teeth.

8. An area of a tooth that touches an adjacent tooth in the same arch is the _____.

332

9. An object is _____ if it is moving or lying in the same plane and is always separated by the same distance.

10. _____ means to cut across or through.

11. Something is _____ if it intersects at or forms a right angle.

12. A 90-degree angle formed by two lines perpendicular to each other is a _____.

13. The _____ is an imaginary line that divides the tooth longitudinally into two equal halves.

14. The _____ is the central portion of the primary beam of radiation.

MULTIPLE-CHOICE QUESTIONS

Complete each question by circling the best answer.

1. What technique is used for exposing dental images?
   a. Digressive
   b. Parallel
   c. Bisection of angle
   d. b and c

2. Which exposure technique do the American Academy of Oral and Maxillofacial Radiology and the American Association of Dental Schools recommend?
   a. Bisection of angle
   b. Parallel
   c. Intersection
   d. Dissection

3. Why is an exposure sequence important?
   a. So areas of the mouth are not missed or retaken
   b. To follow guidelines
   c. For proper mounting of film
   d. To keep up with them in the processing

4. When you are exposing images, in which area of the mouth should you begin?
   a. Maxillary right
   b. Mandibular anterior
   c. Mandibular left
   d. Maxillary anterior

5. Which exposure should be the first for the posterior regions?
   a. Maxillary molar
   b. Mandibular premolar
   c. Maxillary premolar
   d. Mandibular molar

6. Why is it not recommended to have the patient hold the image receptor during exposure?
   a. The patient's finger will get in the way of the image.
   b. The dental assistant must position the film or sensor properly.
   c. The patient receives unnecessary radiation.
   d. It does not meet with infection control standards.

7. What type of film holder can be used in the bisecting angle technique?
   a. BAI
   b. EeZee Grip
   c. Stabe
   d. All of the above

8. What error occurs when the horizontal angulation is incorrect?
   a. Elongation
   b. Overlapping
   c. Blurring
   d. Herringbone pattern

9. Which of the following can occur when the vertical angulation is incorrect?
   a. Elongation
   b. Overlapping
   c. Foreshortening
   d. a and c

10. In the bisecting angle technique, how is the image receptor placed in relation to the teeth?
    a. Parallel
    b. Far from the teeth
    c. Close to the teeth
    d. On the opposite side of the arch

11. What is the purpose of bitewing images?
    a. To view the occlusal third of the teeth
    b. To view the gingival third of the teeth
    c. To view the apices of the teeth
    d. To view the interproximal surfaces

12. What vertical angulation should be used for bitewing images?
    a. −10 degrees
    b. −15 degrees
    c. +10 degrees
    d. +15 degrees

13. What film size is used in the occlusal technique for an adult?
    a. 1
    b. 2
    c. 3
    d. 4

14. When are occlusal radiographs indicated?
    a. To show a wide view of the arch
    b. To view the sinus
    c. To detect interproximal decay
    d. To view the apex

15. For partially edentulous patients, how can you modify the technique for using a bite-block?
    a. Use a larger size of film or sensor
    b. Use a cotton roll
    c. Use the patient's partial denture
    d. Use a custom tray

16. When you are exposing films for a pediatric patient, what analogy can you use to describe the tubehead?
    a. Space gun
    b. Alien machine
    c. Camera
    d. Tubehead

17. What changes must be made in the exposure factors when dental images from a pediatric patient are exposed?
    a. No changes are made.
    b. Exposure factors must be reduced.
    c. Exposure factors must be increased.
    d. It depends on whether the patient is male or female.

18. What film size is recommended for a pediatric patient with all primary dentition?
    a. 0
    b. 1
    c. 2
    d. 3

19. Where would you begin making exposures for a patient with a severe gag reflex?
    a. Maxillary anterior
    b. Mandibular molar
    c. Maxillary molar
    d. Mandibular anterior

20. What is a good diagnostic quality image for endodontics?
    a. One that allows you to see an impaction
    b. One that allows you to see interproximally
    c. One that allows you to see 5 mm beyond the apex
    d. One that allows you to see the incisal edge

21. When radiographs are mounted, where is the dot placed?
    a. It does not matter
    b. Facing away from you
    c. Facing down
    d. Facing up

22. Why is it important for the dental assistant to recognize normal anatomic landmarks?
    a. For diagnostic purposes
    b. For mounting of x-ray films
    c. For quality control
    d. For identification of the patient

23. Why is it important to avoid retakes?
    a. The dentist will deduct it from your pay.
    b. To avoid unnecessary radiation exposure
    c. To avoid wasting film
    d. Insurance will not pay for retakes.

MULTIMEDIA PROCEDURES RECOMMENDED REVIEW

- Assembling XCP Instruments
- Bisecting Technique (8 videos)
- Bitewing Technique (2 videos)
- Mounting Dental Radiographs
- Occlusal Technique
- Paralleling Technique (8 videos)
- Positioning the Patient for Radiographs
- Preparing the Operatory and Equipment to Take Radiographs

334

Access the *Interactive Dental Office on Evolve* and click on the patient case file for Christopher Brooks.
■ Review Christopher's file.
■ Mount his radiographs.
■ Answer the following questions.

1. What types of projections were used for his radiographic survey?

2. What sizes of film were used for each projection?

Access the *Interactive Dental Office on Evolve* and click on the patient case file for Antonio DeAngelis.
■ Review Mr. DeAngelis's file.
■ Mount his radiographs.
■ Answer the following questions.

1. What technique error occurred on the mandibular left premolar exposure?

2. What is wrong with the maxillary left molar projection?

3. What is wrong with the right premolar bitewing, and what would be the correction?

With the first patient, allow yourself 5 minutes. Time yourself and note how many errors you make when you are placing these on the mount. Continue this practice until you have your mounting skills down to 2 minutes with no errors.

COMPETENCY 41-1: PREPARING THE PATIENT FOR DENTAL IMAGES

Performance Objective

By following a routine procedure that meets stated protocols, the student will demonstrate the proper technique for preparing a patient for intraoral x-ray imaging procedures.

Evaluation and Grading Criteria

__3__ Student competently met the stated criteria without assistance.
__2__ Student required assistance in order to meet the stated criteria.
__1__ Student showed uncertainty when performing the stated criteria.
__0__ Student was not prepared and needs to repeat the step.
__N/A__ No evaluation of this step.
Instructor shall define grades for each point range earned on completion of each performance-evaluated task.

Performance Standards

The minimum number of satisfactory performances required before final evaluation is _____.

Instructor shall identify by * those steps considered critical. If step is missed or minimum competency is not met, the evaluated procedure fails and must be repeated.

PERFORMANCE CRITERIA	*	SELF	PEER	INSTRUCTOR	COMMENT
1. Explained the x-ray procedure to the patient, and asked whether he or she had any questions.					
2. Adjusted the chair with the patient positioned upright. Adjusted the level of the chair to a comfortable working height for the operator.					
3. Adjusted the headrest to support and position the patient's head so that the upper arch was parallel to the floor and the midsagittal (midline) plane was perpendicular to the floor.					
4. Placed and secured the lead apron with thyroid collar on the patient. Asked patient to remove eyeglasses and bulky earrings.					
5. Asked the patient to remove all objects from the mouth, including dentures, retainers, chewing gum, and pierced tongue or pierced lip objects. Placed any objects into the plastic container.					

ADDITIONAL COMMENTS

Total number of points earned _____

Grade _____ Instructor's initials _____

COMPETENCY 41-2: ASSEMBLING THE XCP (EXTENSION-CONE PARALLELING) INSTRUMENTS

Performance Objective

By following a routine procedure that meets stated protocols, the student will demonstrate the proper technique for assembling a localizer ring film- or sensor-holding instrument.

Evaluation and Grading Criteria

 3   Student competently met the stated criteria without assistance.
 2   Student required assistance in order to meet the stated criteria.
 1   Student showed uncertainty when performing the stated criteria.
 0   Student was not prepared and needs to repeat the step.
 N/A   No evaluation of this step.

Instructor shall define grades for each point range earned on completion of each performance-evaluated task.

Performance Standards

The minimum number of satisfactory performances required before final evaluation is _____.

Instructor shall identify by * those steps considered critical. If step is missed or minimum competency is not met, the evaluated procedure fails and must be repeated.

PERFORMANCE CRITERIA	*	SELF	PEER	INSTRUCTOR	COMMENT
1. Personal protective equipment placed according to procedure.					
2. Assembled the instruments for the area to be radiographed.					
3. Placed the film or sensor into the backing plate.					
4. Used the entire horizontal length of the bite-block.					
5. Placed the anterior edge of the bite-block on the incisal or occlusal surfaces of the teeth being radiographed.					
6. Instructed the patient to close the mouth slowly but firmly.					
7. Placed a cotton roll between the bite-block and the teeth of the opposite arch.					
8. Moved the localizer ring down the indicator rod into position.					

Continued

9. Aligned the position indicator device.				
10. Exposed the image, then removed the film- or sensor-holding device from the patient's mouth.				

ADDITIONAL COMMENTS

Total number of points earned _____

Grade _____ Instructor's initials _____

COMPETENCY 41-3: PRODUCING A FULL-MOUTH RADIOGRAPHIC SURVEY USING THE PARALLELING TECHNIQUE

Performance Objective

By following a routine procedure that meets stated protocols, the student will produce a full-mouth radiographic survey using the proper paralleling technique.

Evaluation and Grading Criteria

3   Student competently met the stated criteria without assistance.
2   Student required assistance in order to meet the stated criteria.
1   Student showed uncertainty when performing the stated criteria.
0   Student was not prepared and needs to repeat the step.
N/A   No evaluation of this step.

Instructor shall define grades for each point range earned on completion of each performance-evaluated task.

Performance Standards

The minimum number of satisfactory performances required before final evaluation is _____.

Instructor shall identify by * those steps considered critical. If step is missed or minimum competency is not met, the evaluated procedure fails and must be repeated.

PERFORMANCE CRITERIA	*	SELF	PEER	INSTRUCTOR	COMMENT
Preparation					
1. Personal protective equipment placed according to procedure.					
2. Determined the numbers and types of images to be exposed.					
3. Labeled a paper cup, plastic bag, or transfer box and placed it outside the room where the x-ray machine was used.					
4. Turned on the x-ray machine and checked the basic settings.					
5. Washed hands.					
6. If using conventional film or PSPs, dispensed the desired number of films and stored them outside the room where the x-ray machine was used.					
7. Placed all necessary barriers.					
8. Adjusted the chair with the patient positioned upright. Adjusted the level of the chair to a comfortable working height for the operator.					
9. Adjusted the headrest to support and position the patient's head so that the upper arch was parallel to the floor and the midsagittal (midline) plane was perpendicular to the floor.					

Continued

10. Asked the patient to remove eyeglasses and bulky earrings.				
11. Draped the patient with a lead apron and thyroid collar.				
12. Washed hands, and put on clean examination gloves.				
13. Asked the patient to remove any removable prosthetic appliances from his or her mouth.				
14. Opened the package, and assembled the sterile film or sensor-holding instruments.				
15. Used a mouth mirror to inspect the oral cavity.				
Maxillary Central or Lateral Incisor Region				
16. Inserted the film packet or sensor vertically into the anterior block.				
17. Positioned the film or sensor.				
18. Instructed the patient to close the mouth slowly but firmly.				
19. Positioned the localizing ring and the position indicator device (PID), and then exposed the film or sensor.				
Maxillary Canine Region				
20. Inserted the film packet or sensor vertically into the anterior bite-block.				
21. Positioned the film packet or sensor with the canine and first premolar centered.				
22. Instructed the patient to close the mouth slowly but firmly.				
23. Positioned the localizing ring and the PID, and then exposed the film or sensor.				
Maxillary Premolar Region				
24. Inserted the film packet or sensor horizontally into the posterior bite-block.				
25. Centered the film packet or sensor on the second premolar.				
26. With the instrument and film or sensor in place, instructed the patient to close the mouth slowly but firmly.				

27. Positioned the localizing ring and PID, and then exposed the film or sensor.				
Maxillary Molar Region				
28. Inserted the film packet or sensor horizontally into the posterior bite-block.				
29. Centered the film packet or sensor on the second molar.				
30. With the instrument and film or sensor in place, instructed the patient to close the mouth slowly but firmly.				
31. Positioned the localizing ring and PID, then exposed the film or sensor.				
Mandibular Incisor Region				
32. Inserted the film packet or sensor vertically into the anterior bite-block.				
33. Centered the film packet or sensor between the central incisors.				
34. With the instrument and film or sensor in place, instructed the patient to close the mouth slowly but firmly.				
35. Positioned the localizing ring and PID, then exposed the film or sensor.				
Mandibular Canine Region				
36. Inserted the film packet or sensor vertically into the anterior bite-block.				
37. Centered the film or sensor on the canine.				
38. Used a cotton roll between the maxillary teeth and the bite-block, if necessary.				
39. With the instrument and film or sensor in place, instructed the patient to close the mouth slowly but firmly.				
40. Positioned the localizing ring and PID, then exposed the film or sensor.				

Continued

Mandibular Premolar Region					
41. Inserted the film or sensor horizontally into the posterior bite-block.					
42. Centered the film or sensor on the contact point between the second premolar and the first molar.					
43. With the instrument and film or sensor in place, instructed the patient to close the mouth slowly but firmly.					
44. Positioned the localizing ring and PID, then exposed the film or sensor.					
Mandibular Molar Region					
45. Inserted the film or sensor horizontally into the posterior bite-block.					
46. Centered the film or sensor on the second molar.					
47. With the instrument and film in place, instructed the patient to close slowly but firmly.					
48. Positioned the localizing ring and PID, then exposed the film or sensor.					
49. Procedure documented in patient record.					
ADDITIONAL COMMENTS					

Total number of points earned _____

Grade _____ Instructor's initials _____

COMPETENCY 41-4: PRODUCING A FULL-MOUTH RADIOGRAPHIC SURVEY USING THE BISECTING TECHNIQUE

Performance Objective
By following a routine procedure that meets stated protocols, the student will produce a full-mouth radiographic survey using the proper bisecting technique.

Evaluation and Grading Criteria
__3__   Student competently met the stated criteria without assistance.
__2__   Student required assistance in order to meet the stated criteria.
__1__   Student showed uncertainty when performing the stated criteria.
__0__   Student was not prepared and needs to repeat the step.
__N/A__   No evaluation of this step.
Instructor shall define grades for each point range earned on completion of each performance-evaluated task.

Performance Standards
The minimum number of satisfactory performances required before final evaluation is _____.

Instructor shall identify by * those steps considered critical. If step is missed or minimum competency is not met, the evaluated procedure fails and must be repeated.

PERFORMANCE CRITERIA	*	SELF	PEER	INSTRUCTOR	COMMENT
1. Personal protective equipment placed according to procedure.					
2. Prepared the operatory with all infection control barriers.					
3. Determined the numbers and types of films to be exposed through a review of the patient's chart, directions from the dentist, or both.					
4. Labeled a paper cup or transfer box with the patient's name and the date, and placed it outside the room where the radiograph machine was used.					
5. Turned on the x-ray machine, and checked the basic settings (kilovoltage, milliamperage, exposure time).					
6. Washed and dried hands.					
7. Dispensed the desired number of films or PSPs, and stored them outside the room where the x-ray machine was used.					
Maxillary Canine Exposure					
8. Positioned the patient so that the occlusal plane was positioned parallel to the floor and the sagittal plane of the patient's face is perpendicular to the floor.					
9. Centered the film packet or sensor on the canine.					

Continued

10. Positioned the lower edge of the holder to the occlusal plane so that 1/8 inch extended below the incisal edge of the canine.					
11. Instructed the patient to exert light but firm pressure on the lower edge of the holder.					
12. Established the correct vertical angulation by bisecting the angle and directing the central ray perpendicular to the imaginary bisector.					
13. Established the correct horizontal angulation by directing the central ray between the contacts of the canine and the first premolar.					
14. Centered the PID over the film packet or sensor to avoid cone cutting.					
15. Exposed the film or sensor.					
Maxillary Incisor Exposure					
16. Centered the film packet or sensor on the contact between the two central incisors.					
17. Positioned the lower edge of the film or sensor holder to the occlusal plane so that 1/8 extended below the incisal edge of the canine.					
18. Instructed the patient to exert light but firm pressure on the lower edge of the holder.					
19. Established the correct vertical angulation by bisecting the angle and directing the central ray perpendicular to the imaginary bisector.					
20. Established the correct horizontal angulation by directing the central ray between the contacts of central incisors.					
21. Centered the PID over the film or sensor to avoid cone cutting.					
22. Exposed the film or sensor.					
Mandibular Canine Exposure					
23. Centered the film packet or sensor on the canine.					

24. Positioned the lower edge of the film or sensor holder to the occlusal plane so that 1/8 inch extended above the incisal edge of the canine.				
25. Instructed the patient to exert light but firm pressure on the lower edge of the holder.				
26. Established the correct vertical angulation by bisecting the angle and directing the central ray perpendicular to the imaginary bisector.				
27. Established the correct horizontal angulation by directing the central ray between the contacts of the canine and the first premolar.				
28. Centered the PID over the film or sensor to avoid cone cutting.				
29. Exposed the film or sensor.				
Mandibular Incisor Exposure				
30. Centered the film packet or sensor on the contact between the two central incisors.				
31. Positioned the upper edge of the holder to the occlusal plane so that 1/8 inch extended above the incisal edges of the teeth.				
32. Instructed the patient to exert light but firm pressure on the lower edge of the holder.				
33. Established the correct vertical angulation by bisecting the angle and directing the central ray perpendicular to the imaginary bisector.				
34. Established the correct horizontal angulation by directing the central ray between the contacts of the central incisors.				
35. Centered the PID over the film or sensor to avoid cone cutting.				
36. Exposed the film or sensor.				
Maxillary Premolar Exposure				
37. Centered the film packet or sensor on the second premolar, with the front edge of the film or sensor aligned with the midline of the canine.				

Continued

38. Positioned the lower edge of the film or sensor parallel to the occlusal plane so that 1/8 inch extended below the occlusal edges of the teeth.					
39. Instructed the patient to close gently on the holder.					
40. Established the correct vertical angulation by bisecting the angle and directing the central ray perpendicular to the imaginary bisector.					
41. Established the correct horizontal angulation by directing the central ray between the contacts of the premolars.					
42. Centered the PID over the film or sensor to avoid cone cutting.					
43. Exposed the film or sensor.					
Maxillary Molar Exposure					
44. Centered the film or sensor holder and film packet or sensor on the second molar, with the front edge of the film or sensor aligned with the midline of the second premolar.					
45. Positioned the lower edge of the holder parallel to the occlusal plane so that 1/8 inch extended below the occlusal surfaces of the teeth.					
46. Instructed the patient to bite firmly on the holder. *Note:* You may have to ask the patient to lower the chin so that the occlusal surfaces are parallel with the floor.					
47. Established the correct vertical angulation by bisecting the angle and directing the central ray perpendicular to the imaginary bisector.					
48. Established the correct horizontal angulation by directing the central ray between the contacts of the molars.					
49. Centered the PID over the film or sensor to avoid cone cutting.					
50. Exposed the film or sensor.					

Mandibular Premolar Exposure					
51. Centered the film packet or sensor on the second premolar, with the front edge of the film or sensor aligned with the mesial aspect of the canine.					
52. Positioned the upper edge of the film or sensor parallel to the occlusal plane so that 1/8 inch extended above the occlusal edges of the teeth.					
53. Instructed the patient to close the mouth gently on the holder.					
54. Established the correct vertical angulation by bisecting the angle and directing the central ray perpendicular to the imaginary bisector.					
55. Established the correct horizontal angulation by directing the central ray between the contacts of the premolars.					
56. Centered the PID over the film or sensor to avoid cone cutting.					
57. Exposed the film or sensor.					
Mandibular Molar Exposure					
58. Centered the film or sensor holder and film packet on the second molar, with the front edge of the film or sensor aligned with the midline of the second premolar.					
59. Positioned the upper edge of the holder parallel to the occlusal plane so that 1/8 inch extended above the occlusal surfaces of the teeth.					
60. Instructed the patient to bite firmly on the holder.					
61. Established the correct vertical angulation by bisecting the angle and directing the central ray perpendicular to the imaginary bisector.					
62. Established the correct horizontal angulation by directing the central ray between the contacts of the molars.					
63. Centered the PID over the film or sensor to avoid cone cutting.					

Continued

64. Exposed the film or sensor.					
65. Procedure documented in patient record.					

ADDITIONAL COMMENTS

Total number of points earned _____

Grade _____ Instructor's initials _____

COMPETENCY 41-5: PRODUCING A FOUR-FILM RADIOGRAPHIC SURVEY USING THE BITEWING TECHNIQUE

Performance Objective

By following a routine procedure that meets stated protocols, the student will produce a full-mouth radiographic survey using the proper bitewing technique.

Evaluation and Grading Criteria

<u>3</u>   Student competently met the stated criteria without assistance.
<u>2</u>   Student required assistance in order to meet the stated criteria.
<u>1</u>   Student showed uncertainty when performing the stated criteria.
<u>0</u>   Student was not prepared and needs to repeat the step.
<u>N/A</u>   No evaluation of this step.
Instructor shall define grades for each point range earned on completion of each performance-evaluated task.

Performance Standards

The minimum number of satisfactory performances required before final evaluation is _____.

Instructor shall identify by * those steps considered critical. If step is missed or minimum competency is not met, the evaluated procedure fails and must be repeated.

PERFORMANCE CRITERIA	*	SELF	PEER	INSTRUCTOR	COMMENT
1. Personal protective equipment placed according to procedure.					
2. Placed the film or sensor in the patient's mouth for a premolar film.					
3. Positioned the film or sensor in proper position.					
4. Set the vertical angulation.					
5. Positioned horizontal angulation.					
6. Positioned the position indicator device.					
7. Directed the central ray through the contact areas.					
8. Pressed the exposure button.					
9. Procedure documented in patient record.					
ADDITIONAL COMMENTS					

Total number of points earned _____

Grade _____ Instructor's initials _____

COMPETENCY 41-6: PRODUCING MAXILLARY AND MANDIBULAR RADIOGRAPHS USING THE OCCLUSAL TECHNIQUE

Performance Objective

By following a routine procedure that meets stated protocols, the student will produce maxillary and mandibular occlusal radiographs using the proper occlusal technique.

Evaluation and Grading Criteria

3   Student competently met the stated criteria without assistance.
2   Student required assistance in order to meet the stated criteria.
1   Student showed uncertainty when performing the stated criteria.
0   Student was not prepared and needs to repeat the step.
N/A No evaluation of this step.
Instructor shall define grades for each point range earned on completion of each performance-evaluated task.

Performance Standards

The minimum number of satisfactory performances required before final evaluation is _____.

Instructor shall identify by * those steps considered critical. If step is missed or minimum competency is not met, the evaluated procedure fails and must be repeated.

PERFORMANCE CRITERIA	*	SELF	PEER	INSTRUCTOR	COMMENT
Maxillary Occlusal Technique					
1. Personal protective equipment placed according to procedure.					
2. Asked the patient to remove prosthetic appliances or objects from the mouth.					
3. Placed the lead apron and thyroid collar.					
4. Positioned the patient's head so the film plane was parallel to the floor.					
5. Placed the film packet in the patient's mouth with the white side of the film on the occlusal surfaces of the maxillary teeth.					
6. Placed the film as far posterior as possible.					
7. Positioned the position indicator device (PID) so that the central ray was directed at a 65-degree angle through the bridge of the nose to the center of the film packet.					
8. Pressed the x-ray machine–activating button, and made the exposure.					
9. Procedure documented in patient record.					

Continued

Mandibular Occlusal Technique					
10. Tilted the patient's head back to a comfortable position, ensuring that the midsagittal plane was vertical.					
11. Placed the film packet in the patient's mouth with the white side of the film on the occlusal surfaces of the mandibular teeth.					
12. Positioned the film as far posterior as possible.					
13. Positioned the PID so that the central ray was directed at 90 degrees (a right angle) to the center of the film packet.					
14. Pressed the x-ray machine–activating button, and made the exposure.					
15. Procedure documented in patient record.					

ADDITIONAL COMMENTS

Total number of points earned _____

Grade _____ Instructor's initials _____

COMPETENCY 41-7: MOUNTING DENTAL RADIOGRAPHS

Performance Objective

By following a routine procedure that meets stated protocols, the student will demonstrate the proper technique for mounting a full-mouth series of radiographs.

Evaluation and Grading Criteria

 3   Student competently met the stated criteria without assistance.
 2   Student required assistance in order to meet the stated criteria.
 1   Student showed uncertainty when performing the stated criteria.
 0   Student was not prepared and needs to repeat the step.
 N/A   No evaluation of this step.
Instructor shall define grades for each point range earned on completion of each performance-evaluated task.

Performance Standards

The minimum number of satisfactory performances required before final evaluation is _____.

Instructor shall identify by * those steps considered critical. If step is missed or minimum competency is not met, the evaluated procedure fails and must be repeated.

PERFORMANCE CRITERIA	*	SELF	PEER	INSTRUCTOR	COMMENT
1. Ensured that hands were clean and dry before handling radiographs. Grasped films only at the edges, not on the front or back.					
2. Selected the appropriately sized mount, and labeled it with the patient's name and the date the radiographs were exposed.					
3. Arranged the dried radiographs in anatomic order on a piece of clean white paper or on a flat view box.					
4. Once the films were arranged properly, placed them neatly in the mount.					
ADDITIONAL COMMENTS					

Total number of points earned _____

Grade _____ Instructor's initials _____

42 Extraoral Imaging

SHORT-ANSWER QUESTIONS

1. Describe the purpose and uses of panoramic imaging.

2. Describe the purpose and uses of cone beam computed tomography.

3. Describe the equipment used in panoramic imaging.

4. Describe the steps for patient preparation and positioning in panoramic imaging.

5. Discuss the advantages and disadvantages of panoramic imaging.

6. Describe the errors caused during patient preparation and positioning during panoramic imaging.

7. Describe the equipment used in extraoral imaging.

8. Identify the specific purpose of each of the extraoral film projections.

9. Describe the purposes and uses of extraoral imaging.

10. Describe the advantages of 3D imaging.

FILL-IN-THE-BLANK STATEMENTS

Select the best term from the list below and complete the following statements.

cone beam computed tomography
extraoral images
focal trough
Frankfort plane

magnetic resonance imaging (MRI)
midsagittal plane
temporomandibular
tomography

357

1. An imaginary three-dimensional curved zone that is horseshoe shaped and is used to focus panoramic radiographs is the _____.

2. The _____ is the imaginary plane that passes through the top of the ear canal and the bottom of the eye socket.

3. The imaginary line that divides the patient's face into right and left sides is the _____.

4. _____ is a radiographic technique that allows imaging of one layer or section of the body while blurring images from structures in other planes.

5. _____ is a three-dimensional digital imaging method that uses a cone-shaped beam of radiation that rotates around the patient.

6. _____ are taken when large areas of the skull or jaw must be examined.

7. _____ is the use of magnetic resonance to create images of the body.

8. _____ is the joint on each side of the head that allows movement of the mandible.

MULTIPLE-CHOICE QUESTIONS

Complete each question by circling the best answer.

1. What type of additional images are no longer necessary to supplement a panoramic radiograph when the new full-featured digital panoramic units are used?
   a. Periapical
   b. Bitewing
   c. Occlusal
   d. All of the above

2. A focal trough is _____.
   a. the area where the patient bites down
   b. an imaginary horseshoe-shaped area used for jaw placement
   c. where the patient looks during the process
   d. earpieces used for positioning

3. Which of the following is NOT an advantage of extraoral radiographs?
   a. They show a close-up image of something.
   b. They minimize radiation to the patient.
   c. They provide an overview of the skull and jaws.
   d. They prevent the patient from gagging.

4. What type of device is included on a panoramic unit?
   a. Cephalostat
   b. Hemostat
   c. Periapical film holder
   d. Bitewing holder

5. The purpose of a grid is to _____.
   a. increase the size of the image
   b. reduce the amount of scatter radiation
   c. hold the patient's head still
   d. hold the film in place

6. What type of imaging is best for soft tissues of the temporomandibular joint?
   a. Panorex
   b. Digital x-ray examination
   c. Cephalometric
   d. Computed tomographic scan

7. On new full-featured digital panoramic units, which of the following can now be detected on a panoramic radiograph?
   a. Location of impacted teeth
   b. Lesions in the mandible
   c. Interproximal caries
   d. All of the above

8. What type of technology is used in panoramic units?
   a. Conventional film-based technology
   b. Digital technology
   c. Both a and b

9. Which of the following is (are) a component of a panoramic unit?
   a. Chin rest
   b. Notched bite-block
   c. Forehead rest
   d. All of the above

10. Which of the following can cause "ghost images" on a panoramic image?
   a. Eyeglasses
   b. Earrings
   c. Necklaces
   d. All of the above

CASE STUDY

Sixteen-year-old Jeremy Davis is scheduled for an examination and consultation today. Some of the problems that Jeremy exhibits are class III occlusion, crowding, recurrent decay, and slight gingivitis. In order for the dentist to proceed with treatment, a more detailed evaluation is required with the use of radiographs.

1. What type of image would reveal a class III occlusion?

2. What type of image would reveal crowding?

3. To what specialist should Jeremy be referred for his class III occlusion and crowding?

4. What type of image would reveal recurrent decay?

5. What type of image would reveal gingivitis?

MULTIMEDIA PROCEDURES RECOMMENDED REVIEW

- Panoramic Imaging (2 videos)

INTERACTIVE DENTAL OFFICE PATIENT CASE EXERCISES

Access the *Interactive Dental Office on Evolve* and click on the patient case file for Cindy Valladares.
- Review the patient's panoramic radiograph.
- Answer the following questions.

1. Were the dark areas over the roots of the mandibular teeth most likely caused by a processing error or by a positioning error?

2. Is this radiograph diagnostically acceptable? Why or why not?

Chapter **42** **Extraoral Imaging**

Access the *Interactive Dental Office on Evolve* and click on the patient case file for Ingrid Pedersen.
- Review the patient's panoramic radiograph.
- Answer the following question.

3. Why are the images of the posterior teeth overlapped? Is this a positioning error?

Access the *Interactive Dental Office on Evolve* and click on the patient case file for Tiffany Cole.
- Review the patient's panoramic radiograph.
- Answer the following question.

4. Based on the development of Tiffany's teeth, how old do you think she is?

5. The panoramic radiograph indicates that tooth #27 is impacted. Click on tooth #27.

COMPETENCY 42-1: PREPARING EQUIPMENT FOR PANORAMIC IMAGING

Performance Objective

By following a routine procedure that meets stated protocols, the student will demonstrate the proper technique for preparing equipment for a panoramic radiograph.

Evaluation and Grading Criteria

<u>_3_</u>   Student competently met the stated criteria without assistance.
<u>_2_</u>   Student required assistance in order to meet the stated criteria.
<u>_1_</u>   Student showed uncertainty when performing the stated criteria.
<u>_0_</u>   Student was not prepared and needs to repeat the step.
<u>N/A</u>   No evaluation of this step.
Instructor shall define grades for each point range earned on completion of each performance-evaluated task.

Performance Standards

The minimum number of satisfactory performances required before final evaluation is _____.

Instructor shall identify by * those steps considered critical. If step is missed or minimum competency is not met, the evaluated procedure fails and must be repeated.

PERFORMANCE CRITERIA	*	SELF	PEER	INSTRUCTOR	COMMENT
1. Personal protective equipment placed according to procedure.					
2. Loaded the panoramic cassette in the darkroom under safelight conditions. Handled the film only by its edges to avoid fingerprints.					
3. Placed all infection control barriers and containers.					
4. Covered the bite-block with a disposable plastic barrier. If the bite-block was not covered, sterilized it before using it on the next patient.					
5. Covered or disinfected (or both) any part of the machine that came in contact with the patient.					
6. Set the exposure factors (kilovoltage, milliamperage) according to the manufacturer's recommendations.					
7. Adjusted the machine to accommodate the height of the patient, and aligned all movable parts properly.					
8. Loaded the cassette into the carrier of the panoramic unit.					

Continued

ADDITIONAL COMMENTS

Total number of points earned _____

Grade _____ Instructor's initials _____

COMPETENCY 42-2: PREPARING THE PATIENT FOR PANORAMIC IMAGING

Performance Objective

By following a routine procedure that meets stated protocols, the student will demonstrate the proper technique for preparing a patient for panoramic imaging.

Evaluation and Grading Criteria

 3 Student competently met the stated criteria without assistance.
 2 Student required assistance in order to meet the stated criteria.
 1 Student showed uncertainty when performing the stated criteria.
 0 Student was not prepared and needs to repeat the step.
N/A No evaluation of this step.
Instructor shall define grades for each point range earned on completion of each performance-evaluated task.

Performance Standards

The minimum number of satisfactory performances required before final evaluation is _____.

Instructor shall identify by * those steps considered critical. If step is missed or minimum competency is not met, the evaluated procedure fails and must be repeated.

PERFORMANCE CRITERIA	*	SELF	PEER	INSTRUCTOR	COMMENT
1. Explained the procedure to the patient. Gave the patient the opportunity to ask questions.					
2. Personal protective equipment placed according to procedure.					
3. Asked the patient to remove all objects from the head and neck area, including eyeglasses, earrings, lip piercing and tongue piercing objects, necklaces, napkin chains, hearing aids, hairpins, and complete and partial dentures. Placed objects in separate containers.					
4. Placed a double-sided (for protecting the front and back of the patient) lead apron on the patient, or used the style of lead apron recommended by the manufacturer.					
ADDITIONAL COMMENTS					

Total number of points earned _____

Grade _____ Instructor's initials _____

COMPETENCY 42-3: POSITIONING THE PATIENT FOR PANORAMIC IMAGING

Performance Objective

By following a routine procedure that meets stated protocols, the student will demonstrate the proper technique for positioning a patient for panoramic imaging.

Evaluation and Grading Criteria

3   Student competently met the stated criteria without assistance.
2   Student required assistance in order to meet the stated criteria.
1   Student showed uncertainty when performing the stated criteria.
0   Student was not prepared and needs to repeat the step.
N/A   No evaluation of this step.
Instructor shall define grades for each point range earned on completion of each performance-evaluated task.

Performance Standards

The minimum number of satisfactory performances required before final evaluation is _____.

Instructor shall identify by * those steps considered critical. If step is missed or minimum competency is not met, the evaluated procedure fails and must be repeated.

PERFORMANCE CRITERIA	*	SELF	PEER	INSTRUCTOR	COMMENT
1. Personal protective equipment placed according to procedure.					
2. Instructed the patient to sit or stand "as tall as possible" with the back straight and erect.					
3. Instructed the patient to bite on the plastic bite-block, and slid the upper and lower teeth into the notch (groove) on the end of the bite-block.					
4. Positioned the midsagittal plane perpendicular to the floor.					
5. Positioned the Frankfort plane parallel to the floor.					
6. Instructed the patient to position the tongue on the roof of the mouth and then to close the lips around the bite-block.					
7. After the patient was positioned, instructed the patient to remain still while the machine rotated during exposure.					
8. Exposed the film and proceeded with film processing.					
9. Procedure documented in patient record.					

Continued

ADDITIONAL COMMENTS

Total number of points earned _____

Grade _____ Instructor's initials _____

43 Restorative and Esthetic Dental Materials

SHORT-ANSWER QUESTIONS

1. Describe how a dental material is evaluated before it can be marketed to the profession.

2. List the properties of dental materials, and explain how these properties affect their application.

3. Differentiate between direct and indirect restorative materials.

4. Describe the factors that affect how dental materials are manufactured for the oral cavity.

5. Give the composition of amalgam and describe the application used in the restoration of teeth.

6. Give the composition of composite resin materials and the application in the restoration of teeth.

7. Give the properties of glass ionomers and their application in the restoration of teeth.

8. Give the properties of temporary restorative materials and their application in the restoration of teeth.

9. Discuss the composition and variety of tooth-whitening products.

10. Describe the properties of gold alloys and their application in the restoration of teeth.

11. Describe the properties of porcelain and its application in the restoration of teeth.

FILL-IN-THE-BLANK STATEMENTS

Select the best term from the list below and complete the following statements.

adhere
alloy
amalgam
auto-cure
ceramic
cured
esthetic
filler
galvanic
gold

microleakage
palladium
pestle
porcelain
restorative
retention
spherical
strain
stress
viscosity

1. A(n) _____ reaction is the effect of an electrical shock that results when two metals touch.

2. A type of dental restorative material that is hard, brittle, and resistant to heat and corrosion and that resembles clay is _____.

3. For a material to become hardened or set, it is said to be _____.

4. To bond or attach two items together is to _____.

5. _____ is a soft, silvery white metallic chemical element that resembles platinum.

6. _____ is a process that brings a tooth or teeth back to their natural appearance.

7. An object within the amalgam capsule used for pounding or pulverizing is the _____.

8. _____ is a solid white, translucent ceramic material made by firing pure clay and then glazing it.

9. An artistically pleasing and beautiful appearance is said to be _____.

10. _____ is a soft, yellow, corrosion-resistant metal used in the making of indirect restorations.

11. The property of a liquid that prevents it from flowing easily is the _____.

12. _____ is a mixture of alloys triturated with mercury.

13. _____ refers to how a material hardens or sets through a chemical reaction of two materials.

14. A(n) _____ is a minute area where moisture and contaminants can enter.

15. A(n) _____ is a combination of two or more metals.

16. _____ is the ability to retain or hold something in place.

17. Something that is round is said to be _____.

18. _____ is the distortion or change produced as a result of stress.

19. The internal reaction or resistance to an externally applied force is added _____.

20. _____ is an inorganic material that adds strength and other characteristics to composite resins.

MULTIPLE-CHOICE QUESTIONS

Complete each question by circling the best answer.

1. Which professional organization evaluates a new dental material?
   a. FDA
   b. DDS
   c. ADA
   d. MDA

2. What type of reaction does a dental material undergo when a person is chewing?
   a. Thermal change
   b. Compressive stress
   c. Galvanic reaction
   d. Corrosion

3. What happens to a dental material when it is exposed to extreme temperatures of hot and then cold?
   a. Contraction and expansion
   b. Melting and hardening
   c. Galvanic reaction
   d. Strain and stress

4. Which is an example of how galvanic action can occur?
   a. Salt within saliva
   b. Leakage of a material
   c. Touching of two metals
   d. a and c

5. How does an auto-cured material harden or set?
   a. It air-dries
   b. By chemical reaction
   c. With light
   d. With heat

6. Select the correct makeup of the alloy powder in amalgam.
   a. Porcelain, glass, zinc, and composite
   b. Gold, tin, silver, and aluminum
   c. Mercury, silver, zinc, and tin
   d. Silver, tin, copper, and zinc

7. Why is dental amalgam not placed in anterior teeth?
   a. Esthetics
   b. It is not strong enough
   c. It is difficult to finish
   d. Retention

8. Most amalgams have a high copper content. What does copper provide to amalgam restorations?
   a. Strength
   b. Malleability
   c. Corrosion resistance
   d. a and c

9. Where are amalgam scraps disposed of?
   a. In the garbage
   b. Down the sink
   c. Underwater or in a fixer solution
   d. In a biohazard bag

10. What is used to triturate amalgam?
    a. Mortar and pestle
    b. Amalgamator
    c. Paper pad and spatula
    d. Bowl and spatula

11. The term commonly used to refer to dimethacrylate is

    _____.
    a. alloy
    b. composite resin
    c. mercury
    d. BIS-GMA

12. Which filler type of composite resin has the strongest makeup and has been used most commonly for posterior restorations?
    a. Macrofilled
    b. Microfilled
    c. Monofilled
    d. Autofilled

13. When light-curing composite resins, which factor can affect curing time of the material?
    a. Type of tooth
    b. Depth or extent of restoration
    c. Surface that is being restored
    d. Type of composite

14. What is used to determine the color of composite resin material for a procedure?
    a. Color palate
    b. Picture
    c. Shade guide
    d. Radiograph

15. The final step in finishing a composite resin is

    _____.
    a. using a diamond bur
    b. using a sandpaper strip
    c. using a rubber cup and polishing paste
    d. using a white stone

16. The acronym *IRM* stands for _____.
    a. inside the restorative matrix
    b. intermediate restorative material
    c. interdental resin material
    d. international restorative material

369

17. What temporary restorative material would most likely be selected for a class II cavity preparation?
    a. Acrylic resin
    b. Amalgam
    c. Glass ionomer
    d. IRM

18. Which material would most likely be selected for provisional coverage?
    a. IRM
    b. Acrylic resin
    c. Amalgam
    d. Glass ionomer

19. The three noble metals used in making indirect restorations are _____.
    a. gold, palladium, and platinum
    b. silver, tin, and zinc
    c. mercury, copper, and tin
    d. glass, porcelain, and fillers

20. What type of restoration is made in the dental laboratory?
    a. Direct restoration
    b. Provisional coverage
    c. Indirect restoration
    d. Temporary restoration

CASE STUDY

You are assisting in a restorative procedure. The patient record indicates that the decay is located on the gingival third on the facial surface of teeth #10 and #11. The dentist informs you that you will be using the dental dam for this procedure.

1. What cavity classification would this type of decay represent?

2. What type of restorative material would most likely be selected for this procedure?

3. Why do you think the dentist has requested the use of the dental dam for this procedure?

4. What specific instrument would be on the tray for the placement of the restorative dental material?

5. What additional piece of equipment will be used for the hardening of the restorative material?

6. How will the dentist finish or carve this material?

7. How would this procedure be charted on a patient record?

MULTIMEDIA PROCEDURES RECOMMENDED REVIEW

- Mixing and Transferring Amalgam

COMPETENCY 43-1: MIXING AND TRANSFERRING DENTAL AMALGAM

Performance Objective

By following a routine procedure that meets stated protocols, the student will demonstrate the proper skills for mixing and transferring amalgam.

Evaluation and Grading Criteria

3   Student competently met the stated criteria without assistance.

2   Student required assistance in order to meet the stated criteria.

1   Student showed uncertainty when performing the stated criteria.

0   Student was not prepared and needs to repeat the step.

N/A   No evaluation of this step.

Instructor shall define grades for each point range earned on completion of each performance-evaluated task.

Performance Standards

The minimum number of satisfactory performances required before final evaluation is _____.

Instructor shall identify by * those steps considered critical. If step is missed or minimum competency is not met, the evaluated procedure fails and must be repeated.

PERFORMANCE CRITERIA	*	SELF	PEER	INSTRUCTOR	COMMENT
1. Selected the proper equipment and supplies.					
2. Personal protective equipment placed according to procedure.					
3. Activated the capsule in the amalgamator.					
4. Placed the capsule in the amalgamator.					
5. Adjusted settings for the specific type of amalgam.					
6. Closed the cover on the amalgamator, and began trituration.					
7. Removed the capsule, and dispensed amalgam in the well.					
8. Filled the small end of the carrier, and transferred it to the dentist.					
9. Ensured that the carrier was directed toward the preparation.					
10. Continued delivery until the preparation was overfilled.					
ADDITIONAL COMMENTS					

Total number of points earned _____

Grade _____ Instructor's initials _____

COMPETENCY 43-2: PREPARING COMPOSITE RESIN MATERIALS

Performance Objective

By following a routine procedure that meets stated protocols, the student will assemble the necessary supplies, then prepare composite resin for a restorative procedure.

Evaluation and Grading Criteria

 3   Student competently met the stated criteria without assistance.
 2   Student required assistance in order to meet the stated criteria.
 1   Student showed uncertainty when performing the stated criteria.
 0   Student was not prepared and needs to repeat the step.
 N/A   No evaluation of this step.
Instructor shall define grades for each point range earned on completion of each performance-evaluated task.

Performance Standards

The minimum number of satisfactory performances required before final evaluation is _____.

Instructor shall identify by * those steps considered critical. If step is missed or minimum competency is not met, the evaluated procedure fails and must be repeated.

PERFORMANCE CRITERIA	*	SELF	PEER	INSTRUCTOR	COMMENT
1. Selected the proper equipment and supplies.					
2. Personal protective equipment placed according to procedure.					
3. Selected the shade of composite resin to match the tooth color using a shade guide and natural light.					
4. Expressed composite material onto treatment pad or in a light-protected well.					
5. Transferred the composite instrument and material to the dentist in the transfer zone.					
6. Had gauze available for the dentist to clean composite instrument.					
7. Had the curing light readied or positioned the light correctly on the tooth.					
8. When finished, cared for supplies and materials appropriately.					
ADDITIONAL COMMENTS					

Total number of points earned _____

Grade _____ Instructor's initials _____

COMPETENCY 43-3: MIXING INTERMEDIATE RESTORATIVE MATERIALS (IRM)

Performance Objective
By following a routine procedure that meets stated protocols, the student will assemble the necessary supplies, then correctly manipulate the material for placement into a class I cavity preparation.

Evaluation and Grading Criteria
3   Student competently met the stated criteria without assistance.
2   Student required assistance in order to meet the stated criteria.
1   Student showed uncertainty when performing the stated criteria.
0   Student was not prepared and needs to repeat the step.
N/A   No evaluation of this step.
Note: In states where it is legal, the assistant may place the temporary restoration in a prepared tooth.
Instructor shall define grades for each point range earned on completion of each performance-evaluated task.

Performance Standards
The minimum number of satisfactory performances required before final evaluation is _____.

Instructor shall identify by * those steps considered critical. If step is missed or minimum competency is not met, the evaluated procedure fails and must be repeated.

PERFORMANCE CRITERIA	*	SELF	PEER	INSTRUCTOR	COMMENT
1. Selected the proper material, and assembled the appropriate supplies.					
2. Personal protective equipment placed according to procedure.					
3. Dispensed materials in the proper sequence and quantity; then immediately recapped the containers.					
4. Incorporated the powder and liquid according to the manufacturer's instructions.					
5. Completed the mix within the appropriate working time.					
6. Ensured that completed mix was of the appropriate consistency for a temporary restoration.					
7. When finished, cared for supplies and materials appropriately.					

ADDITIONAL COMMENTS

Total number of points earned _____

Grade _____ Instructor's initials _____

COMPETENCY 43-4: MIXING ACRYLIC RESIN FOR PROVISIONAL COVERAGE

Performance Objective

By following a routine procedure that meets stated protocols, the student will demonstrate the proper technique for preparing acrylic resin for the fabrication of provisional coverage.

Evaluation and Grading Criteria

3   Student competently met the stated criteria without assistance.
2   Student required assistance in order to meet the stated criteria.
1   Student showed uncertainty when performing the stated criteria.
0   Student was not prepared and needs to repeat the step.
N/A   No evaluation of this step.
Instructor shall define grades for each point range earned on completion of each performance-evaluated task.

Performance Standards

The minimum number of satisfactory performances required before final evaluation is _____.

Instructor shall identify by * those steps considered critical. If step is missed or minimum competency is not met, the evaluated procedure fails and must be repeated.

PERFORMANCE CRITERIA	*	SELF	PEER	INSTRUCTOR	COMMENT
1. Selected the proper material, and assembled the appropriate supplies.					
2. Personal protective equipment placed according to procedure.					
3. Used the dropper to dispense the liquid monomer in the dappen dish. Used 10 drops per unit.					
4. Dispensed the powder (polymer) into the liquid quickly until the liquid was overfilled.					
5. "Dumped" out any extra powder onto a towel.					
6. Used a small spatula to blend the powder and liquid.					
7. Allowed the material to sit and achieve a doughlike state.					
8. Placed the material in a tray or impression, and transferred to the dentist for placement.					

ADDITIONAL COMMENTS

Total number of points earned _____

Grade _____ Instructor's initials _____

44 Dental Liners, Bases, and Bonding Systems

SHORT-ANSWER QUESTIONS

1. Describe how the sensitivity of a tooth determines what types of supplemental dental materials are selected for placement.

2. Describe how and why cavity liners are used in the restoration process.

3. Describe how and why varnishes are used in the restoration process.

4. Describe how and why dentin sealers are used in the restoration process.

5. Describe how and why dental bases are used in the restoration process.

6. Describe the etching process of a tooth and its importance in the bonding procedure.

7. Describe the bonding system, and explain how this procedure provides better adaptation of a dental material to the tooth structure.

FILL-IN-THE-BLANK STATEMENTS

Select the best term from the list below and complete the following statements.

desiccate	obliterating
etching	polymerization
eugenol	retention
hybrid	sedative
insulating	smear layer
micromechanical	thermal

1. The _____ is a very thin layer of debris on newly prepared dentin.

2. _____ refers to the temperature of something.

3. A composite material made up of a combination of particles of various sizes is referred to as a(n) _____.

4. _____ is a method of preventing the passage of heat or electricity.

379

5. _____ is the process of breaking down or removing enamel rods with the use of an acid product.

6. _____ is the process of bonding two or more monomers.

7. A liquid made from clove oil that is used for its soothing qualities is _____.

8. To _____ means to remove all moisture from an item.

9. _____ refers to the union of a material and a structure with the use of minute cuttings.

10. _____ is the process of removing completely.

11. Some dental materials have a _____ effect, which provides a soothing or calming effect.

12. _____ is a way of holding a restoration in place.

MULTIPLE-CHOICE QUESTIONS

Complete each question by circling the best answer.

1. The purpose of a dental liner is to _____.
   a. make the restorative material look natural
   b. protect the pulp from any type of irritation
   c. create a mechanical lock of the dental material
   d. cover the smear layer

2. On what tooth structure is calcium hydroxide placed?
   a. Enamel
   b. Cementum
   c. Dentin
   d. Pulp

3. Which is not a unique characteristic of calcium hydroxide?
   a. Protects the tooth from chemical irritation
   b. Produces reparative dentin
   c. Is compatible with all restorative materials
   d. Replaces the need for a dentin sealer

4. The main ingredient in varnish is _____.
   a. resin
   b. acid
   c. eugenol
   d. sealant

5. Which supplemental material is contraindicated under composite resins and glass ionomer restorations?
   a. Etchant
   b. Calcium hydroxide
   c. Dentin sealer
   d. Varnish

6. Another name for dentin sealer is _____.
   a. cement
   b. desensitizer
   c. etchant
   d. base

7. What does the dentin sealer seal?
   a. Enamel rods
   b. Etched tags
   c. Dentin tubules
   d. Pulpal chambers

8. An insulating base _____.
   a. protects the pulp from thermal shock
   b. protects the pulp from moisture
   c. helps soothe the pulp
   d. protects the pulp from the restoration

9. What effect does eugenol have on the pulp?
   a. Regenerative
   b. Soothing
   c. Irritant
   d. Restorative

10. A base is placed in or on the _____ in a cavity preparation.
    a. proximal box
    b. cavity walls
    c. enamel margin
    d. pulpal floor

11. What dental instrument is used to adapt a base into a cavity preparation?
    a. Explorer
    b. Hollenback
    c. Condenser
    d. Burnisher

12. The purpose of a dental bonding material is to _____.
    a. seal the dentinal tubules
    b. bond restorative materials to the tooth structure
    c. etch the tooth structure
    d. act as a permanent restorative material

13. An example of an enamel bonding procedure is _____.
    a. orthodontic brackets
    b. sealants
    c. amalgam
    d. a and b

14. What must be removed from tooth structure before bonding material can be placed on dentin?
    a. Enamel
    b. Decay
    c. Smear layer
    d. Dentin tubules

15. Which sequence is recommended for the application of supplementary materials for a deep restoration?
    a. Liner, base, dentin sealer, bonding system
    b. Base, liner, dentin sealer, bonding system
    c. Bonding system, base, liner, dentin sealer
    d. Dentin sealer, base, bonding system, liner

CASE STUDY

Dr. Clark has completed the preparation of a class III restoration on the distal surface of tooth #7. She has asked you to prepare and ready the supplemental materials for placement. You inquire about the depth of the preparation, and Dr. Clark indicates that it is moderately deep.

1. What type of direct restorative material would most likely be selected for a class III restoration on tooth #7?

2. What supplemental materials should be set up for this procedure?

3. What types of instruments and mixing pad or slab will be set out?

4. How many steps will be required to complete the application of these supplemental materials?

5. What type of moisture control is commonly placed for this type of restoration, and for the application of these materials?

6. Is the application of any of these materials legal for the expanded-functions assistant in your state? If so, which ones?

MULTIMEDIA PROCEDURES RECOMMENDED REVIEW

■ Liners, Bases, and Bonding Systems (3 videos)

381

Chapter **44** Dental Liners, Bases, and Bonding Systems

COMPETENCY 44-1: APPLYING CALCIUM HYDROXIDE (EXPANDED FUNCTION)

Performance Objective

By following a routine procedure that meets stated protocols, the student will assemble the necessary supplies and then will correctly manipulate and place the cavity liner in a prepared tooth.

Evaluation and Grading Criteria

 3 Student competently met the stated criteria without assistance.
 2 Student required assistance in order to meet the stated criteria.
 1 Student showed uncertainty when performing the stated criteria.
 0 Student was not prepared and needs to repeat the step.
 N/A No evaluation of this step.
Instructor shall define grades for each point range earned on completion of each performance-evaluated task.

Performance Standards

The minimum number of satisfactory performances required before final evaluation is _____.

Instructor shall identify by * those steps considered critical. If step is missed or minimum competency is not met, the evaluated procedure fails and must be repeated.

PERFORMANCE CRITERIA	*	SELF	PEER	INSTRUCTOR	COMMENT
1. Selected the proper material and assembled the appropriate supplies.					
2. Personal protective equipment placed according to procedure.					
3. Identified preparation and where material is to be placed.					
4. Dispensed small, equal quantities of the catalyst and the base pastes onto the paper mixing pad.					
5. Used a circular motion to mix the material over a small area of the paper pad with the spatula.					
6. Used gauze to clean the spatula.					
7. With the tip of the applicator, picked up a small amount of the material and applied a thin layer at the deepest area of the preparation.					
8. Used an explorer to remove any excess material from the enamel before drying.					

Continued

9. Cleaned and disinfected the equipment.				
10. Procedure documented in patient record.				

ADDITIONAL COMMENTS

Total number of points earned _____

Grade _____ Instructor's initials _____

COMPETENCY 44-2: APPLYING DENTAL VARNISH (EXPANDED FUNCTION)

Performance Objective
By following a routine procedure that meets stated protocols, the student will assemble the necessary supplies and then will correctly apply dental varnish to a prepared tooth surface.

Evaluation and Grading Criteria
<u>3</u>   Student competently met the stated criteria without assistance.
<u>2</u>   Student required assistance in order to meet the stated criteria.
<u>1</u>   Student showed uncertainty when performing the stated criteria.
<u>0</u>   Student was not prepared and needs to repeat the step.
<u>N/A</u>   No evaluation of this step.
Instructor shall define grades for each point range earned on completion of each performance-evaluated task.

Performance Standards
The minimum number of satisfactory performances required before final evaluation is _____.

Instructor shall identify by * those steps considered critical. If step is missed or minimum competency is not met, the evaluated procedure fails and must be repeated.

PERFORMANCE CRITERIA	*	SELF	PEER	INSTRUCTOR	COMMENT
1. Selected the proper material and assembled the appropriate supplies.					
2. Personal protective equipment placed according to procedure.					
3. Identified cavity preparation and where material is to be placed.					
4. Retrieved the applicator or sterile cotton pellets in cotton pliers.					
5. Opened the bottle of varnish and placed the tip of the applicator or cotton pellet into the liquid, making sure not to wet the cotton pliers.					
6. Replaced the cap on the bottle immediately.					
7. Placed a coating of the varnish on the walls, floor, and margin of the cavity preparation.					
8. Applied a second coat.					
9. Cleaned and disinfected the equipment.					
10. Procedure documented in patient record.					
ADDITIONAL COMMENTS					

Total number of points earned _____

Grade _____ Instructor's initials _____

Chapter **44** Dental Liners, Bases, and Bonding Systems

COMPETENCY 44-3: APPLYING A DESENSITIZER (EXPANDED FUNCTION)

Performance Objective

By following a routine procedure that meets stated protocols, the student will assemble the necessary supplies and then will correctly apply dentin sealer to a prepared tooth surface.

Evaluation and Grading Criteria

 3 Student competently met the stated criteria without assistance.
 2 Student required assistance in order to meet the stated criteria.
 1 Student showed uncertainty when performing the stated criteria.
 0 Student was not prepared and needs to repeat the step.
 N/A No evaluation of this step.

Instructor shall define grades for each point range earned on completion of each performance-evaluated task.

Performance Standards

The minimum number of satisfactory performances required before final evaluation is _____.

Instructor shall identify by * those steps considered critical. If step is missed or minimum competency is not met, the evaluated procedure fails and must be repeated.

PERFORMANCE CRITERIA	*	SELF	PEER	INSTRUCTOR	COMMENT
1. Selected the proper material and assembled the appropriate supplies.					
2. Personal protective equipment placed according to procedure.					
3. Identified cavity outline and where material is placed					
4. Rinsed the area with water not over drying the preparation.					
5. Applied the dentin sealer with the applicator over all surfaces of the dentin.					
6. Waited 30 seconds and dried the area thoroughly.					
7. Repeated application of sealer if sensitivity was a problem for the patient.					
8. Cleaned and disinfected the equipment.					
9. Procedure documented in patient record.					
ADDITIONAL COMMENTS					

Total number of points earned _____

Grade _____ Instructor's initials _____

COMPETENCIES 44-4 TO 44-6: MIXING A SELECTED TYPE OF CEMENT AS A BASE

Performance Objective
By following a routine procedure that meets stated protocols, the student will select the appropriate cement, assemble the necessary supplies, and correctly manipulate the material for use as a base.

Evaluation and Grading Criteria
<u>3</u>   Student competently met the stated criteria without assistance.
<u>2</u>   Student required assistance in order to meet the stated criteria.
<u>1</u>   Student showed uncertainty when performing the stated criteria.
<u>0</u>   Student was not prepared and needs to repeat the step.
<u>N/A</u> No evaluation of this step.
Instructor shall define grades for each point range earned on completion of each performance-evaluated task.

Performance Standards
The minimum number of satisfactory performances required before final evaluation is _____.

Instructor shall identify by * those steps considered critical. If step is missed or minimum competency is not met, the evaluated procedure fails and must be repeated.

PERFORMANCE CRITERIA	*	SELF	PEER	INSTRUCTOR	COMMENT
As a Base					
Name of Material					
1. Selected the proper material for the procedure and assembled the appropriate supplies.					
2. Personal protective equipment placed according to procedure.					
3. Dispensed materials in the proper sequence and quantity, then immediately recapped the containers.					
4. Incorporated the powder and liquid according to the manufacturer's instructions.					
5. Completed the mix within the appropriate working time.					
6. Ensured that the completed mix was the appropriate consistency for use as a base.					
7. When finished, cared for supplies and materials appropriately.					
8. Procedure documented in patient record.					
ADDITIONAL COMMENTS					

Total number of points earned _____

Grade _____ Instructor's initials _____

COMPETENCY 44-7: APPLYING AN ETCHANT MATERIAL (EXPANDED FUNCTION)

Performance Objective

By following a routine procedure that meets stated protocols, the student will assemble the necessary supplies and then will correctly apply etchant to a prepared tooth surface.

Evaluation and Grading Criteria

__3__   Student competently met the stated criteria without assistance.
__2__   Student required assistance in order to meet the stated criteria.
__1__   Student showed uncertainty when performing the stated criteria.
__0__   Student was not prepared and needs to repeat the step.
__N/A__ No evaluation of this step.
Instructor shall define grades for each point range earned on completion of each performance-evaluated task.

Performance Standards

The minimum number of satisfactory performances required before final evaluation is _____.

Instructor shall identify by * those steps considered critical. If step is missed or minimum competency is not met, the evaluated procedure fails and must be repeated.

PERFORMANCE CRITERIA	*	SELF	PEER	INSTRUCTOR	COMMENT
1. Selected the proper material and assembled the appropriate supplies.					
2. Personal protective equipment placed according to procedure.					
3. Identified cavity outline and where material is placed.					
4. Used a dental dam or cotton rolls to isolate the prepared tooth.					
5. Ensured that the surface of the tooth structure was clean and free of any debris, plaque, or calculus before etching.					
6. Carefully dried (but did not desiccate) the surface.					
7. Applied etchant to the enamel or dentin.					
8. Etched the tooth structure for the time recommended by the manufacturer.					
9. After etching, thoroughly rinsed and dried the surface for 15 to 30 seconds.					
10. Ensured that the etched surface had a frosty-white appearance.					
11. When finished, cared for supplies and materials appropriately.					
12. Procedure documented in patient record.					

Continued

COMPETENCY 44-8: APPLYING A BONDING SYSTEM (EXPANDED FUNCTION)

Performance Objective
By following a routine procedure that meets stated protocols, the student will assemble the necessary supplies and then will correctly apply a bonding system to a prepared tooth surface.

Evaluation and Grading Criteria
 3 Student competently met the stated criteria without assistance.
 2 Student required assistance in order to meet the stated criteria.
 1 Student showed uncertainty when performing the stated criteria.
 0 Student was not prepared and needs to repeat the step.
 N/A No evaluation of this step.
Instructor shall define grades for each point range earned on completion of each performance-evaluated task.

Performance Standards
The minimum number of satisfactory performances required before final evaluation is _____.

Instructor shall identify by * those steps considered critical. If step is missed or minimum competency is not met, the evaluated procedure fails and must be repeated.

PERFORMANCE CRITERIA	*	SELF	PEER	INSTRUCTOR	COMMENT
1. Selected the proper material and assembled the appropriate supplies.					
2. Personal protective equipment placed according to procedure.					
3. Identified cavity outline and placement of material.					
4. If a metal matrix band was required, prepared the band with cavity varnish or wax before placement around the tooth.					
5. Etched the cavity preparation and the enamel margins according to the manufacturer's instructions.					
6. If a primer was part of the system, applied a primer to the entire preparation in one or multiple coats, depending on the manufacturer's instructions.					
7. Placed the dual-cured bonding resin in the entire cavity preparation and lightly air-thinned the material. The resin should have appeared unset or semiset.					
8. When finished, cared for supplies and materials appropriately.					
9. Procedure documented in patient record.					

Continued

Total number of points earned _____

Grade _____ Instructor's initials _____

Dental Cements

SHORT-ANSWER QUESTIONS

1. Describe luting cements and the difference between permanent and temporary cements.

2. Discuss the factors that influence luting cements.

3. List the five cements discussed in the chapter, and describe their similarities and differences.

FILL-IN-THE-BLANK STATEMENTS

Select the best term from the list below and complete the following statements.

cement	provisional
exothermic	retard
luting agent	spatulate

1. _____ is the process of mixing by using a flat flexible metal or plastic instrument.

2. _____ refers to the process of releasing heat.

3. A(n) _____ refers to a temporary type of tooth coverage used for a short time.

4. A dental material that can be used temporarily or permanently to hold an indirect restoration in place is a(n) _____.

5. To _____ is to slow down the process of something.

6. Another name for dental cement is _____.

MULTIPLE-CHOICE QUESTIONS

Complete each question by circling the best answer.

1. Another name used to describe permanent cement is _____.
   a. liner
   b. luting agent
   c. resin
   d. base

2. For which of the following procedures would you include temporary cement on the tray setup?
   a. Composite restoration
   b. Sealants
   c. Amalgam restoration
   d. Provisional coverage

3. Which variable can affect the addition or loss of water in a material?
   a. Time
   b. Speed of spatulation
   c. Humidity
   d. Moisture control

4. What type of zinc oxide–eugenol (ZOE) is used for permanent cementation?
   a. Type I
   b. Type II
   c. Type III
   d. Type IV

395

5. On what type of mixing pad is ZOE mixed?
   a. Treated paper pad
   b. Glass
   c. Plastic
   d. Tile

6. Temp bond is supplied as _____.
   a. powder and liquid
   b. paste and powder
   c. two tubes of paste
   d. two liquids

7. The main component in the liquid of zinc phosphate
   is _____.
   a. hydrogen peroxide
   b. zinc oxide
   c. resin
   d. phosphoric acid

8. How do you dissipate the heat from zinc phosphate
   in the mixing process?
   a. Cool the spatula
   b. Use a cool glass slab
   c. Decrease the temperature in the room
   d. Chill the material

9. If the powder of a dental material is dispersed in
   increments, which size of the increment is commonly
   brought into the liquid first?
   a. Smallest
   b. Medium
   c. Half of the material
   d. Largest

10. How would you place permanent cement in a gold
    crown?
    a. Overfill
    b. Fill level
    c. Line the interior surface
    d. Line the occlusal surface only

11. How is polycarboxylate cement liquid supplied?
    a. Tube
    b. Squeeze bottle
    c. Calibrated syringe
    d. b and c

12. How should polycarboxylate cement appear after the
    mixing process?
    a. Dull
    b. Glossy
    c. Streaky
    d. Clear

13. Can glass ionomer material be used for a restoration?
    a. Yes
    b. No

14. What ingredient in the powder of glass ionomer
    cement helps in inhibiting recurrent decay?
    a. Zinc
    b. Composite resin
    c. Iron
    d. Calcium

15. Can resin cement be used under metal castings?
    a. Yes
    b. No

CASE STUDY

Dr. Matthews will be cementing four stainless steel crowns on four primary molars of a 10-year-old patient. He has indicated that "Duralon" will be the cement of choice.

1. Are stainless steel crowns for this procedure considered permanent or provisional?

2. What type of cement is Duralon?

3. List what is needed for the cementation setup.

4. Describe the mixing technique for this cement.

5. How would the excess cement be removed from around the cemented crown?

MULTIMEDIA PROCEDURES RECOMMENDED REVIEW

- Mixing Glass Ionomer for Permanent Cementation
- Mixing Zinc Oxide-Eugenol for Temporary Cementation

COMPETENCY 45-1: MIXING GLASS IONOMER FOR PERMANENT CEMENTATION

Performance Objective
By following a routine procedure that meets stated protocols, the student will assemble the necessary supplies and will correctly manipulate the material for use in the cementation of a cast crown.

Evaluation and Grading Criteria
 _3_   Student competently met the stated criteria without assistance.
 _2_   Student required assistance in order to meet the stated criteria.
 _1_   Student showed uncertainty when performing the stated criteria.
 _0_   Student was not prepared and needs to repeat the step.
 _N/A_   No evaluation of this step.
Instructor shall define grades for each point range earned on completion of each performance-evaluated task.

Performance Standards
The minimum number of satisfactory performances required before final evaluation is _____.

Instructor shall identify by * those steps considered critical. If step is missed or minimum competency is not met, the evaluated procedure fails and must be repeated.

PERFORMANCE CRITERIA	*	SELF	PEER	INSTRUCTOR	COMMENT
1. Selected the proper material and assembled the appropriate supplies.					
2. Personal protective equipment placed according to procedure.					
3. Dispensed the manufacturer's recommended proportion of the *liquid* on one half of the paper pad.					
4. Dispensed the manufacturer's recommended proportion of the *powder* on the other half of the pad; this usually is divided into two or three increments.					
5. Incorporated the powder into the liquid for the recommended mixing time until the material had a glossy appearance.					
6. Lined inside of crown with cement.					
7. Turned the casting over in the palm and transferred it to the dentist.					
8. Transferred a cotton roll so the patient could bite down on it, to help seat the crown and displace the excess cement.					
9. When finished, cared for supplies and materials appropriately.					

Continued

ADDITIONAL COMMENTS

Total number of points earned _____

Grade _____ Instructor's initials _____

COMPETENCY 45-2: MIXING COMPOSITE RESIN FOR PERMANENT CEMENTATION

Performance Objective
By following a routine procedure that meets stated protocols, the student will assemble the necessary supplies and will correctly manipulate the material for use in the cementation of a cast crown.

Evaluation and Grading Criteria
 3 Student competently met the stated criteria without assistance.
 2 Student required assistance in order to meet the stated criteria.
 1 Student showed uncertainty when performing the stated criteria.
 0 Student was not prepared and needs to repeat the step.
N/A No evaluation of this step.
Instructor shall define grades for each point range earned on completion of each performance-evaluated task.

Performance Standards
The minimum number of satisfactory performances required before final evaluation is _____.

Instructor shall identify by * those steps considered critical. If step is missed or minimum competency is not met, the evaluated procedure fails and must be repeated.

PERFORMANCE CRITERIA	*	SELF	PEER	INSTRUCTOR	COMMENT
1. Selected the proper material and assembled the appropriate supplies.					
2. Personal protective equipment placed according to procedure.					
3. Applied etchant to enamel and dentin for 15 seconds, then rinsed. Blotted excess water with a moist cotton pellet, leaving the tooth moist.					
4. Applied a bond adhesive to the enamel and dentin and dried gently. Avoided excess adhesive on all prepared surfaces.					
5. Light-cured each surface for 10 seconds.					
6. Applied primer to etched porcelain or roughened metal surfaces. Dried for 5 seconds.					
7. Dispensed a 1:1 ratio of powder/liquid onto a mixing pad and mixed for 10 seconds. Applied a thin layer of cement to the bonding surface of the restoration.					
8. After the crown was seated, light-cured the margins for 40 seconds or allowed to self-cure for 10 minutes from the start of the mixing.					
9. When finished, cared for supplies and materials appropriately.					

Continued

Total number of points earned _____

Grade _____ Instructor's initials _____

COMPETENCY 45-3: MIXING ZINC OXIDE–EUGENOL FOR TEMPORARY CEMENTATION

Performance Objective

By following a routine procedure that meets stated protocols, the student will assemble the necessary supplies and will correctly manipulate ZOE for temporary cementation.

Evaluation and Grading Criteria

 3 Student competently met the stated criteria without assistance.
 2 Student required assistance in order to meet the stated criteria.
 1 Student showed uncertainty when performing the stated criteria.
 0 Student was not prepared and needs to repeat the step.
 N/A No evaluation of this step.
Instructor shall define grades for each point range earned on completion of each performance-evaluated task.

Performance Standards

The minimum number of satisfactory performances required before final evaluation is _____.

Instructor shall identify by * those steps considered critical. If step is missed or minimum competency is not met, the evaluated procedure fails and must be repeated.

PERFORMANCE CRITERIA	*	SELF	PEER	INSTRUCTOR	COMMENT
1. Selected the proper material and assembled the appropriate supplies.					
2. Personal protective equipment placed according to procedure.					
3. Measured the pastes onto the mixing pad at equal lengths, approximately ½ inch per unit of restoration.					
4. Replaced the caps immediately.					
5. Incorporated the two pastes together.					
6. Mixed while wiping the material over an area of the mixing pad.					
7. Ensured that the material was smooth and creamy and that the process was completed within 20 to 30 seconds.					
8. Filled the temporary coverage with the cement immediately.					

Continued

9. Inverted crown in palm and readied for transfer.					
10. When finished, cared for supplies and materials appropriately.					

ADDITIONAL COMMENTS

Total number of points earned _____

Grade _____ Instructor's initials _____

COMPETENCY 45-4: MIXING ZINC OXIDE–EUGENOL FOR PERMANENT CEMENTATION

Performance Objective

By following a routine procedure that meets stated protocols, the student will assemble the necessary supplies and will correctly manipulate ZOE for permanent cementation.

Evaluation and Grading Criteria

 3 Student competently met the stated criteria without assistance.
 2 Student required assistance in order to meet the stated criteria.
 1 Student showed uncertainty when performing the stated criteria.
 0 Student was not prepared and needs to repeat the step.
 N/A No evaluation of this step.
Instructor shall define grades for each point range earned on completion of each performance-evaluated task.

Performance Standards

The minimum number of satisfactory performances required before final evaluation is _____.

Instructor shall identify by * those steps considered critical. If step is missed or minimum competency is not met, the evaluated procedure fails and must be repeated.

PERFORMANCE CRITERIA	*	SELF	PEER	INSTRUCTOR	COMMENT
1. Selected the proper material and assembled the appropriate supplies.					
2. Personal protective equipment placed according to procedure.					
3. Measured the powder and placed it onto the mixing pad. Replaced the cap on the powder immediately.					
4. Dispensed the liquid near the powder on the mixing pad. Replaced the cap on the liquid container immediately.					
5. Incorporated the powder and liquid all at once, and mixed them with the spatula for 30 seconds.					
6. After ensuring a putty-like consistency of the initial mix, mixed for an additional 30 seconds until it became more fluid for loading into a casting.					
7. Lined the crown with the permanent cement.					
8. Inverted crown in the palm and readied for transfer.					
9. When finished, cared for supplies and materials appropriately.					

Continued

Chapter **45** **Dental Cements**

ADDITIONAL COMMENTS

Total number of points earned _____

Grade _____ Instructor's initials _____

COMPETENCY 45-5: MIXING POLYCARBOXYLATE FOR PERMANENT CEMENTATION

Performance Objective

By following a routine procedure that meets stated protocols, the student will assemble the necessary supplies and will correctly manipulate the material for use in cementation.

Evaluation and Grading Criteria

 3   Student competently met the stated criteria without assistance.
 2   Student required assistance in order to meet the stated criteria.
 1   Student showed uncertainty when performing the stated criteria.
 0   Student was not prepared and needs to repeat the step.
N/A   No evaluation of this step.
Instructor shall define grades for each point range earned on completion of each performance-evaluated task.

Performance Standards

The minimum number of satisfactory performances required before final evaluation is _____.

Instructor shall identify by * those steps considered critical. If step is missed or minimum competency is not met, the evaluated procedure fails and must be repeated.

PERFORMANCE CRITERIA	*	SELF	PEER	INSTRUCTOR	COMMENT
For Cementation					
1. Selected the proper material and assembled the appropriate supplies.					
2. Personal protective equipment placed according to procedure.					
3. Gently shook the powder to fluff the ingredients.					
4. Measured the powder onto the mixing pad and immediately recapped the container.					
5. Dispensed the liquid and then recapped the container.					
6. Used the flat side of the spatula to incorporate all the powder quickly into the liquid at one time. The mix was completed within 30 seconds.					
7. Ensured that the mix was somewhat thick with a shiny, glossy surface.					
8. Lined inside of crown with cement.					
9. Turned the casting over in the palm and transferred it to the dentist.					

Continued

10. Transferred a cotton roll so the patient could bite down on it to help seat the crown and displace the excess cement.				
11. When finished, cared for supplies and materials appropriately.				

ADDITIONAL COMMENTS

Total number of points earned _____

Grade_____ Instructor's initials _____

COMPETENCY 45-6: MIXING ZINC PHOSPHATE FOR PERMANENT CEMENTATION

Performance Objective

By following a routine procedure that meets stated protocols, the student will assemble the necessary supplies and will correctly manipulate the material for use in the cementation of a cast crown.

Evaluation and Grading Criteria

<u>3</u>   Student competently met the stated criteria without assistance.

<u>2</u>   Student required assistance in order to meet the stated criteria.

<u>1</u>   Student showed uncertainty when performing the stated criteria.

<u>0</u>   Student was not prepared and needs to repeat the step.

<u>N/A</u> No evaluation of this step.

Instructor shall define grades for each point range earned on completion of each performance-evaluated task.

Performance Standards

The minimum number of satisfactory performances required before final evaluation is _____.

Instructor shall identify by * those steps considered critical. If step is missed or minimum competency is not met, the evaluated procedure fails and must be repeated.

PERFORMANCE CRITERIA	*	SELF	PEER	INSTRUCTOR	COMMENT
Preparing the Mix					
1. Selected the proper material and assembled the appropriate supplies.					
2. Personal protective equipment placed according to procedure.					
3. Cooled and dried glass slab for mixing.					
4. Dispensed the powder toward one end of the slab and the liquid at the opposite end. Recapped the containers.					
5. Divided the powder into small increments as directed by the manufacturer.					
6. Incorporated each powder increment into the liquid, beginning with smaller increments.					
7. Spatulated the mix thoroughly, using broad strokes or a figure-eight movement over a large area of the slab.					
8. Tested the material for appropriate cementation consistency. (The cement should string up and break about 1 inch from the slab.)					

Continued

9. Held the casting with the inner portion facing upward.				
10. Retrieved the cement onto the spatula. Scraped the edge of the spatula along the margin to cause the cement to flow from the spatula into the casting.				
11. Placed the tip of the spatula or a black spoon into the bulk of the cement and moved the material so that it covered all internal walls with a thin lining of cement.				
12. Turned the casting over in the palm and transferred it to the dentist.				
13. Transferred a cotton roll so the patient could bite down on it to help seat the crown and displace the excess cement.				
14. When finished, cared for supplies and materials appropriately.				

ADDITIONAL COMMENTS

Total number of points earned _____

Grade _____ Instructor's initials _____

COMPETENCY 45-7: REMOVING CEMENT FROM A PERMANENT OR TEMPORARY CEMENTATION (EXPANDED FUNCTION)

Performance Objective

By following a routine procedure that meets stated protocols, in states where it is legal, the student will remove excess cement from the coronal surfaces of a cast restoration.

Evaluation and Grading Criteria

3	Student competently met the stated criteria without assistance.
2	Student required assistance in order to meet the stated criteria.
1	Student showed uncertainty when performing the stated criteria.
0	Student was not prepared and needs to repeat the step.
N/A	No evaluation of this step.

Instructor shall define grades for each point range earned on completion of each performance-evaluated task.

Performance Standards

The minimum number of satisfactory performances required before final evaluation is _____.

Instructor shall identify by * those steps considered critical. If step is missed or minimum competency is not met, the evaluated procedure fails and must be repeated.

PERFORMANCE CRITERIA	*	SELF	PEER	INSTRUCTOR	COMMENT
1. Assembled the appropriate setup.					
2. Personal protective equipment placed according to procedure.					
3. Determined that the cement had set by testing with explorer. Removed cotton rolls.					
4. Established a firm fulcrum for the hand holding the explorer.					
5. Placed the tip of the instrument at the gingival edge of the cement and used overlapping horizontal strokes (away from the gingiva) to remove the bulk of the cement.					
6. Applied slight lateral pressure (toward the tooth surface) to remove the remaining cement.					
7. Passed a length of dental floss, with knots tied in it, through the mesial and distal contact areas to remove excess cement from interproximal areas.					
8. Used overlapping strokes with an explorer to examine all tooth surfaces.					
9. Completed the procedure without scratching the cast restoration.					

Continued

10. Removed any remaining cement particles and performed a complete mouth rinse.					
11. Maintained patient comfort and followed appropriate infection-control measures throughout the procedure.					

ADDITIONAL COMMENTS

Total number of points earned _____

Grade _____ Instructor's initials _____

46 Impression Materials

1. List the three types of impressions that would be taken in a dental office.

2. Describe the types of impression trays and their characteristics of use.

3. Discuss hydrocolloid impression materials, and describe their use, mixing techniques, and application of material.

4. Discuss elastomeric impression materials, and describe their use, mixing techniques, and application of material.

5. Describe the importance of an occlusal registration and its use.

FILL-IN-THE-BLANK STATEMENTS

Select the best term from the list below and complete the following statements.

agar
alginate
base
border molding
catalyst
centric
colloid
elastomeric

hydro-
hysteresis
imbibition
occlusal registration
syneresis
tempering
viscosity

1. A(n) _____ is a gelatinous material used to obtain impressions.

2. _____ is the process of using your fingers to achieve a closer adaptation of the edges of an impression.

3. A(n) _____ material has elastic properties and is made from rubber.

4. A foundation or basic ingredient of a material is the _____.

5. To have something _____ is to have it centered, such as your maxillary teeth centered over your mandibular teeth.

6. _____ is a gelatin-type material derived from seaweed.

7. _____ is the loss of water, causing shrinkage.

8. _____ is to bring a material to a desired temperature and consistency.

9. _____ describes a property of fluids with a high resistance to flow.

10. _____ is the material of choice in dentistry for preliminary impressions.

11. _____ is to transform a material from one physical state to another.

12. _____ means water.

13. A(n) _____ is a reproduction of someone's bite with the use of wax or elastomeric material.

14. A(n) _____ is a substance that modifies or increases the rate of a chemical reaction.

15. _____ is the absorption of water, causing an object to swell.

MULTIPLE-CHOICE QUESTIONS

Complete each question by circling the best answer.

1. An impression would be considered a _____.
   a. negative reproduction
   b. mirror image
   c. positive reproduction
   d. duplication

2. Of the three classifications of impressions, which of these would be considered an expanded function(s) for the certified dental assistant?
   a. Irreversible hydrocolloid
   b. Final
   c. Bite registration
   d. a and c

3. Which of the three classifications of impressions would be used by the dental lab tech for the occlusal relationship?
   a. Irreversible hydrocolloid
   b. Final
   c. Bite registration
   d. Reversible hydrocolloid

4. Which type of stock tray would you select to cover half of an arch?
   a. Anterior
   b. Quadrant
   c. Full
   d. Custom

5. Which type of tray allows impression material to mechanically lock on?
   a. Metal
   b. Plastic
   c. Custom
   d. Perforated

6. Which type of tray is constructed to fit the mouth of a specific patient?
   a. Metal
   b. Plastic
   c. Custom
   d. Perforated

7. _____ is used to extend the length of a tray to accommodate third molars.
   a. Rope wax
   b. Impression material
   c. Border molding
   d. Boxing wax

8. The organic substance of hydrocolloid material is _____.
   a. tree bark
   b. volcanic ash
   c. seaweed
   d. mud

9. Why would a fast-set alginate be selected for taking a preliminary impression?
   a. The patient is late for the appointment.
   b. The patient has a strong gag reflex.
   c. The patient does not like the taste.
   d. The patient must be kept from talking.

10. Give the powder/water ratio for a maxillary impression.
    a. 1 scoop of powder to 1 measure of water
    b. 2 scoops of powder to 2 measures of water
    c. 3 scoops of powder to 3 measures of water
    d. 4 scoops of powder to 4 measures of water

11. Hydro means _____.
    a. air
    b. mass
    c. water
    d. temperature

12. Another name for irreversible hydrocolloid is _____.
    a. alginate
    b. elastomeric
    c. polyether
    d. polysulfide

13. How is irreversible hydrocolloid mixed?
    a. Glass slab
    b. Mixing bowl
    c. Paper pad
    d. Automix system

14. Where is the reversible hydrocolloid material placed before the impression is taken?
    a. Refrigerator
    b. Autoclave
    c. Patient tray
    d. Conditioning bath

15. Elastomeric materials would be selected for what type(s) of impression?
    a. Final
    b. Preliminary
    c. Bite registration
    d. a and c

16. How are elastomeric materials supplied?
    a. Paste
    b. Cartridge
    c. Putty
    d. All of the above

17. Which viscosity of a final impression material is applied first to the prepared tooth or teeth?
    a. Light body
    b. Medium body
    c. Heavy body

18. Another name for polysulfide is _____.
    a. polyether
    b. rubber base
    c. silicone
    d. alginate

19. What would the dentist use to express the light-body impression material around a prepared tooth?
    a. Extruder with tip
    b. Air-water syringe
    c. COE syringe
    d. a or c

20. What system accomplishes the mixing of final impression material for the assistant?
    a. Vibrator
    b. Spatula and pad
    c. Triturator
    d. Automix

21. _____ is the material universally used for taking a bite registration.
    a. Baseplate wax
    b. Alginate
    c. Silicone
    d. Rubber base

22. What tray type is most commonly selected when polysiloxane bite registration material is used?
    a. Perforated tray
    b. Metal tray
    c. Gauze tray
    d. Water-cooled tray

23. Baseplate wax is _____ before placement in the patient's mouth for a bite registration.
    a. molded
    b. cooled
    c. placed in a tray
    d. warmed

24. While the dentist is dispensing the syringe material around the prepared tooth, what should the dental assistant be doing during a final impression procedure?
    a. Suctioning
    b. Preparing the provisional coverage
    c. Readying the tray with heavy-body material
    d. Triturating the restorative material

25. A preliminary impression is _____ before transport to the lab to pour up.
    a. immersed in a disinfectant solution
    b. rinsed, disinfected, wrapped in a moist paper towel, and placed in a precautionary bag
    c. placed in a rubber mixing bowl and filled with cold water
    d. left on the patient tray to dry completely

Dr. Clark asks you to take a maxillary and mandibular preliminary impression on the next patient for the fabrication of bleaching trays.

1. What impression material will you select to take preliminary impressions?

2. What type of trays will you select for the procedure?

3. How do you know which size tray to use? How are the trays prepared for the impression material?

4. Describe the setup that is required for taking these impressions.

5. Describe the mixing technique used for taking this type of impression.

6. Which impression will you take first, and why?

7. Is there any specific area in the mouth that is most critical when taking this type of impression?

8. What will you do with these impressions once they are taken?

MULTIMEDIA PROCEDURES RECOMMENDED REVIEW ⊖volve
learning system

- Mixing alginate and taking preliminary impressions

COMPETENCY 46-1: MIXING ALGINATE IMPRESSION MATERIAL

Performance Objective

By following a routine procedure that meets stated protocols, the student will mix alginate impression material.

Evaluation and Grading Criteria

 3 Student competently met the stated criteria without assistance.
 2 Student required assistance in order to meet the stated criteria.
 1 Student showed uncertainty when performing the stated criteria.
 0 Student was not prepared and needs to repeat the step.
 N/A No evaluation of this step.
Instructor shall define grades for each point range earned on completion of each performance-evaluated task.

Performance Standards

The minimum number of satisfactory performances required before final evaluation is _____.

Instructor shall identify by * those steps considered critical. If step is missed or minimum competency is not met, the evaluated procedure fails and must be repeated.

PERFORMANCE CRITERIA	*	SELF	PEER	INSTRUCTOR	COMMENT
1. Gathered appropriate supplies.					
2. Personal protective equipment placed according to procedure.					
3. Placed the appropriate amount of water into the bowl using the calibrated measure.					
4. Shook the can of alginate to "fluff" the contents. After fluffing, carefully lifted the lid to prevent the particles from flying into the air.					
5. Using the correct scoop, sifted the powder into the water.					
6. Used the spatula to mix with a stirring action to wet the powder until it was all moistened.					
7. Firmly spread the alginate between the spatula and the side of the rubber bowl.					
8. Spatulated material for the appropriate length of time, until the mixture appeared smooth and creamy.					

Continued

9. Wiped the alginate mix into one mass on the inside edge of the bowl.				
10. When finished, cared for supplies and materials appropriately.				

ADDITIONAL COMMENTS

Total number of points earned _____

Grade _____ Instructor's initials _____

COMPETENCIES 46-2 AND 46-3: TAKING A MANDIBULAR AND/OR MAXILLARY PRELIMINARY IMPRESSION (EXPANDED FUNCTION)

Performance Objective

By following a routine procedure that meets stated protocols, the student will take a mandibular and maxillary alginate impression of diagnostic quality.

Evaluation and Grading Criteria

__3__   Student competently met the stated criteria without assistance.
__2__   Student required assistance in order to meet the stated criteria.
__1__   Student showed uncertainty when performing the stated criteria.
__0__   Student was not prepared and needs to repeat the step.
_N/A_   No evaluation of this step.
Instructor shall define grades for each point range earned on completion of each performance-evaluated task.

Performance Standards

The minimum number of satisfactory performances required before final evaluation is _____.

Instructor shall identify by * those steps considered critical. If step is missed or minimum competency is not met, the evaluated procedure fails and must be repeated.

PERFORMANCE CRITERIA	*	SELF	PEER	INSTRUCTOR	COMMENT
1. Gathered all necessary supplies.					
2. Personal protective equipment placed according to procedure.					
3. Seated and prepared the patient.					
4. Explained the procedure to the patient.					
Taking the Mandibular Impression					
5. Selected and prepared the mandibular impression tray.					
6. Obtained two measures of room temperature water with two scoops of alginate, and mixed the material.					
7. Gathered half the alginate in the bowl onto the spatula, then wiped alginate into one side of the tray from the lingual side. Quickly pressed the material down to the base of the tray.					
8. Gathered the remaining half of the alginate in the bowl onto the spatula, and then loaded the other side of the tray in the same way.					
9. Smoothed the surface of the alginate by wiping a moistened finger along the surface.					
10. Placed additional material over the occlusal surfaces of the mandibular teeth.					
11. Retracted the patient's cheek with the index finger.					

Continued

12. Turned the tray slightly sideways when placing it into the mouth.				
13. Centered the tray over the teeth.				
14. Seated the tray from the posterior border first.				
15. Instructed the patient to breathe normally while the material set.				
16. Observed the alginate around the tray to determine when the material had set.				
17. Placed fingers on top of the impression tray and gently broke the seal between the impression and the peripheral tissues by moving the inside of the patient's cheeks or lips with the finger.				
18. Grasped the handle of the tray with the thumb and index finger and used a firm lifting motion to break the seal.				
19. Snapped up the tray and impression from the dentition.				
20. Instructed the patient to rinse with water to remove excess alginate material.				
21. Evaluated the impression for accuracy.				
22. Procedure documented in patient record.				
Taking the Maxillary Impression.				
Loading the Maxillary Impression Tray				
1. For a maxillary impression, mixed 3 measures of water and 3 scoops of powder.				
2. Loaded the maxillary tray in one large increment and used a wiping motion to fill the tray from the posterior end.				
3. Placed the bulk of the material toward the anterior palatal area of the tray.				
4. Moistened fingertips with tap water and smoothed the surface of the alginate.				
5. Used the index finger to retract the patient's cheek.				
6. Turned the tray slightly sideways to position the tray into the mouth.				
7. Centered the tray over the patient's teeth.				
8. Seated the posterior border (back) of the tray up against the posterior border of the hard palate to form a seal.				
9. Directed the anterior portion of the tray upward over the teeth.				

10. Gently lifted the patient's lips out of the way as the tray was seated, and instructed the patient to tilt head forward.					
11. Checks the posterior border of the tray to ensure that no material was flowing into the patient's throat. If necessary, wiped excess material away with a cotton-tipped applicator.					
12. Held the tray firmly in place while the alginate set.					
13. To avoid injury to the impression and the patient's teeth, places a finger along the lateral borders of the tray to push down and break the palatal seal.					
14. Used a straight, downward snapping motion to remove the tray from the teeth.					
15. Instructed the patient to rinse with water to remove any excess alginate impression material.					
16. Gently rinsed the impression under cold tap water to remove any blood or saliva.					
17. Sprayed the impression with an approved disinfectant.					
18. Wrapped the impression in a damp paper towel and stored it in a covered container or a plastic biohazard bag labeled with the patient's name.					
19. Examines the patient's mouth for any remaining fragments of alginate and removed them using an explorer and dental floss.					
20. Used a moist facial tissue to remove any alginate from the patient's face and lips.					
21. Procedure documented in patient record.					

ADDITIONAL COMMENTS

Total number of points earned _____

Grade _____ Instructor's initials _____

COMPETENCY 46-4: MIXING A TWO-PASTE FINAL IMPRESSION MATERIAL

Performance Objective

By following a routine procedure that meets stated protocols, the student will prepare and mix a two-paste final impression material.

Evaluation and Grading Criteria

_3_ Student competently met the stated criteria without assistance.
_2_ Student required assistance in order to meet the stated criteria.
_1_ Student showed uncertainty when performing the stated criteria.
_0_ Student was not prepared and needs to repeat the step.
_N/A_ No evaluation of this step.
Instructor shall define grades for each point range earned on completion of each performance-evaluated task.

Performance Standards

The minimum number of satisfactory performances required before final evaluation is _____.

Instructor shall identify by * those steps considered critical. If step is missed or minimum competency is not met, the evaluated procedure fails and must be repeated.

PERFORMANCE CRITERIA	*	SELF	PEER	INSTRUCTOR	COMMENT
1. Gathered appropriate supplies.					
2. Personal protective equipment placed according to procedure.					
Preparing Light-Bodied Syringe Material					
1. Dispensed approximately 1½ to 2 inches of equal lengths of the base and catalyst of the light-bodied material onto the top third of the pad, ensuring that the materials were not too close to each other.					
2. Wiped the tube openings clean with gauze, and recapped immediately.					
3. Placed the tip of the spatula blade into the catalyst and base and mixed in a swirling direction for approximately 5 seconds.					
4. Gathered the material onto the flat portion of the spatula and placed it on a clean area of the pad, preferably the center.					
5. Spatulated smoothly, wiping back and forth and trying to use only one side of the spatula during the mixing process.					
6. To obtain a more homogenous mix, picked the material up by the spatula blade and wiped it onto the pad.					

Continued

7. Gathered the material together, took the syringe tube, and began "cookie cutting" the material into the syringe. Inserted the plunger, and expressed a small amount of the material to ensure that the syringe was in working order.				
8. Transferred the syringe to the dentist, ensuring that the tip of the syringe was directed toward the tooth.				
Preparing Heavy-Bodied Tray Material				
1. Dispensed equal lengths of the base and catalyst of the heavy-bodied material on the top third of the pad for a quadrant tray.				
2. Placed the tip of the spatula blade into the catalyst and base and mixed in a swirling direction for approximately 5 seconds.				
3. Gathered the material onto the flat portion of the spatula, and placed it onto a clean area of the pad.				
4. Spatulated smoothly, wiping back and forth using only one side of the spatula during the mixing process.				
5. To get a more homogenous mix, picked the material up with the spatula blade and wiped it onto the pad.				
6. Gathered the bulk of the material with the spatula and loaded the material into the tray.				
7. Using the tip of the spatula, spread the material evenly from one end of the tray to the other without picking up the material.				
8. Retrieved the syringe from the dentist and transferred the tray, ensuring that the dentist could grasp the handle of the tray properly.				
9. When finished, cared for supplies and materials appropriately.				
10. Procedure documented in patient record.				

ADDITIONAL COMMENTS

Total number of points earned _____

Grade _____ Instructor's initials _____

COMPETENCY 46-5: PREPARING AN AUTOMIX FINAL IMPRESSION MATERIAL

Performance Objective

By following a routine procedure that meets stated protocols, the student will prepare an automix final impression material.

Evaluation and Grading Criteria

  3   Student competently met the stated criteria without assistance.
  2   Student required assistance in order to meet the stated criteria.
  1   Student showed uncertainty when performing the stated criteria.
  0   Student was not prepared and needs to repeat the step.
 N/A   No evaluation of this step.
 Instructor shall define grades for each point range earned on completion of each performance-evaluated task.

Performance Standards

The minimum number of satisfactory performances required before final evaluation is _____.

Instructor shall identify by * those steps considered critical. If step is missed or minimum competency is not met, the evaluated procedure fails and must be repeated.

PERFORMANCE CRITERIA	*	SELF	PEER	INSTRUCTOR	COMMENT
1. Gathered appropriate supplies.					
2. Personal protective equipment placed according to procedure.					
3. Loaded the extruder with dual cartridges of the base and the catalyst of light-bodied material.					
4. Removed the caps from the tube and extruded a small amount of unmixed material onto the gauze pad.					
5. Attached a mixing tip on the extruder, along with a syringe tip for light-bodied application by the dentist.					
6. When the dentist signaled, began squeezing the trigger until the material reached the tip.					
7. Transferred the extruder to the dentist, directing the tip toward the area of the impression.					
8. Placed the heavy-bodied cartridges in the extruder, expressing a small amount as before with the light-bodied material. Attached the mixing tip to the cartridge.					
9. When the dentist signaled, began squeezing the trigger, mixing the heavy-bodied material.					

Continued

10. Loaded the impression tray with heavy-bodied material, making sure not to trap air in the material.				
11. Transferred the tray, ensuring that the dentist could grasp the handle of the tray.				
12. Disinfected the impression, placed it in a biohazard bag, labeled it with the patient's name, and readied it for the laboratory.				
13. Procedure documented in patient record.				

ADDITIONAL COMMENTS

Total number of points earned _____

Grade _____ Instructor's initials _____

COMPETENCY 46-6: TAKING A WAX BITE REGISTRATION (EXPANDED FUNCTION)

Performance Objective
By following a routine procedure that meets stated protocols, the student will take a wax-bite registration.

Evaluation and Grading Criteria
 3   Student competently met the stated criteria without assistance.
 2   Student required assistance in order to meet the stated criteria.
 1   Student showed uncertainty when performing the stated criteria.
 0   Student was not prepared and needs to repeat the step.
 N/A   No evaluation of this step.
Note: Mandibular and maxillary impressions have already been taken for this patient.
Instructor shall define grades for each point range earned on completion of each performance-evaluated task.

Performance Standards
The minimum number of satisfactory performances required before final evaluation is _____.

Instructor shall identify by * those steps considered critical. If step is missed or minimum competency is not met, the evaluated procedure fails and must be repeated.

PERFORMANCE CRITERIA	*	SELF	PEER	INSTRUCTOR	COMMENT
1. Gathered appropriate supplies.					
2. Personal protective equipment placed according to procedure.					
3. Explained the procedure to the patient.					
4. Instructed the patient to practice opening and closing his or her mouth normally.					
5. Placed the wax over the biting surfaces of the teeth and checked the length. Used the laboratory knife to shorten the length of the wax if needed.					
6. Used a heat source to soften the wax.					
7. Placed the softened wax against the biting surfaces of the teeth.					
8. Instructed the patient to bite gently and naturally into the wax.					
9. Allowed the wax to cool.					
10. Removed the wax-bite registration carefully to avoid distortion.					
11. Wrote the patient's name on a piece of paper and kept it with the wax-bite registration.					

Continued

12. Stored the wax-bite registration with the impressions or casts until it was needed during the trimming of the casts.				
13. Maintained patient comfort and followed appropriate infection control measures throughout the procedure.				
14. Procedure documented in patient record.				

ADDITIONAL COMMENTS

Total number of points earned _____

Grade _____ Instructor's initials _____

COMPETENCY 46-7: MIXING POLYSILOXANE MATERIAL FOR A BITE REGISTRATION

Performance Objective
By following a routine procedure that meets stated protocols, the student will mix and prepare polysiloxane material for a bite registration.

Evaluation and Grading Criteria
 3   Student competently met the stated criteria without assistance.
 2   Student required assistance in order to meet the stated criteria.
 1   Student showed uncertainty when performing the stated criteria.
 0   Student was not prepared and needs to repeat the step.
 N/A No evaluation of this step.
Note: Mandibular and maxillary impressions have already been taken for this patient.
Instructor shall define grades for each point range earned on completion of each performance-evaluated task.

Performance Standards
The minimum number of satisfactory performances required before final evaluation is _____.

Instructor shall identify by * those steps considered critical. If step is missed or minimum competency is not met, the evaluated procedure fails and must be repeated.

PERFORMANCE CRITERIA	*	SELF	PEER	INSTRUCTOR	COMMENT
1. Gathered appropriate supplies.					
2. Personal protective equipment placed according to procedure.					
3. Mixed the material and dispensed it using an extruder.					
4. Extruded the material directly onto the tray, making sure to fill both sides of the tray.					
5. Instructed the patient to close in proper occlusion.					
6. After the material was set (about 1 minute), removed the impression and had dentist check for accuracy.					
7. Rinsed, disinfected, and dried the impression and sent it to the laboratory with the written prescription and other impressions.					
8. When finished, cared for supplies and materials appropriately.					
9. Procedure documented in patient record.					
ADDITIONAL COMMENTS					

Total number of points earned _____

Grade _____ Instructor's initials _____

COMPETENCY 46-8: MIXING ZINC OXIDE–EUGENOL BITE REGISTRATION MATERIAL

Performance Objective
By following a routine procedure that meets stated protocols, the student will mix and prepare zinc oxide–eugenol material for a bite registration.

Evaluation and Grading Criteria
3   Student competently met the stated criteria without assistance.
2   Student required assistance in order to meet the stated criteria.
1   Student showed uncertainty when performing the stated criteria.
0   Student was not prepared and needs to repeat the step.
N/A   No evaluation of this step.
Note: Mandibular and maxillary impressions have already been taken for this patient.
Instructor shall define grades for each point range earned on completion of each performance-evaluated task.

Performance Standards
The minimum number of satisfactory performances required before final evaluation is _____.

Instructor shall identify by * those steps considered critical. If step is missed or minimum competency is not met, the evaluated procedure fails and must be repeated.

PERFORMANCE CRITERIA	*	SELF	PEER	INSTRUCTOR	COMMENT
1. Gathered appropriate supplies.					
2. Personal protective equipment placed according to procedure.					
3. Dispensed 1 to 2 inches of base and catalyst paste onto the pad.					
4. Mixed the material thoroughly for 45 seconds.					
5. Gathered half the material on the spatula and wiped the material onto one side of the gauze tray. Gathered the remaining half and wiped it onto the other side of the tray.					
6. Placed the tray in the patient's mouth over the desired areas and instructed the patient to bite down. The material should set within 1 minute.					
7. Instructed the patient to open the mouth, and then removed the tray.					
8. Rinsed, dried, and disinfected the bite registration and sent it to the laboratory with the written prescription and other impressions.					

Continued

9. When finished, cared for supplies and materials appropriately.				
10. Procedure documented in patient record.				

ADDITIONAL COMMENTS

Total number of points earned _____

Grade _____ Instructor's initials _____

47 Laboratory Materials and Procedures

SHORT-ANSWER QUESTIONS

1. Discuss the types of safety precautions that should be taken when working in the dental laboratory.

2. List the types of equipment commonly found in a dental laboratory, and describe their use.

3. Define dental models, and explain their use in dentistry.

4. Discuss gypsum products and their use in fabricating dental models.

5. Describe the three types of custom impression trays and their use in dentistry.

6. Describe the types of dental waxes and their use in dentistry.

FILL-IN-THE-BLANK STATEMENTS

Select the best term from the list below and complete the following statements.

anatomic portion	homogeneous
articulator	lathe
crystallization	model
dihydrate	monomer
dimensionally stable	polymer
facebow	slurry
gypsum	volatile
hemihydrate	

1. A material that is uniform in quality and consistent throughout is said to be _____.

2. A(n) _____ is a machine used for cutting or polishing dental appliances.

3. _____ is the mineral used in the formation of plaster of Paris and stone.

4. A substance is said to be _____ if it has an explosive property.

5. When referring to a gypsum product, a(n) _____ indicates that there are two parts of water to every one part of calcium sulfate.

6. If an object is resistant to change in width, height, and length, it is said to be _____.

7. The _____ is the portion of an articulator used to measure the upper teeth and compare with the temporomandibular joint.

8. A(n) _____ is the compound of many molecules.

9. _____ is a chemical process in which crystals form into a structure.

10. _____ is the removal of one-half part water to one part calcium sulfate to form the powder product of gypsum.

11. A(n) _____ is a replica of the maxillary and mandibular arches made from an impression.

12. _____ refers to the structural portion of a dental model.

13. A(n) _____ is a dental laboratory device that simulates the movement of the mandible and the temporomandibular joint when models of the dental arches are attached.

14. A(n) _____ is a molecule that when combined with others forms a polymer.

15. _____ is a mixture of gypsum and water used in the finishing of models.

MULTIPLE-CHOICE QUESTIONS

Complete each question by circling the best answer.

1. Where would you commonly find the dental lab in a dental office?
   a. In the treatment area
   b. In the reception area
   c. In a separate space away from patient care
   d. In the dentist's office

2. Which specialty practice(s) might have a more extensive laboratory setup?
   a. Oral surgery
   b. Fixed prosthodontics
   c. Orthodontics
   d. b and c

3. An example of a contaminated item that could be found in the dental lab would be (a)n _____.
   a. explorer
   b. x-ray
   c. impression
   d. high-speed handpiece

4. Which piece of lab equipment would be used to grind away plaster or stone?
   a. Model trimmer
   b. Lathe
   c. Bunsen burner
   d. Laboratory handpiece

5. Which piece of lab equipment would the dentist use to determine centric relation from a diagnostic model?
   a. Vibrator
   b. Model trimmer
   c. Articulator
   d. Bunsen burner

6. The size of the wax spatula most commonly used in the laboratory is a _____.
   a. #1
   b. #3
   c. #5
   d. #7

7. Another name for a dental model is _____.
   a. dental die
   b. dental impression
   c. dental cast
   d. dental wax-up

8. What dental material would be selected to fabricate a dental model?
   a. Hydrocolloid
   b. Gypsum
   c. Elastomeric
   d. Wax

9. Which form of gypsum is used to fabricate a die for making an indirect restoration?
   a. Plaster
   b. Stone
   c. High-strength stone
   d. Thermoplastic resin

10. The powder/water ratio of plaster for pouring a dental model is _____.
   a. 50/100
   b. 75/50
   c. 100/50
   d. 150/30

11. When a gypsum material is mixed, how is the powder and water incorporated?
   a. Add water and powder at the same time.
   b. Add water to the powder.
   c. Add powder to the water.
   d. It does not matter.

12. How are gypsum materials mixed?
   a. Using a spatula and rubber bowl
   b. Using a spatula and paper pad
   c. Using an automix syringe
   d. Using an amalgamator

13. Which of the following is a section of a dental model?
   a. Anatomic
   b. Art
   c. Skeletal
   d. a and b

14. When pouring an impression, where would you begin placing the gypsum material in a mandibular impression?
   a. Anterior teeth
   b. Palatal area
   c. Most posterior tooth
   d. Premolar teeth

15. How long should you wait before you separate a model from its impression?
   a. 15 to 20 minutes
   b. 30 to 45 minutes
   c. 40 to 60 minutes
   d. 24 hours

16. Which of the two models (maxillary or mandibular) do you begin trimming first?
   a. Maxillary
   b. Smallest model
   c. Mandibular
   d. Largest model

17. What is the one specific area of a dental model in which the maxillary and mandibular models are trimmed differently?
   a. Heels
   b. Buccal surfaces
   c. Base
   d. Anterior portion

18. What should be placed between the two models when they are trimmed together?
   a. Tongue depressor
   b. Wax bite
   c. Hydrocolloid material
   d. Cotton rolls

19. Of the three types of custom trays discussed in the chapter, which technique uses a volatile hazardous material?
   a. Acrylic resin
   b. Light-cured resin
   c. Thermoplastic resin
   d. Composite resin

20. What type of custom tray would be made for a vital bleaching procedure?
   a. Acrylic resin
   b. Light-cured resin
   c. Thermoplastic resin
   d. Composite resin

21. How is self-cured Acrylic resin supplied for the fabrication of custom trays?
   a. Powder and liquid
   b. Tubes of paste
   c. Putty
   d. a and c

22. What type of wax is used to form a wall around a preliminary impression when it is poured up?
   a. Rope wax
   b. Boxing wax
   c. Inlay wax
   d. Baseplate wax

23. To extend an impression tray, what type of wax is used?
   a. Rope utility wax
   b. Boxing wax
   c. Inlay wax
   d. Baseplate wax

24. What type of wax is used to get a patient's bite?
   a. Rope wax
   b. Boxing wax
   c. Inlay wax
   d. Baseplate wax

25. What is placed to prevent a tray from seating too deeply onto the arch or quadrant?
    a. Undercut
    b. Separating medium
    c. Spacer stops
    d. Finisher

CASE STUDY

It is 4:30 PM, and Dr. Campbell has asked you to take preliminary impressions on the patient in Room 3. The study models from these impressions will be used for a case presentation at a scheduled appointment.

1. What type of impression material will be used for this impression?

2. What type of tray is commonly selected for this procedure?

3. Is this a procedure that the dental assistant can complete independently? If so, how and why?

4. How are preliminary impressions cared for before they are taken to the dental laboratory?

5. Because of the time of day, can you wait until tomorrow morning to pour them up?

6. Because these models will be used for a case presentation, which gypsum material would provide a more professional presentation?

7. How will you prepare the models for a more professional appearance?

8. How will you polish the finished model?

MULTIMEDIA PROCEDURES RECOMMENDED REVIEW

- Constructing a vacuum-formed tray
- Pouring dental models using the inverted-pour method

COMPETENCY 47-1: TAKING A FACE-BOW REGISTRATION (EXPANDED FUNCTION)

Performance Objective

By following a routine procedure that meets stated protocols, the student will take a facebow registration that will be used by the dentist or dental laboratory technician in the mounting of the study cast.

Evaluation and Grading Criteria

 3   Student competently met the stated criteria without assistance.
 2   Student required assistance in order to meet the stated criteria.
 1   Student showed uncertainty when performing the stated criteria.
 0   Student was not prepared and needs to repeat the step.
 N/A   No evaluation of this step.

Instructor shall define grades for each point range earned on completion of each performance-evaluated task.

Performance Standards

The minimum number of satisfactory performances required before final evaluation is _____.

Instructor shall identify by * those steps considered critical. If step is missed or minimum competency is not met, the evaluated procedure fails and must be repeated.

PERFORMANCE CRITERIA	*	SELF	PEER	INSTRUCTOR	COMMENT
1. Gathered appropriate supplies and materials.					
2. Personal protective equipment placed according to procedure.					
3. Attached the vertical indicator rod to the analyzer bow.					
4. Attached either a disposable index tray or a bite-fork to the analyzer bow.					
5. Prepared the bite-fork with either a disposable index tray or compound bite tabs.					
6. Made sure the patient bit slowly when the bite-fork was positioned in the mouth.					
7. Aligned the vertical indicator rod with the patient's facial midline.					
8. Positioned the analyzer bow until the lateral wings were level.					
9. Removed the tray or bite-fork from the bow.					

Continued

10. Procedure documented in patient record.					
ADDITIONAL COMMENTS					

Total number of points earned _____

Grade _____ Instructor's initials _____

COMPETENCY 47-2: MIXING DENTAL PLASTER

Performance Objective

By following a routine procedure that meets stated protocols, the student will mix dental plaster in preparation for pouring a dental model.

Evaluation and Grading Criteria

 3 Student competently met the stated criteria without assistance.
 2 Student required assistance in order to meet the stated criteria.
 1 Student showed uncertainty when performing the stated criteria.
 0 Student was not prepared and needs to repeat the step.
 N/A No evaluation of this step.
Note: Mandibular and maxillary impressions have already been taken.
Instructor shall define grades for each point range earned on completion of each performance-evaluated task.

Performance Standards

The minimum number of satisfactory performances required before final evaluation is _____.

Instructor shall identify by * those steps considered critical. If step is missed or minimum competency is not met, the evaluated procedure fails and must be repeated.

PERFORMANCE CRITERIA	*	SELF	PEER	INSTRUCTOR	COMMENT
1. Gathered appropriate supplies.					
2. Personal protective equipment placed according to procedure.					
3. Measured 50 mL of room-temperature water into a clean rubber mixing bowl.					
4. Weighed out 100 g of dental plaster.					
5. Added the powder to the water in steady increments. Allowed the powder to settle into the water for about 30 seconds.					
6. Used the spatula to incorporate the powder slowly into the water.					
7. Achieved a smooth and creamy mix in about 20 seconds.					
8. Turned the vibrator to low or medium speed, and placed the bowl of plaster mix on the vibrator platform.					
9. Lightly pressed and rotated the bowl on the vibrator until air bubbles rose to the surface.					

Continued

10. Completed mixing and vibration of the plaster in 2 minutes or less.					
11. When finished, cared for supplies and materials appropriately.					

ADDITIONAL COMMENTS

Total number of points earned _____

Grade _____ Instructor's initials _____

COMPETENCY 47-3: POURING DENTAL MODELS USING THE INVERTED-POUR METHOD

Performance Objective

By following a routine procedure that meets stated protocols, the student will pour a maxillary and mandibular dental model using the inverted-pour method.

Evaluation and Grading Criteria

 3 Student competently met the stated criteria without assistance.
 2 Student required assistance in order to meet the stated criteria.
 1 Student showed uncertainty when performing the stated criteria.
 0 Student was not prepared and needs to repeat the step.
 N/A No evaluation of this step.
Instructor shall define grades for each point range earned on completion of each performance-evaluated task.

Performance Standards

The minimum number of satisfactory performances required before final evaluation is _____.

Instructor shall identify by * those steps considered critical. If step is missed or minimum competency is not met, the evaluated procedure fails and must be repeated.

PERFORMANCE CRITERIA	*	SELF	PEER	INSTRUCTOR	COMMENT
1. Gathered the appropriate supplies.					
2. Personal protective equipment placed according to procedure.					
3. Used air to remove excess moisture from the impression.					
4. Used a laboratory knife or laboratory cutters to remove any excess impression material that would interfere with pouring of the model.					
5. Mixed the plaster, then set the vibrator at low to medium speed.					
6. Held the impression tray by the handle, and placed the edge of the tray onto the vibrator.					
7. Placed small increments of plaster in the impression near the most posterior tooth.					
8. Continued to place small increments in the same area as the first increment, and allowed the plaster to flow toward the anterior teeth.					
9. Turned the tray on its side to provide continuous flow of material forward into each tooth impression.					

Continued

10. When all teeth in the impression were covered, added larger increments until the entire impression was filled.				
11. Placed the additional material onto a glass slab (or tile), and shaped the base to approximately 2×2 inches and 1 inch thick.				
12. Inverted the impression onto the new mix without pushing the impression into the base.				
13. Used a spatula to smooth the plaster base mix up onto the margins of the initial pour.				
Pouring the Maxillary Cast				
1. Repeated steps 3 to 5 using clean equipment for the fresh mix of plaster.				
2. Placed a small increment of plaster at the posterior area of the impression. Guided the material as it flowed down into the impression of the most posterior tooth.				
3. Continued to place small increments in the same area as the first increment, and allowed the plaster to flow toward the anterior teeth.				
4. Rotated the tray on its side to provide continuous flow of material into each tooth impression.				
5. When all teeth in the impression were covered, added larger increments until the entire impression was filled.				
6. Placed the mix onto a glass slab (or tile), and shaped the base to approximately 2×2 inches and 1 inch thick.				
7. Inverted the impression onto the new mix.				
8. Used a spatula to smooth the stone base mix up onto the margins of the initial pour.				

9. Placed the impression tray on the base so the handle and the occlusal plane of the teeth on the cast were parallel with the surface of the glass slab (or tile).					
Separating the Casts from the Impression					
1. Waited 45 to 60 minutes after the base was poured before separating the impression from the model.					
2. Used the laboratory knife to gently separate the margins of the tray.					
3. Applied firm, straight, upward pressure on the handle of the tray to remove the impression.					
4. Pulled the tray handle straight up from the model.					
5. The models were ready for trimming and polishing.					
6. When finished, cared for supplies and materials appropriately.					

ADDITIONAL COMMENTS

Total number of points earned _____

Grade _____ Instructor's initials _____

COMPETENCY 47-4: TRIMMING AND FINISHING DENTAL MODELS

Performance Objective
By following a routine procedure that meets stated protocols, the student will trim and finish a set of dental models to be used for diagnostic purposes.

Evaluation and Grading Criteria
 3 Student competently met the stated criteria without assistance.
 2 Student required assistance in order to meet the stated criteria.
 1 Student showed uncertainty when performing the stated criteria.
 0 Student was not prepared and needs to repeat the step.
 N/A No evaluation of this step.
Instructor shall define grades for each point range earned on completion of each performance-evaluated task.

Performance Standards
The minimum number of satisfactory performances required before final evaluation is _____.

Instructor shall identify by * those steps considered critical. If step is missed or minimum competency is not met, the evaluated procedure fails and must be repeated.

PERFORMANCE CRITERIA	*	SELF	PEER	INSTRUCTOR	COMMENT
1. Gathered appropriate supplies.					
2. Personal protective equipment placed according to procedure.					
3. Soaked the art portion of the model in a bowl of water for at least 5 minutes.					
4. Placed the maxillary model on a flat countertop with the teeth resting on the table.					
5. Measured up 1¼ inches from the counter and drew a line around the model.					
6. Turned on the trimmer, held the model firmly against the trimmer, and trimmed the bottom of the base to the line drawn.					
7. Drew a line ¼ inch behind the maxillary tuberosities. With the base flat on the trimmer, removed excess plaster in the posterior area of the model to the marked line.					
8. Drew a line through the center of the occlusal ridges on one side of the model. Measured out ¼ inch from the line, and drew a line parallel to the line drawn.					
9. Repeated these measurements on the other side of the model.					

Continued

10. Trimmed the sides of the cast to the lines drawn.				
11. Trimmed maxillary heel cuts by drawing a line behind the tuberosity that was perpendicular to the opposite canine.				
12. Made the final cut by drawing a line from the canine to the midline at an angle (completed this on both sides, and trimmed to the line).				
13. Occluded the mandibular model with the maxillary model using the wax bite.				
14. With the mandibular base on the trimmer, trimmed the posterior portion of the mandibular model until even with the maxillary model.				
15. Placed the models upside down (maxillary base on the table), measured 3 inches from the surface up, and marked a line around the base of the mandibular model.				
16. Trimmed the mandibular model base to the line drawn.				
17. With the models in occlusion with the wax bite, placed the mandibular model on the trimmer and trimmed the lateral cuts to match the maxillary lateral cuts.				
18. Trimmed the back and heel cuts to match the maxillary heel cuts.				
19. Checked that the mandibular anterior cut was a rounded circle from mandibular canine to mandibular canine.				
20. Mixed a slurry of gypsum and filled any voids.				
21. Used a laboratory knife to remove any extra gypsum that appeared as beads on the occlusion or model.				

22. When finished, cared for supplies and materials appropriately.					
ADDITIONAL COMMENTS					

Total number of points earned _____

Grade _____ Instructor's initials _____

COMPETENCY 47-5: CONSTRUCTING AN ACRYLIC RESIN CUSTOM TRAY

Performance Objective
By following a routine procedure that meets stated protocols, the student will construct an acrylic resin custom tray.

Evaluation and Grading Criteria
3	Student competently met the stated criteria without assistance.
2	Student required assistance in order to meet the stated criteria.
1	Student showed uncertainty when performing the stated criteria.
0	Student was not prepared and needs to repeat the step.
N/A	No evaluation of this step.

Instructor shall define grades for each point range earned on completion of each performance-evaluated task.

Performance Standards
The minimum number of satisfactory performances required before final evaluation is _____.

Instructor shall identify by * those steps considered critical. If step is missed or minimum competency is not met, the evaluated procedure fails and must be repeated.

PERFORMANCE CRITERIA	*	SELF	PEER	INSTRUCTOR	COMMENT
1. Gathered appropriate supplies.					
2. Personal protective equipment placed according to procedure.					
Preparing the Model					
1. Filled the undercuts on the diagnostic model.					
2. Outlined the tray in pencil.					
3. Placed the baseplate wax spacer, trimmed the wax, and luted it to the cast.					
4. Cut the appropriate stops in the spacer.					
5. Painted the spacer and surrounding area with separating medium.					
Mixing the Acrylic Resin					
1. Used the manufacturer's measuring devices to measure the powder into the mixing container. Then added an equal part of liquid and recapped the container immediately.					
2. Used the tongue blade to mix the powder and liquid until the mix appeared thin and sticky.					
3. Set the mix aside for 2 to 3 minutes to allow polymerization.					

Continued

Forming the Tray					
1. When the mix reached a "doughy" stage, removed it from the container with the spatula or tongue blade.					
2. Lubricated the palms of the hands with petroleum jelly and kneaded the resin to form a flat patty approximately the size of the wax spacer.					
3. Placed the material on the cast to cover the wax spacer. Adapted it to extend 1 to 1.5 mm beyond the edges of the wax spacer.					
4. Used an instrument or laboratory knife to trim away the excess tray material quickly while it was still soft.					
Creating the Handle					
1. Used the excess material to shape the handle.					
2. Placed a drop of monomer on the handle and on the tray, where they join.					
3. Attached the handle so it extended out of the mouth and was parallel with the occlusal surfaces of the teeth.					
4. Held the handle in place until it was firm.					
Finishing the Tray					
1. After the initial set (7 to 10 minutes), removed the spacer and returned the tray to the cast.					
2. Cleaned the wax completely from the inside of the tray after the tray resin had reached final cure.					
3. Finished the edges, then cleaned and disinfected the tray.					

4. When finished, cared for supplies and materials appropriately.					

ADDITIONAL COMMENTS

Total number of points earned _____

Grade _____ Instructor's initials _____

COMPETENCY 47-6: CREATING A LIGHT-CURED CUSTOM TRAY

Performance Objective

By following a routine procedure that meets stated protocols, the student will construct a light-cured custom tray.

Evaluation and Grading Criteria

- __3__   Student competently met the stated criteria without assistance.
- __2__   Student required assistance in order to meet the stated criteria.
- __1__   Student showed uncertainty when performing the stated criteria.
- __0__   Student was not prepared and needs to repeat the step.
- __N/A__   No evaluation of this step.

Instructor shall define grades for each point range earned on completion of each performance-evaluated task.

Performance Standards

The minimum number of satisfactory performances required before final evaluation is _____.

Instructor shall identify by * those steps considered critical. If step is missed or minimum competency is not met, the evaluated procedure fails and must be repeated.

PERFORMANCE CRITERIA	*	SELF	PEER	INSTRUCTOR	COMMENT
1. Gathered appropriate supplies.					
2. Personal protective equipment placed according to procedure.					
3. Completed a model before tray construction.					
4. Used a pencil to outline the vestibular area and posterior tray border on the stone model.					
5. Painted separating medium on the model before placement of the material.					
6. Adapted precut sections of the custom tray material for use on the maxillary model with full palatal coverage, and on the mandibular model without full palatal coverage.					
7. Molded the sheet of tray material to conform to the study model using the thumb and forefinger with minimal pressure.					
8. Trimmed away excess tray material with a laboratory knife. *Note:* If desired, the excess material can be used to form a handle on the tray.					
9. Placed the model and tray in a light-curing unit. Cured the tray for 2 minutes.					

Continued

10. After curing, placed the model and tray in cool water to solidify the wax spacer and facilitate separation of the tray from the model.				
11. Used the acrylic extruded through the holes in the spacer to create occlusal stops on the inside of the tray.				
12. Removed the wax spacer from the tray using a #7 wax spatula.				
13. Placed the tray in hot water to remove any remnants of wax from the inside.				
14. Trimmed the borders of the tray using an acrylic laboratory bur.				
15. Used a thin acrylic bur to perforate the custom tray.				
16. Using a laboratory acrylic bur, trimmed the borders of the edentulous tray to 2 mm short of the vestibule to allow for border molding material.				
17. When finished, cared for supplies and materials appropriately.				

ADDITIONAL COMMENTS

Total number of points earned _____

Grade _____ Instructor's initials _____

COMPETENCY 47-7: CONSTRUCTING A VACUUM-FORMED CUSTOM TRAY

Performance Objective
By following a routine procedure that meets stated protocols, the student will construct a vacuum-formed custom tray.

Evaluation and Grading Criteria
 3   Student competently met the stated criteria without assistance.
 2   Student required assistance in order to meet the stated criteria.
 1   Student showed uncertainty when performing the stated criteria.
 0   Student was not prepared and needs to repeat the step.
N/A   No evaluation of this step.
Instructor shall define grades for each point range earned on completion of each performance-evaluated task.

Performance Standards
The minimum number of satisfactory performances required before final evaluation is _____.

Instructor shall identify by * those steps considered critical. If step is missed or minimum competency is not met, the evaluated procedure fails and must be repeated.

PERFORMANCE CRITERIA	*	SELF	PEER	INSTRUCTOR	COMMENT
1. Gathered appropriate supplies.					
2. Personal protective equipment placed according to procedure.					
3. Readied a set of completed models.					
4. Trimmed the model so it extended 3 to 4 mm past the gingival border.					
5. To extend the tray from the teeth for the purpose of holding bleaching solution, placed a spacer material on the facial surfaces of the teeth on the model.					
6. Using a vacuum former, heated a tray sheet until it sagged 1/2 to 1 inch.					
7. Lowered the sheet over the model and turned on the vacuum for 10 seconds.					
8. Removed the sheet after allowing it to cool completely.					
9. Using scissors, cut the excess material from the tray.					
10. Used small, sharp scissors to trim the tray approximately 0.5 mm away from the gingival margin.					

Continued

11. Placed the tray onto the original model, and checked gingival extensions.				
12. If necessary, applied a thin coat of petroleum jelly to the facial surface. Using a low flame, gently heated and readapted the margins on the model so that all of the teeth were covered, taking care to avoid overlapping onto the gingiva.				
13. After readaptation of all the margins, retrimmed excess material.				
14. Left the tray on the model until the delivery appointment, at which time it was washed in cold, soapy water and then cold-sterilized.				
15. When finished, cared for supplies and materials appropriately.				

ADDITIONAL COMMENTS

Total number of points earned _____

Grade _____ Instructor's initials _____

48 General Dentistry

1. Describe the process and principles of cavity preparation.

2. Discuss the differences in assisting with an amalgam and with a composite procedure.

3. Discuss why retention pins would be selected for a complex restoration.

4. Describe the need for placing an intermediate restoration.

5. Describe the procedure for composite veneers.

6. Describe the role of the dental assistant in tooth whitening.

FILL-IN-THE-BLANK STATEMENTS

Select the best term from the list below and complete the following statements.

axial wall	operative dentistry
cavity	outline form
cavity wall	pulpal wall
convenience form	restoration
diastema	retention form
line angle	veneer

1. The dentist will place a direct _____ to replace decayed tooth structure.

2. An internal surface of a cavity preparation is the _____.

3. The dentist will place _____ within a cavity preparation to help retain and support the restorative material.

4. A space between two teeth is a(n) _____.

5. A(n) _____ is a thin layer of restorative material used to correct the facial surface of a tooth.

6. _____ is another term for decay.

7. _____ is the cavity preparation step that allows the dentist easier access when restoring a tooth.

8. The _____ is an internal wall of the cavity preparation that is perpendicular to the long axis of the tooth.

9. The _____ is the design and specific shape of the cavity preparation used by the dentist to restore a tooth.

10. A common term used when describing restorative and esthetic dentistry is _____.

11. The junction of two walls in a cavity preparation forms a(n) _____.

12. A(n) _____ is an internal wall of a cavity preparation that runs parallel to the long axis of the tooth.

MULTIPLE-CHOICE QUESTIONS

Complete each question by circling the best answer.

1. Restorative dentistry is often referred to as _____.
   a. fillings
   b. operative dentistry
   c. prosthetic dentistry
   d. surgical dentistry

2. Another term for decay is _____.
   a. abscess
   b. hole
   c. preparation
   d. cavity

3. The process of removing decay is known as _____.
   a. cavity preparation
   b. drill and fill
   c. extraction
   d. restoration

4. Which wall of the cavity preparation is perpendicular to the long axis of the tooth?
   a. Proximal wall
   b. Pulpal floor
   c. External wall
   d. Marginal wall

5. Where would you find a class I restoration in the mouth?
   a. Occlusal surface
   b. Buccal pit of posterior teeth
   c. Lingual pit of anterior teeth
   d. All of the above

6. How many surfaces could a class II restoration affect?
   a. One
   b. Two
   c. Three
   d. b and c

7. Which tooth could have a class II restoration?
   a. Tooth #8
   b. Tooth #13
   c. Tooth #22
   d. Tooth #26

8. What restorative material would be set up for a class IV restorative procedure?
   a. Composite resin
   b. Amalgam
   c. Veneer
   d. Bleaching

9. What kind of moisture control is recommended for class III and IV procedures?
   a. Cotton rolls
   b. 2 × 2-inch gauze
   c. Dental dam
   d. Saliva ejector

10. What population has a higher incidence of class V lesions?
    a. Children
    b. Teenagers
    c. Adults
    d. Older adults

11. Why would an intermediate restoration be placed?
    a. Health of a tooth
    b. Waiting for a permanent restoration
    c. Financial reasons
    d. All of the above

12. What tooth surface would receive a veneer?
    a. Lingual
    b. Facial
    c. Distal
    d. Incisal

13. The types of veneers commonly placed are
    _____.
    a. direct composite resin
    b. indirect porcelain
    c. amalgam
    d. a and b

14. Indications for tooth whitening are _____.
    a. extrinsic stains
    b. aged teeth
    c. intrinsic stains
    d. All of the above

15. What is used to hold tooth-whitening gel on the teeth?
    a. Thermoplastic tray
    b. Toothbrush
    c. Gauze tray
    d. Molded wax

16. An ingredient of the tooth-whitening strip is
    _____.
    a. carbamide peroxide
    b. phosphoric acid
    c. hydrogen peroxide
    d. toothpaste

17. What adverse effect may a patient experience during tooth whitening?
    a. Nausea
    b. Fever
    c. Hypersensitivity
    d. Decay

18. What classification would an MOD on tooth #14 be referred to as?
    a. Class I
    b. Class II
    c. Class III
    d. Class IV

19. What classification would a lingual pit on tooth #8 be referred to as?
    a. Class I
    b. Class II
    c. Class III
    d. Class IV

20. What classification would require the use of a matrix system?
    a. Class I
    b. Class II
    c. Class III
    d. b and c

CASE STUDY

Your next patient is scheduled to have an MO restoration on tooth #19.

1. What surfaces of the tooth are M and O?

2. What type of restorative material could be selected for this specific tooth?

3. Are there any expanded functions that could be delegated to you in this procedure? If so, what are they?

4. You will be preparing the dental dam for this procedure. Dr. Campbell prefers to isolate one tooth distal to the opposite canine. Which teeth will be involved in the isolation?

5. Will a matrix system be used for the procedure? If so, how many wedges will be placed?

6. The preparation is moderately deep. What supplemental materials besides the restorative material will you set out for this procedure? (Remember, this will depend on the restorative material.)

7. After the procedure has been completed, how is this charted in the patient record?

MULTIMEDIA PROCEDURES RECOMMENDED REVIEW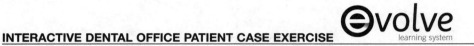

- Assisting in a Class II amalgam restoration
- Placing an intermediate restoration

INTERACTIVE DENTAL OFFICE PATIENT CASE EXERCISE

Access the *Interactive Dental Office* on *Evolve* and click on the patient case file for Crystal Malone.
- Review Ms. Malone's file.
- Complete all exercises on Evolve for Ms. Malone's case.
- Answer the following questions.

1. Define the number of teeth that have the following classifications restored: class I, II, III, IV.

2. Does Ms. Malone have any composite restorations in place at this time?

3. For what restorative procedure should Ms. Malone be scheduled?

4. Ms. Malone discovers that her insurance does not cover whitening, and she cannot afford to have the procedure completed at this time. What would be an alternative that the dental team could educate Ms. Malone about?

5. Ms. Malone had tooth #19 restored with a root canal and porcelain-fused-to-metal crown. What dental specialists might have been involved in this restoration process?

COMPETENCIES 48-1 AND 48-2: ASSISTING IN AN AMALGAM RESTORATION

Performance Objective

By following a routine procedure that meets stated protocols, the student will demonstrate the proper techniques when assisting with the preparation, placement, and finishing of an amalgam restoration.

Evaluation and Grading Criteria

_3_   Student competently met the stated criteria without assistance.
_2_   Student required assistance in order to meet the stated criteria.
_1_   Student showed uncertainty when performing the stated criteria.
_0_   Student was not prepared and needs to repeat the step.
_N/A_   No evaluation of this step.
Instructor shall define grades for each point range earned on completion of each performance-evaluated task.

Performance Standards

The minimum number of satisfactory performances required before final evaluation is _____.

Instructor shall identify by * those steps considered critical. If step is missed or minimum competency is not met, the evaluated procedure fails and must be repeated.

PERFORMANCE CRITERIA	*	SELF	PEER	INSTRUCTOR	COMMENT
1. Gathered the appropriate setup.					
2. Personal protective equipment placed according to procedure.					
3. Ensured dental materials were placed and readied.					
4. Assisted during administration of topical and local anesthetic solution.					
5. Assisted in placement of the dental dam or other moisture control devices.					
Preparing the Tooth					
6. Transferred the mirror and explorer.					
7. During cavity preparation, used the HVE and air-water syringe, adjusted the light, and retracted as necessary to maintain a clear field.					
8. Transferred the explorer, excavators, and hand cutting instruments as needed throughout cavity preparation.					
Placing the Matrix Band and Wedge (if Required)					
9. Prepared the universal retainer and matrix band according to preparation.					
10. Assisted in placement or performed complete placement of the matrix band.					

Continued

11. Assisted in placement or performed complete insertion of wedges using #110 pliers.				
Placing Dental Materials				
12. Rinsed and dried the preparation for evaluation.				
13. Mixed and transferred the base, liner, sealer, etchant, and bonding materials in the proper sequence.				
Mixing the Amalgam				
14. Activated the capsule, placed it in the amalgamator, and set the correct time for trituration.				
15. Placed mixed amalgam in the well.				
16. Reassembled the capsule and discarded it properly.				
Placing, Condensing, and Carving the Amalgam				
17. Filled the amalgam carrier and transferred it to the dentist.				
18. Transferred restorative instruments to the dentist as needed.				
19. Transferred the carving instruments.				
20. Assisted with removal of the wedge, retainer, matrix band, and dental dam.				
21. Assisted during final carving and occlusal adjustment.				
22. Gave postoperative instructions to the patient.				
23. Maintained patient comfort and followed appropriate infection control measures throughout the procedure.				
24. When finished, cared for supplies and materials appropriately.				
25. Procedure documented in patient record.				
ADDITIONAL COMMENTS				

Total number of points earned _____

Grade _____ Instructor's initials _____

COMPETENCIES 48-3 AND 48-4: ASSISTING IN A COMPOSITE RESTORATION

Performance Objective

By following a routine procedure that meets stated protocols, the student will demonstrate the proper techniques when assisting with the preparation, placement, and finishing of a composite restoration.

Evaluation and Grading Criteria

 3 Student competently met the stated criteria without assistance.
 2 Student required assistance in order to meet the stated criteria.
 1 Student showed uncertainty when performing the stated criteria.
 0 Student was not prepared and needs to repeat the step.
 N/A No evaluation of this step.
Instructor shall define grades for each point range earned on completion of each performance-evaluated task.

Performance Standards

The minimum number of satisfactory performances required before final evaluation is _____.

Instructor shall identify by * those steps considered critical. If step is missed or minimum competency is not met, the evaluated procedure fails and must be repeated.

PERFORMANCE CRITERIA	*	SELF	PEER	INSTRUCTOR	COMMENT
1. Gathered the appropriate setup.					
2. Personal protective equipment placed according to procedure.					
3. Dental materials were placed and readied.					
4. Assisted during administration of the topical and local anesthetic solutions.					
5. Assisted in selection of the shade of composite material.					
6. Assisted in placement of the dental dam or other moisture control devices.					
Preparing the Tooth					
1. Transferred the mirror and explorer.					
2. During cavity preparation, used the HVE and air-water syringe, adjusted the light, and retracted as necessary to maintain a clear field.					
3. Transferred the explorer, excavators, and hand cutting instruments as needed throughout cavity preparation.					
Placing the Matrix Band and Wedge (if Required)					
1. Prepared a clear strip and wedge according to the preparation.					
2. Assisted in placement or performed complete placement of matrix band.					

Continued

463

Chapter **48** General Dentistry

3. Assisted in placement or performed complete insertion of wedges using #110 pliers.					
Placing Dental Materials					
1. Rinsed and dried the preparation for evaluation.					
2. Mixed and transferred the base, liner, sealer, etchant, and bonding materials in proper sequence.					
Preparing the Composite					
1. Dispensed the composite material on the paper pad, and transferred it to the dentist.					
2. Transferred restorative instruments to the dentist as needed.					
3. Assisted in light-curing of the material.					
Finishing the Restoration					
1. Assisted with the transfer of burs or diamonds for the high-speed handpiece.					
2. Transferred finishing strips.					
3. Assisted with removal of the wedge, matrix band, and dental dam.					
4. Assisted during final polishing and occlusal adjustment.					
5. Gave postoperative instructions to the patient.					
6. Maintained patient comfort and followed appropriate infection control measures throughout the procedure.					
7. When finished, cared for supplies and materials appropriately.					
8. Procedure documented in patient record.					

ADDITIONAL COMMENTS

Total number of points earned _____

Grade _____ Instructor's initials _____

COMPETENCY 48-5: PLACING AND CARVING AN INTERMEDIATE RESTORATION (EXPANDED FUNCTION)

Performance Objective

By following a routine procedure that meets stated protocols, the student will demonstrate the proper technique for placing and carving an intermediate restoration.

Evaluation and Grading Criteria

 3   Student competently met the stated criteria without assistance.
 2   Student required assistance in order to meet the stated criteria.
 1   Student showed uncertainty when performing the stated criteria.
 0   Student was not prepared and needs to repeat the step.
 N/A   No evaluation of this step.
Instructor shall define grades for each point range earned on completion of each performance-evaluated task.

Performance Standards

The minimum number of satisfactory performances required before final evaluation is _____.

Instructor shall identify by * those steps considered critical. If step is missed or minimum competency is not met, the evaluated procedure fails and must be repeated.

PERFORMANCE CRITERIA	*	SELF	PEER	INSTRUCTOR	COMMENT
1. Gathered the appropriate setup.					
2. Personal protective equipment placed according to procedure.					
3. Cleaned, dried, and isolated the site with cotton rolls or a dental dam.					
4. Examined the tooth and preparation.					
5. If the preparation included a proximal wall, assembled and placed a matrix band and wedge.					
6. Mixed the IRM to the appropriate consistency.					
7. Used a plastic instrument or FP1 and took increments of the materials to the preparation. If there was an interproximal box, began filling this area first.					
8. After each increment, condensed the material using the small end of the condenser or nib first.					
9. Continued filling the preparation until it was overfilled.					
10. While the material was still in the putty form, used an explorer to remove excess material from the marginal ridge and the proximal box.					

Continued

11. Removed any excess material from the occlusal surface using the discoid-cleoid carver.				
12. If a matrix system was used, removed it at this time, leaving the wedge in place.				
13. Completed the final carving of the occlusal surface with the discoid-cleoid carver, making sure to carve back to the tooth's normal anatomy.				
14. If interproximal surface involved, uses the Hollenback carver to remove excess material from the interproximal area, making sure not to create an overhang or indentation in the material.				
15. Removed the wedge when carving was completed.				
16. Instructed the patient to bite down gently on articulating paper to check the occlusion.				
17. After the final carving, used a wet cotton pellet to wipe over the restoration.				
18. Informed the patient that the restoration was "short term," and instructed him or her not to chew sticky foods on that side.				
19. When finished, cared for supplies and materials appropriately.				
20. Procedure documented in patient record.				

ADDITIONAL COMMENTS

Total number of points earned _____

Grade _____ Instructor's initials _____

COMPETENCY 48-6: ASSISTING IN THE PLACEMENT OF A VENEER

Performance Objective

By following a routine procedure that meets stated protocols, the student will demonstrate the proper techniques when assisting in the placement of a veneer.

Evaluation and Grading Criteria

 3 Student competently met the stated criteria without assistance.
 2 Student required assistance in order to meet the stated criteria.
 1 Student showed uncertainty when performing the stated criteria.
 0 Student was not prepared and needs to repeat the step.
 N/A No evaluation of this step.
Instructor shall define grades for each point range earned on completion of each performance-evaluated task.

Performance Standards

The minimum number of satisfactory performances required before final evaluation is _____.

Instructor shall identify by * those steps considered critical. If step is missed or minimum competency is not met, the evaluated procedure fails and must be repeated.

PERFORMANCE CRITERIA	*	SELF	PEER	INSTRUCTOR	COMMENT
1. Gathered the appropriate setup.					
2. Personal protective equipment placed according to procedure.					
3. Assisted in administration of topical and local anesthetic solutions.					
4. Assisted with shade selection of the composite material.					
5. Assisted in placement of cotton rolls or placement of the dental dam.					
6. Assisted in measurement of the appropriate crown form size.					
7. Assisted in tooth preparation by maintaining moisture control and retraction for better visibility.					
8. Assisted in the placement of liners, etchant and matrix.					
9. If veneers were being placed to cover dark stains, prepared an opaque material.					
10. Transferred restorative instruments throughout the procedure.					
11. Assisted with light-curing for the time recommended by the manufacturer.					

Continued

12. Assisted with sandpaper discs, strips, and finishing burs to trim and smooth the veneer.				
13. Assisted as needed for each tooth to receive a veneer.				
14. When finished, cared for supplies and materials appropriately.				
15. Procedure documented in patient record.				

ADDITIONAL COMMENTS

Total number of points earned _____

Grade _____ Instructor's initials _____

49 Matrix Systems for Restorative Dentistry

SHORT-ANSWER QUESTIONS

1. Describe why a matrix system is required for the restoration of a class II, III, and IV.

2. Give the most common type of matrix system used for posterior restorations.

3. Describe the types of matrices used for composite restorations.

4. Discuss the purpose and use of a wedge.

5. Discuss alternative methods of matrix systems used in restorative dentistry.

FILL-IN-THE-BLANK STATEMENTS

Select the best term from the list below and complete the following statements.

automatrix   overhang
celluloid strip   palodent
cupping   universal retainer
matrix   wedge
Mylar

1. _____ and _____ are other names for a clear plastic strip that is used to provide a temporary wall for the restoration of an anterior tooth.

2. Excess restorative material that extends beyond the cavity margin because of improper wedge placement is referred to as a(n) _____.

3. _____ is a term that is used when a restoration on a tooth surface is concave and has not been contoured properly.

4. A(n) _____ is placed in the embrasure to provide the contour needed when the interproximal surfaces of a class II, III, or IV restoration are restored.

5. A(n) _____ is a band that acts as a temporary wall for a tooth structure in restoring proximal contours and contracting to its normal shape and function.

6. A(n) _____ is a small, oval-shaped matrix made of a polished stainless steel that can be used for posterior amalgam and composite materials.

7. The _____ is a matrix system designed to establish a temporary wall for the restoration of a class II restoration without the need to use it as a retainer.

8. The _____ is used to keep a matrix band in place during a class II restoration.

MULTIPLE-CHOICE QUESTIONS

Complete each question by circling the best answer.

1. Which classification would require using a matrix system?
   a. I
   b. II
   c. V
   d. VI

2. The plural word for matrix is _____.
   a. matrixes
   b. martinis
   c. matrices
   d. martins

3. Which would be used to hold a posterior matrix band in position?
   a. Cotton pliers
   b. #110 pliers
   c. Wedge
   d. Universal retainer

4. In what direction is the smaller circumference of the posterior matrix band positioned when placed properly?
   a. Gingival
   b. Occlusal
   c. Facial
   d. Lingual

5. Which instrument could be selected to thin and contour a matrix band?
   a. Carver
   b. Explorer
   c. #110 pliers
   d. Burnisher

6. What additional item is placed for a posterior matrix system to reestablish proper interproximal contact of the newly placed material?
   a. Retraction cord
   b. Wedge
   c. Cotton roll
   d. Articulating paper

7. What could improper wedge placement result in?
   a. Overfilling
   b. Cupping
   c. Overhang
   d. b and c

8. Which matrix system could be an alternative to the universal retainer?
   a. Celluloid strip
   b. Dental dam
   c. T-band
   d. Automatrix

9. Why are metal matrix bands contraindicated with the use of composite resin materials?
   a. They do not fit around anterior teeth properly.
   b. They cannot contour a metal band properly.
   c. The metal can scratch some composite resins.
   d. They keep the dentist from seeing the preparation.

10. Another term(s) for the clear matrix is _____.
   a. celluloid
   b. sandpaper strip
   c. Mylar strip
   d. a and c

CASE STUDY

You are assisting in an MOD amalgam restoration on tooth #29. During preparation of the tooth, the dentist removes an extensive amount of tooth structure on the mesial facial cusp. The cavity preparation is now below the gingival margin, creating a large preparation.

1. Have the surfaces of the restoration changed because of the final preparation? If so, what surfaces are now involved?

2. You have been asked to place the matrix system. What type of matrix system should you prepare?

3. Because the preparation has changed, are there any changes that have to be made in the setup? If so, what are they?

4. How will the matrix band be adapted for the preparation just described?

5. Which surfaces of the preparation are most critical for stabilizing the newly placed amalgam before carving?

6. How many wedges will be used, and from what direction will they be inserted?

7. Could any other matrix system have been used for this procedure? If so, what would it be?

MULTIMEDIA PROCEDURES RECOMMENDED REVIEW

- Assembling a matrix band and universal retainer
- Placing a matrix band and wedge for a Class II restoration

INTERACTIVE DENTAL OFFICE PATIENT CASE EXERCISE

Access the *Interactive Dental Office* on *Evolve* and click on the patient case file for Miguel Ricardo.
- Review Mr. Ricardo's record.
- Complete all exercises on Evolve for Mr. Ricardo's case.
- Answer the following questions.

1. Which teeth received a matrix in the restoration process?

2. Does Mr. Ricardo have any composite restorations in place at this time?

3. For what restorative procedure should Mr. Ricardo be scheduled?

4. Which tooth will be restored?

5. What type of matrix system will be prepared for the procedure?

COMPETENCY 49-1: ASSEMBLING A MATRIX BAND AND UNIVERSAL RETAINER

Performance Objective

By following a routine procedure that meets stated protocols, the student will demonstrate the proper technique for assembling a matrix band and Tofflemire retainer for each quadrant of the dental arch.

Evaluation and Grading Criteria

 3   Student competently met the stated criteria without assistance.
 2   Student required assistance in order to meet the stated criteria.
 1   Student showed uncertainty when performing the stated criteria.
 0   Student was not prepared and needs to repeat the step.
 N/A   No evaluation of this step.
Instructor shall define grades for each point range earned on completion of each performance-evaluated task.

Performance Standards

The minimum number of satisfactory performances required before final evaluation is _____.

Instructor shall identify by * those steps considered critical. If step is missed or minimum competency is not met, the evaluated procedure fails and must be repeated.

PERFORMANCE CRITERIA	*	SELF	PEER	INSTRUCTOR	COMMENT
1. Gathered the appropriate supplies.					
2. Personal protective equipment placed according to procedure.					
3. Stated which guide slot would be used for each quadrant.					
4. Determined the tooth to be treated, and selected the appropriate band.					
5. Placed the middle of the band on the paper pad, and burnished the band with a ball burnisher.					
6. Held the retainer so that the diagonal slot was visible, and turned the outer knob clockwise until the end of the spindle was visible in the diagonal slot in the vise.					
7. Turned the inner knob counterclockwise until the vise moved next to the guide slots and the retainer was ready to receive the matrix band.					
8. Identified the occlusal and gingival aspects of the matrix band, and brought the ends of the band together to form a loop.					

Continued

9. Placed the occlusal edge of the band into the retainer first, and then guided the band between the correct guide slots.					
10. Locked the band in the vise.					
11. Used the handle end of the mouth mirror to open and round the loop of the band.					
12. Adjusted the size of the loop to fit the selected tooth.					

ADDITIONAL COMMENTS

Total number of points earned _____

Grade _____ Instructor's initials _____

COMPETENCY 49-2: PLACING AND REMOVING A MATRIX BAND AND WEDGE FOR A CLASS II RESTORATION (EXPANDED FUNCTION)

Performance Objective

By following a routine procedure that meets stated protocols, the student will demonstrate the proper technique for placing a Tofflemire retainer, matrix band, and wedge on a tooth with a class II amalgam preparation. The student will then remove the matrix band, retainer, and wedge.

Evaluation and Grading Criteria

__3__ Student competently met the stated criteria without assistance.
__2__ Student required assistance in order to meet the stated criteria.
__1__ Student showed uncertainty when performing the stated criteria.
__0__ Student was not prepared and needs to repeat the step.
__N/A__ No evaluation of this step.
Instructor shall define grades for each point range earned on completion of each performance-evaluated task.

Performance Standards

The minimum number of satisfactory performances required before final evaluation is _____.

Instructor shall identify by * those steps considered critical. If step is missed or minimum competency is not met, the evaluated procedure fails and must be repeated.

PERFORMANCE CRITERIA	*	SELF	PEER	INSTRUCTOR	COMMENT
1. Personal protective equipment placed according to procedure.					
2. Used mirror and explorer to evaluate tooth for matrix.					
3. Matrix band assembled correctly in retainer for procedure.					
4. Positioned and seated the band's loop over the occlusal surface.					
5. Held the band securely while tightening it by turning the inner knob clockwise.					
6. Used an explorer to check adaptation of the band to determine that it was firm and extended no farther than 1 to 1.5 mm beyond the gingival margin of the cavity preparation.					
7. Selected the correct size and number of wedges.					
8. Used cotton pliers or #110 pliers to insert the wedge from the lingual embrasure so that the flat side of the wedge was toward the gingiva.					
9. Verified proximal contact and sealed the gingival margin.					

Continued

Band Removal					
1. Held the band securely while slowly turning the outer knob of the retainer in a counterclockwise direction.					
2. Carefully slid the retainer toward the occlusal surface.					
3. Used cotton pliers to gently spread open the ends of the matrix band and gently lift the matrix band in an occlusal direction using a seesaw motion.					
4. Removed the wedge using #110 pliers or cotton pliers.					
5. Discarded the used matrix band in the sharps container.					
6. Maintained patient comfort and followed appropriate infection control measures throughout the procedure.					

ADDITIONAL COMMENTS

Total number of points earned _____

Grade _____ Instructor's initials _____

COMPETENCY 49-3: PLACING A PLASTIC MATRIX FOR A CLASS III OR IV RESTORATION (EXPANDED FUNCTION)

Performance Objective

By following a routine procedure that meets stated protocols, the student will demonstrate the proper technique for placing and removing a plastic matrix band.

Evaluation and Grading Criteria

 3   Student competently met the stated criteria without assistance.
 2   Student required assistance in order to meet the stated criteria.
 1   Student showed uncertainty when performing the stated criteria.
 0   Student was not prepared and needs to repeat the step.
 N/A   No evaluation of this step.
Instructor shall define grades for each point range earned on completion of each performance-evaluated task.

Performance Standards

The minimum number of satisfactory performances required before final evaluation is _____.

Instructor shall identify by * those steps considered critical. If step is missed or minimum competency is not met, the evaluated procedure fails and must be repeated.

PERFORMANCE CRITERIA	*	SELF	PEER	INSTRUCTOR	COMMENT
1. Gathered the appropriate setup.					
2. Personal protective equipment placed according to procedure.					
3. Examined the contour of the tooth and preparation site, paying special attention to the outline of the preparation.					
4. Contoured the matrix strip.					
5. Slid the matrix interproximally, ensuring that the gingival edge of the matrix extended beyond the preparation.					
6. Using thumb and forefinger, pulled the band over the prepared tooth on the facial and lingual surfaces.					
7. Using cotton pliers, positioned the wedge into the gingival embrasure.					
8. Removed the matrix after the preparation was filled and light-cured.					
9. Maintained patient comfort and followed appropriate infection control measures throughout the procedure.					

Continued

ADDITIONAL COMMENTS

Total number of points earned _____

Grade _____ Instructor's initials _____

50 Fixed Prosthodontics

1. List the indications and contraindications for a patient to receive a fixed prosthesis.

2. Identify the steps for a diagnostic workup.

3. Describe the role of the laboratory technician.

4. Describe the differences among a full crown, inlay, onlay, and veneer crown.

5. Identify the components of a fixed bridge.

6. Describe the uses of porcelain for fixed prosthodontics.

7. Describe the preparation and placement of a cast crown.

8. Discuss why the use of a core buildup, pin, or post may be required for crown retention.

9. Describe the use of a retraction cord before a final impression is taken.

10. Describe the function of provisional coverage for a crown or fixed bridge.

11. Provide home care instructions for a permanent fixed prosthesis.

FILL-IN-THE-BLANK STATEMENTS

Select the best term from the list below and complete the following statements.

abutment
articulator
cast post
core
die
fixed bridge
full crown
gingival retraction cord
hypertrophied
inlay

investment material
master cast
onlay
opaquer
pontic
Porcelain Fused to Metal
resin-bonded bridge
three-quarter crown
unit
veneer

1. A(n) _____ is a preformed post that is fitted into the canal of an endodontically treated tooth to improve the retention of a cast restoration.

2. The _____ is a buildup of restorative material that provides a larger area of retention for the permanent crown.

3. A(n) _____ is a replica of the prepared portion of a tooth that is used in the laboratory during the making of a cast restoration.

4. A(n) _____ can be a tooth, a root, or an implant used for the retention of a fixed or removable prosthesis.

5. A dental laboratory device that simulates the movements of the mandible and the temporomandibular joint is the

   _____.

6. A fixed prosthetic with artificial teeth that is permanently cemented to natural teeth is called a(n) _____.

7. _____ displaces gingival tissues away from the tooth.

8. A(n) _____ is a cast restoration that covers the entire anatomic portion of a single tooth.

9. A cast restoration designed to restore a conservative class II restoration is a(n) _____.

10. _____ means overgrown tissue.

11. A(n) _____ is a cast that is created from a final impression used to construct baseplates, bite rims, wax setups, and the finished prosthesis.

12. _____ is a special gypsum material that is able to withstand extreme heat.

13. The _____ is an artificial tooth in a bridge that replaces a natural missing tooth.

14. _____ is a type of indirect restoration in which a thin porcelain material is fused to the facial portion of a gold crown.

15. A(n) _____ is a layer of tooth-colored material that is bonded or cemented to the prepared facial surface of a tooth.

16. The _____ is a cast restoration designed to restore the occlusal crown and proximal surfaces of a posterior tooth.

17. A(n) _____, also referred to as a *Maryland bridge,* has winglike projections that are bonded to the lingual surfaces of adjacent teeth.

18. A(n) _____ is a resin material that is placed under a porcelain restoration to prevent discoloration of the tooth from showing.

19. A(n) _____ is a cast restoration that covers the anatomic crown of a tooth except for the facial or buccal portion.

20. Each single component of a fixed bridge is considered a _____.

MULTIPLE-CHOICE QUESTIONS

Complete each question by circling the best answer.

1. Fixed prosthodontics is commonly referred to as _____.
   a. operative
   b. crown and bridge
   c. dentures
   d. prosthetics

2. What could be a contraindication to a patient receiving a fixed prosthesis?
   a. Being overweight
   b. Being over the age of 60
   c. Having poor oral hygiene
   d. Having poor personal hygiene

3. What would the dentist use to reduce the height and contour of a tooth for a casting?
   a. Hand cutting instrument
   b. Sandpaper disk
   c. Model trimmer
   d. Rotary instruments

4. If a tooth is nonvital, what is fabricated and placed into the pulp for better retention of a crown?
   a. Post and core
   b. Root canal filling
   c. Abutment
   d. Pontic

5. A(n) _____ is used during a crown and bridge preparation to displace gingival tissue.
   a. Cotton roll
   b. Dental dam
   c. Gingival retraction cord
   d. Explorer

6. What astringent can be applied to a retraction cord to control bleeding?
   a. Hydrogen peroxide
   b. Hemodent
   c. Disinfectant
   d. Coumadin

7. Another term for overgrown gingival tissue is _____.
   a. hyperthyroid
   b. hyperplasia
   c. hypertrophied
   d. b and c

8. What type of impression is taken to be sent to the dental laboratory for the preparation of a crown?
   a. Preliminary
   b. Final
   c. Secondary
   d. Wax bite

9. How does the dentist convey to the laboratory technician what type of crown is to be made?
   a. Conference call
   b. Fax
   c. Laboratory prescription
   d. Copy of the patient record

10. The laboratory technician prepares an exact replica of the prepared tooth. What is this replica called?
    a. Model
    b. Die
    c. Temporary
    d. Impression

11. What does the patient wear on a prepared tooth while the laboratory is fabricating a crown or a bridge?
    a. Amalgam
    b. Provisional
    c. Wax
    d. Intermediate restorative material

12. Who in the dental office can legally cement a permanent crown or bridge?
    a. Dentist
    b. Hygienist
    c. Assistant
    d. Laboratory technician

13. Which of the following is the minimum number of appointments needed to fabricate a fixed bridge?
    a. One
    b. Two
    c. Three
    d. Four

14. What accessory is used to help in flossing a bridge?
    a. Waterpik
    b. Rubber tip
    c. Floss threader
    d. Electric toothbrush

15. How will the laboratory technician adhere the units of a bridge together?
    a. Permanent cement
    b. Bonding
    c. Light cure
    d. Solder

16. Which is an advantage for the patient of a computer-assisted restoration (CAD/CAM)?
    a. One office visit
    b. No impressions
    c. Reduced tooth sensitivity
    d. All of the above

CASE STUDY

Mandy Moore requires a three-unit bridge for teeth #11, #12, and #13. Because of prolonged neglect of her dental needs, Mandy must first go through a series of dental appointments to correct oral hygiene and restorative problems first before they can start the preparation of the bridge.

1. What hygiene problems might interfere with Mandy's having a bridge placed?

2. What type of bridge might be recommended for the affected teeth?

3. Which teeth are the abutment(s) and which are the pontic(s) for the bridge?

4. What type of impression(s) may be taken through this restoration process?

5. Describe the type of provisional that would best suit this patient.

6. Chart the following procedure for the type of bridge described in question 2.

7. What expanded functions may be possible for you to complete throughout this procedure?

- Placing and Removing Retraction Cord

INTERACTIVE DENTAL OFFICE PATIENT CASE EXERCISE

Access the *Interactive Dental Office* on *Evolve* and click on the patient case file for Jessica Brooks.
- Review Ms. Brooks's record.
- Complete all exercises on Evolve for Ms. Brooks's case.
- Answer the following questions.

1. Does Ms. Brooks have any existing crown and bridge work?

2. If she was charted to have an amalgam, why did the procedure change to that for a crown?

3. Why did Ms. Brooks require a core buildup?

4. What type of crown was prescribed for the preparation?

5. Are there any specific oral hygiene procedures that should be given to Ms. Brooks for the care of a crown?

COMPETENCY 50-1: PLACING AND REMOVING A GINGIVAL RETRACTION CORD (EXPANDED FUNCTION)

Performance Objective

By following a routine procedure that meets stated protocols, the student will demonstrate the proper technique for placing, packing, and removing a gingival retraction cord.

Evaluation and Grading Criteria

<u>3</u>   Student competently met the stated criteria without assistance.
<u>2</u>   Student required assistance in order to meet the stated criteria.
<u>1</u>   Student showed uncertainty when performing the stated criteria.
<u>0</u>   Student was not prepared and needs to repeat the step.
<u>N/A</u> No evaluation of this step.
Instructor shall define grades for each point range earned on completion of each performance-evaluated task.

Performance Standards

The minimum number of satisfactory performances required before final evaluation is _____.

Instructor shall identify by * those steps considered critical. If step is missed or minimum competency is not met, the evaluated procedure fails and must be repeated.

PERFORMANCE CRITERIA	*	SELF	PEER	INSTRUCTOR	COMMENT
1. Gathered the appropriate setup.					
2. Personal protective equipment placed according to procedure.					
3. Rinsed and gently dried the prepared tooth and isolated the quadrant with cotton rolls.					
4. Cut a piece of retraction cord 1 to 1½ inches in length, depending on the size and type of tooth under preparation.					
5. Formed a loose loop of the cord and placed the cord in the cotton pliers.					
6. Slipped the loop of the retraction cord over the tooth so that the overlapping ends were on the facial or buccal surface.					
7. Laid the cord into the sulcus. Then used the packing instrument and, working in a clockwise direction, packed the cord gently but firmly into the sulcus.					
8. Used a gentle rocking movement of the instrument as it moved forward to the next loose section of retraction cord. Repeated this action until the length of cord was packed in place.					

Continued

9. Overlapped the working end of the cord where it met the first end of the cord. Tucked the ends into the sulcus on the facial aspect.				
10. Left the cord in place for no longer than 5 to 7 minutes. During this time, advised the patient to remain still, and kept the area dry.				
Removing the Cord				
11. Grasped the end of the retraction cord with cotton pliers and removed the cord in a counterclockwise direction.				
12. If instructed by the operator, gently dried the area and placed fresh cotton rolls.				
13. Procedure documented in patient record.				
ADDITIONAL COMMENTS				

Total number of points earned _____

Grade _____ Instructor's initials _____

COMPETENCY 50-2: ASSISTING IN A CROWN AND BRIDGE PREPARATION

Performance Objective

By following a routine procedure that meets stated protocols, the student will demonstrate the proper technique when assisting with the preparation for a crown and bridge restoration.

Evaluation and Grading Criteria

  3   Student competently met the stated criteria without assistance.
  2   Student required assistance in order to meet the stated criteria.
  1   Student showed uncertainty when performing the stated criteria.
  0   Student was not prepared and needs to repeat the step.
N/A   No evaluation of this step.
Instructor shall define grades for each point range earned on completion of each performance-evaluated task.

Performance Standards

The minimum number of satisfactory performances required before final evaluation is _____.

Instructor shall identify by * those steps considered critical. If step is missed or minimum competency is not met, the evaluated procedure fails and must be repeated.

PERFORMANCE CRITERIA	*	SELF	PEER	INSTRUCTOR	COMMENT
1. Gathered the appropriate setup.					
2. Personal protective equipment placed according to procedure.					
3. Assisted during administration of topical and local anesthetic solutions.					
4. Took a preliminary impression for making the provisional coverage.					
5. Throughout the preparation, maintained a clear, well-lighted operating field.					
6. Anticipated the dentist's needs. Transferred instruments and changed burs as necessary.					
7. Assisted or placed gingival retraction cord.					
8. Assisted in mixing the impression material and taking the final impression.					
9. Assisted or fabricated the provisional coverage.					
10. Temporarily cemented the provisional coverage.					
11. Provides full mouth rinse.					

Continued

12. Procedure documented in patient record.					
13. Prepared the laboratory prescription to be sent with impression.					
14. Maintained patient comfort and followed appropriate infection control measures throughout the procedure.					

ADDITIONAL COMMENTS

Total number of points earned _____

Grade _____ Instructor's initials _____

COMPETENCY 50-3: ASSISTING IN THE DELIVERY AND CEMENTATION OF A CAST RESTORATION

Performance Objective

By following a routine procedure that meets stated protocols, the student will demonstrate the proper technique when assisting during the cementation of a crown and bridge restoration.

Evaluation and Grading Criteria

<u>3</u>   Student competently met the stated criteria without assistance.
<u>2</u>   Student required assistance in order to meet the stated criteria.
<u>1</u>   Student showed uncertainty when performing the stated criteria.
<u>0</u>   Student was not prepared and needs to repeat the step.
<u>N/A</u> No evaluation of this step.
Instructor shall define grades for each point range earned on completion of each performance-evaluated task.

Performance Standards

The minimum number of satisfactory performances required before final evaluation is _____.

Instructor shall identify by * those steps considered critical. If step is missed or minimum competency is not met, the evaluated procedure fails and must be repeated.

PERFORMANCE CRITERIA	*	SELF	PEER	INSTRUCTOR	COMMENT
1. Determined in advance that the case had been returned from the laboratory.					
2. Gathered the appropriate setup.					
3. Personal protective equipment placed according to procedure.					
4. Assisted during administration of topical and local anesthetic solutions.					
5. Assisted during the removal of provisional coverage. (In a state where it is legal, removed the provisional coverage.)					
6. Anticipated the dentist's needs while the casting was tried and adjusted.					
7. Assisted with placement of or placed cotton rolls to isolate the quadrant and keep the area dry.					
8. Assisted during placement of cavity varnish or desensitizer.					
9. At a signal from the dentist, mixed the cement, lined the internal surface of the casting with a thin coating of cement, and transferred the prepared crown to the dentist.					
10. Instructs patient to bite down on cotton rolls while cement hardens.					

Continued

11. Removed excess cement using explorer, floss and air/water to clean around the crown.				
12. Provided home care instructions to the patient.				
13. Maintained patient comfort and followed appropriate infection control measures throughout the procedure.				
14. Procedure documented in patient record.				

ADDITIONAL COMMENTS

Total number of points earned _____

Grade _____ Instructor's initials _____

COMPETENCY 50-4: ASSISTING IN A CAD/CAM PROCEDURE (EXPANDED FUNCTION)

Performance Objective
By following a routine procedure that meets stated protocols, the student will demonstrate the proper procedures when assisting during a CAD/CAM restoration.

Evaluation and Grading Criteria
  3   Student competently met the stated criteria without assistance.
  2   Student required assistance in order to meet the stated criteria.
  1   Student showed uncertainty when performing the stated criteria.
  0   Student was not prepared and needs to repeat the step.
 N/A No evaluation of this step.
Instructor shall define grades for each point range earned on completion of each performance-evaluated task.

Performance Standards
The minimum number of satisfactory performances required before final evaluation is _____.

Instructor shall identify by * those steps considered critical. If step is missed or minimum competency is not met, the evaluated procedure fails and must be repeated.

PERFORMANCE CRITERIA	*	SELF	PEER	INSTRUCTOR	COMMENT
1. Gathered the appropriate setup.					
2. Personal protective equipment placed according to procedure.					
3. Selected the shade of ceramic to be used.					
4. Assisted during administration of topical and local anesthetic solutions.					
5. Placed cotton rolls, dri-angle, or dental dam to control moisture.					
6. Prepared surrounding teeth with Optispray to obtain photos of the occlusal registration before the removal of tooth structure or restorative material.					
7. Assisted in the removal of tooth structure, exchanging the handpiece and hand cutting instruments.					
8. Completed moisture control throughout the procedure. Rinsed and dried tooth.					
9. Assisted in the placement of gingival retraction if needed.					
10. Prepared the surrounding soft tissue with the Optispray for the taking of an optical impression.					

Continued

11. Took a digital impression using the system camera.				
12. Using the images taken, outlined the new restoration.				
13. Transferred the images to the screen using the toggle switch to view all sides of the restoration to examine the margins.				
14. The contacts and anatomy are viewed and changes are made on the computer screen.				
15. Initiated the computer to mill the restoration from the ceramic block.				
16. The restoration is tried in and readies the finishing burs and disks for adjustment.				
17. Assisted in the etching and bonding agents.				
18. The cement is readied and a thin film is placed in the restoration.				
19. Following the cementation, readies the articulating paper and floss to check the occlusal bite and contacts for accuracy.				
20. Maintained patient comfort and followed appropriate infection control measures throughout the procedure.				
21. Procedure documented in patient record.				
ADDITIONAL COMMENTS				

Total number of points earned _____

Grade _____ Instructor's initials _____

51 Provisional Coverage

SHORT-ANSWER QUESTIONS

1. Discuss the indications for provisional coverage for a crown or a fixed bridge preparation.

2. List the varying types of provisional coverage.

3. Discuss the role of the expanded-functions dental assistant in making a provisional.

4. Identify home care instructions for provisional coverage.

FILL-IN-THE-BLANK STATEMENTS

Select the best term from the list below and complete the following statements.

custom provisional
polycarbonate crown
preformed

provisional
stainless steel crown

1. A(n) _____ is a type of temporary coverage designed from a preliminary impression or a thermoplastic tray that replicates the tooth being prepared.

2. A(n) _____ is the term used for temporary coverage that is to be worn during cast-preparation.

3. An object that is already shaped in the appearance required is termed _____.

4. The _____ is a thin metal material used for provisional coverage of primary molars.

5. A(n) _____ is a provisional that is tooth-colored and used commonly for anterior teeth.

MULTIPLE-CHOICE QUESTIONS

Complete each question by circling the best answer.

1. A temporary covering for a single crown or a bridge is referred to as _____.
   a. an interim
   b. a provisional
   c. a crown
   d. a tray

2. In most cases, how long will a patient normally wear a provisional?
   a. 2 to 4 weeks
   b. 2 to 4 months
   c. 6 months
   d. 1 year

493

3. Who can legally fabricate and temporarily cement a provisional in the dental office?
   a. Dentist
   b. Expanded-functions assistant
   c. Hygienist
   d. All of the above

4. What type of provisional is the most natural looking?
   a. Polycarbonate
   b. Aluminum
   c. Preformed acrylic
   d. Custom

5. What type of provisional could be fabricated for anterior teeth?
   a. Stainless steel
   b. Aluminum
   c. Preformed polycarbonate
   d. a and c

6. What is required before the dentist prepares the tooth for making a custom provisional?
   a. Preliminary impression
   b. Placement of gingival retraction cord
   c. Post and core
   d. Anesthesia

7. What type of dental material would be selected when making a custom provisional?
   a. Hydrocolloid
   b. Silicone
   c. Acrylic resin
   d. Amalgam

8. What would the dentist select to trim or contour a stainless steel crown outside of the mouth?
   a. Sandpaper disk
   b. Curved crown and bridge scissors
   c. Lathe
   d. Model trimmer

9. When using a polycarbonate crown as a provisional, would the crown remain on the prepared tooth as the temporary, or act as a mold for the provisional?
   a. Remains on the prepared tooth
   b. Acts as a mold for the material
   c. Either a or b
   d. Not used as a provisional

10. Where is the acrylic resin extruded when preparing a provisional crown?
    a. Only on the adjacent teeth
    b. In the preliminary impression
    c. In the thermoplastic tray
    d. b or c

CASE STUDY

You have been asked to fabricate a custom provisional for tooth #30.

1. Is there any other type of temporary that could be used for this tooth? If so, what kind?

2. Describe two ways in which you can fabricate a custom provisional.

3. What specific areas of the provisional are the most critical for fit when trimming?

4. What specific instruments will you use in trimming and finishing the provisional?

5. After removing the provisional from the prepared tooth, you notice that the margins are "short" and not within 1 mm of the margin. What is your plan of action in improving the provisional so that it fits properly?

6. Once you have the provisional fitting properly, what is the next step before cementing the provisional?

7. What is set up for cementation of the provisional? Describe the steps in the removal of excess cement around the provisional.

MULTIMEDIA PROCEDURES RECOMMENDED REVIEW

■ Fabricating a Custom Acrylic Provisional Crown

INTERACTIVE DENTAL OFFICE PATIENT CASE EXERCISE

Access the *Interactive Dental Office* on *Evolve* and click on the patient case file for Chester Higgins.
■ Review Mr. Higgins's record.
■ Complete all exercises on Evolve for Mr. Higgins's case.
■ Answer the following questions.

1. What teeth are involved in the three-unit bridge?

2. What type of provisional was selected to fabricate for this case?

3. Besides an alginate impression, what can be used in making a custom provisional?

4. What cement should be used for the cementation of the provisional?

5. What type of home care instructions should be given for provisional coverage?

COMPETENCIES 51-1 AND 51-2: FABRICATING AND CEMENTING A CUSTOM ACRYLIC PROVISIONAL CROWN OR BRIDGE (EXPANDED FUNCTION)

Performance Objective

By following a routine procedure that meets stated protocols, the student will demonstrate the proper technique for preparing and placing temporary coverage for a tooth prepared to receive a crown.

Evaluation and Grading Criteria

3   Student competently met the stated criteria without assistance.
2   Student required assistance in order to meet the stated criteria.
1   Student showed uncertainty when performing the stated criteria.
0   Student was not prepared and needs to repeat the step.
N/A   No evaluation of this step.

Instructor shall define grades for each point range earned on completion of each performance-evaluated task.

Performance Standards

The minimum number of satisfactory performances required before final evaluation is _____.

Instructor shall identify by * those steps considered critical. If step is missed or minimum competency is not met, the evaluated procedure fails and must be repeated.

PERFORMANCE CRITERIA	*	SELF	PEER	INSTRUCTOR	COMMENT
Preliminary Impression					
1. Gathered the appropriate setup.					
2. Personal protective equipment placed according to procedure.					
3. Obtained the preliminary impression.					
4. Isolated and dried the prepared tooth.					
5. If using a separating medium, placed a thin layer on the tooth.					
6. Prepared provisional material according to the manufacturer's directions.					
7. Placed the material in the impression in the area of the tooth. Returned the impression to the mouth and allowed it to set for a minimum of 3 minutes.					
8. Removed the impression from the patient's mouth, and then removed the provisional coverage from the impression.					
9. Located the interproximal contact point and margin of the provisional					
10. Used acrylic burs to trim the temporary coverage.					

Continued

11. Cured the provisional coverage according to the manufacturer's instructions.				
12. After curing, removed any excess material with finishing diamonds, disks, or finishing burs.				
13. Checked the occlusion and made any adjustments using the laboratory burs and disks on the provisional outside of the mouth.				
14. Completed final polishing using rubber disks and polishing lathe and pumice.				
Cementation				
1. Mixed the temporary cement and filled the crown.				
2. Seated the provisional coverage and allowed the cement to set.				
3. Removed any excess cement and checked the occlusion.				
4. Had the dentist check and evaluate the procedure.				
5. Provided the patient with home care instructions.				
6. Maintained patient comfort and followed appropriate infection control measures throughout the procedure.				
7. Procedure documented in patient record.				

ADDITIONAL COMMENTS

Total number of points earned _____

Grade _____ Instructor's initials _____

COMPETENCY 51-3: FABRICATING AND CEMENTING A PREFORMED PROVISIONAL CROWN (EXPANDED FUNCTION)

Performance Objective

By following a routine procedure that meets stated protocols, the student will prepare and temporarily cement a pre-formed provisional crown.

Grading Criteria

__3__   Student competently met the stated criteria without assistance.
__2__   Student required assistance in order to meet the stated criteria.
__1__   Student showed uncertainty when performing the stated criteria.
__0__   Student was not prepared and needs to repeat the step.
__N/A__   No evaluation of this step.
Instructor shall define grades for each point range earned on completion of each performance-evaluated task.

Performance Standards

The minimum number of satisfactory performances required before final evaluation is _____.

Instructor shall identify by * those steps considered critical. If step is missed or minimum competency is not met, the evaluated procedure fails and must be repeated.

PERFORMANCE CRITERIA	*	SELF	PEER	INSTRUCTOR	COMMENT
Preparation					
1. Gathered the appropriate setup.					
2. Personal protective equipment placed according to procedure.					
3. Selected the appropriate shape and size of crown and checked for width, length, and adaptation at the margins.					
4. Used crown and bridge scissors to reduce the height of the crown by trimming the cervical margin.					
5. Smoothed rough edges with an acrylic trimming stone or an acrylic bur.					
6. Polished the edges with a Burlew wheel or on a lathe with pumice.					
Cementation					
1. Mixed the temporary cement and filled the crown.					
2. Seated the provisional coverage and allowed the cement to set.					
3. Removed excess cement with explorer and floss.					

Continued

4. Readied articulating paper to check occlusion.				
5. Provided the patient with home care instructions.				
6. Maintained patient comfort and followed appropriate infection control measures throughout the procedure.				
7. Procedure documented in patient record.				

ADDITIONAL COMMENTS

Total number of points earned _____

Grade _____ Instructor's initials _____

52 Removable Prosthodontics

SHORT-ANSWER QUESTIONS

1. Differentiate between a partial and a full denture.

2. Give indications and contraindications for removable partials and full dentures.

3. List the components of a partial denture.

4. List the components of a full denture.

5. Describe the steps in the construction of a removable partial denture.

6. Describe the steps in the construction of a full denture.

7. Discuss the construction of an overdenture and an immediate denture.

8. Describe home care instructions for removable partial and full dentures.

9. Identify the process of relining or repairing a partial or full denture.

FILL-IN-THE-BLANK STATEMENTS

Select the best term from the list below and complete the following statements.

- border molding
- centric relation
- connectors
- coping
- edentulous
- festooning
- flange

- framework
- full denture
- immediate denture
- lateral excursion
- mastication
- occlusal rim
- partial denture

○ post dam
○ pressure points
○ protrusion

○ relining
○ retainer
○ retrusion

1. _____ is having the maxillary and mandibular arches in a position that produces a centrally related occlusion.

2. A metal bar that joins various parts of the partial denture together is a(n) _____.

3. In _____, you use the fingers to contour a closer adaptation of the margins of an impression while it is still in the mouth.

4. A thin metal covering or cap placed over a prepared tooth in the preparation of a denture is a(n) _____.

5. _____ means without teeth.

6. A procedure to trim or shape a denture to simulate normal tissue appearance is _____.

7. The parts of a full or partial denture that extend from the teeth to the border of the denture are the _____.

8. The _____ is the metal skeleton of the removable partial denture.

9. _____ is the term for chewing.

10. A(n) _____ is a prosthesis that replaces all teeth in one arch.

11. A temporary denture placed after the extraction of anterior teeth is a(n) _____.

12. _____ is the sliding position of the mandible to the left or right of the centric position.

13. The _____ is built on the baseplate to register vertical dimension and occlusal relationship of the mandibular and maxillary arches.

14. The _____ is a seal at the posterior of a full or partial denture that holds it in place.

15. Specific areas in the mouth where a removable prosthesis may rub or apply more force are the _____.

16. _____ is the position of the mandible placed forward as related to the maxilla.

17. A(n) _____ is a removable prosthesis that replaces one or several teeth within the same arch.

18. _____ is the process of resurfacing the tissue side of a partial or full denture so that it fits more accurately.

19. The _____ is a device used to hold something in place, such as the attachments or abutments of a removable prosthesis.

20. _____ is the position of the mandible posterior from the centric position as related to the maxilla.

MULTIPLE-CHOICE QUESTIONS

Complete each question by circling the best answer.

1. The term for a removable prosthesis that replaces one
   or more teeth is a(n) _____.
   a. bridge
   b. denture
   c. partial
   d. custom tray

2. What could affect a person's decision when choosing
   a removable prosthesis?
   a. Increase in salary or promotion
   b. Improve appearance
   c. Build confidence
   d. b and c

3. The presence of a new prosthesis can _____
   the flow of saliva.
   a. increase
   b. decrease
   c. change the texture in
   d. cause no change in

4. Why is it important for the alveolar ridge to be evenly
   contoured for the fitting of a removable prosthesis?
   a. For mastication
   b. For a natural smile
   c. For a better fit
   d. a and c

5. What oral habits can affect the choice of a removable
   prosthesis?
   a. Clenching
   b. Grinding
   c. Mouth breathing
   d. All of the above

6. The metal skeleton of a partial is referred to as the
   _____.
   a. internal partial
   b. framework
   c. clasp
   d. retainer

7. A retainer on a partial can also be called a
   _____.
   a. connector
   b. base
   c. rest
   d. clasp

8. What component of a partial controls the way it is
   seated in the mouth?
   a. Connectors
   b. Base
   c. Rests
   d. Clasp

9. What impression material would be selected and
   prepared for taking a final impression for a partial?
   a. Hydrocolloid
   b. Elastomeric
   c. Silicone
   d. Alginate

10. What dental material would the laboratory technician
    use to set the teeth for the try-in appointment for a
    denture?
    a. Alginate
    b. Plaster
    c. Stone
    d. Wax

11. The suction seal that is created between the denture
    and the mouth is the _____.
    a. post dam
    b. base
    c. border molding
    d. reline

12. How many teeth are in a full set of dentures?
    a. 8
    b. 16
    c. 28
    d. 32

13. What technique does the dentist use to modify the
    borders of an impression?
    a. Relining
    b. Tissue conditioning
    c. Articulating
    d. Border molding

14. What is a "smile line"?
    a. Space between the maxillary and mandibular
       teeth
    b. The portion of the teeth showing when a patient
       smiles
    c. Shape of the teeth when a patient smiles
    d. The patient's degree of happiness with the
       dentures

15. Which position of the jaw does the dentist measure when articulating a denture?
    a. Centric relation
    b. Protrusion
    c. Retrusion
    d. All of the above

16. When is an immediate denture most commonly prescribed?
    a. After a root canal
    b. After extraction of anterior teeth
    c. After extraction of posterior teeth
    d. After periodontal surgery

17. What is the normal length of time for an immediate denture to be worn?
    a. A few days
    b. A few weeks
    c. A few months
    d. A year

18. How is an overdenture supported in the mouth?
    a. Teeth
    b. Implant
    c. Oral mucosa
    d. a and c

19. The term for placing a new layer of resin over the tissue surface of a prosthesis is _____.
    a. border molding
    b. relining
    c. waxing
    d. polishing

20. A complicated denture repair involving the replacement of teeth or a fracture in the framework is usually completed by the _____.
    a. dentist
    b. dental assistant
    c. dental laboratory technician
    d. prosthodontist

CASE STUDY

A friend of the family comes to you for advice. Her dentist has recommended that she have a partial made to replace teeth #19-#21, #28- #30. She is confused as to the options that her dentist discussed with her, and she wants your advice.

1. What is your position in giving family and friend's advice about their dental needs?

2. What are the reasons a dentist would recommend a partial as opposed to two separate bridges?

3. What are the reasons a dentist would recommend a partial versus having the remaining teeth extracted and having a denture made?

4. What are the reasons a dentist would recommend a partial rather than having implants placed?

5. What is the role of the dental laboratory technician in making a partial?

Access the *Interactive Dental Office* on *Evolve* and click on the patient case file for Jose Escobar.
■ Review Mr. Escobar's record.
■ Complete all exercises on Evolve for Mr. Escobar's case.
■ Answer the following questions.

1. How many teeth does Mr. Escobar already have missing?

2. What other specialists might have been involved in the development of the treatment plan?

3. Is Mr. Escobar receiving a full or a partial denture?

4. Why were implants not discussed as a possible treatment?

5. Is it probable that Mr. Escobar will need to have his denture relined? Why is this so?

COMPETENCIES 52-1 TO 52-3: ASSISTING IN THE DELIVERY OF A PARTIAL AND/OR COMPLETE DENTURE

Performance Objective

By following a routine procedure that meets stated protocols, the student will demonstrate the proper technique when assisting with the preparation and placement of a complete and/or partial denture.

Evaluation and Grading Criteria

__3__   Student competently met the stated criteria without assistance.
__2__   Student required assistance in order to meet the stated criteria.
__1__   Student showed uncertainty when performing the stated criteria.
__0__   Student was not prepared and needs to repeat the step.
__N/A__   No evaluation of this step.
Instructor shall define grades for each point range earned on completion of each performance-evaluated task.

Performance Standards

The minimum number of satisfactory performances required before final evaluation is _____.

Instructor shall identify by * those steps considered critical. If step is missed or minimum competency is not met, the evaluated procedure fails and must be repeated.

PERFORMANCE CRITERIA	*	SELF	PEER	INSTRUCTOR	COMMENT
Preliminary Visits					
1. Exposed radiographs as requested.					
2. Prepared diagnostic cast.					
3. Prepared custom tray.					
Preparation Visit					
1. Gathered the appropriate setup.					
2. Personal protective equipment placed according to procedure.					
3. Assisted during preparation of the teeth.					
4. Assisted in obtaining the final impression, opposing arch impression, and intraoral occlusal registration.					
5. Disinfected the completed impressions.					
6. Recorded the shade and type of artificial teeth in the patient's record.					
7. Prepared the case for shipment to the commercial laboratory.					
Try-in Visit(s)					
1. Before the patient's appointment, determined that the case had been returned from the laboratory.					
2. Assisted the dentist during try-in and adjustment of the appliance.					
3. When the appliance was removed, disinfected it and prepared the case to be returned to the laboratory for completion.					

Continued

Delivery Visit				
1. Before the patient's appointment, determined that the completed case had been returned from the laboratory.				
2. Gathered the appropriate setup.				
3. Assisted in making any necessary adjustments.				
4. Provided the patient with home care instructions.				
5. Procedue documented in patient record.				
ADDITIONAL COMMENTS				

Total number of points earned _____

Grade _____ Instructor's initials _____

COMPETENCY 52-4: REPAIRING A FRACTURED DENTURE (EXPANDED FUNCTION)

Performance Objective

By following a routine procedure that meets stated protocols, the student will demonstrate the proper technique for repairing an upper or lower partial or full denture. Infection control protocol must be followed during the procedure.

Evaluation and Grading Criteria

 3   Student competently met the stated criteria without assistance.
 2   Student required assistance in order to meet the stated criteria.
 1   Student showed uncertainty when performing the stated criteria.
 0   Student was not prepared and needs to repeat the step.
 N/A No evaluation of this step.

Instructor shall define grades for each point range earned on completion of each performance-evaluated task.

Performance Standards

The minimum number of satisfactory performances required before final evaluation is _____.

Instructor shall identify by * those steps considered critical. If step is missed or minimum competency is not met, the evaluated procedure fails and must be repeated.

PERFORMANCE CRITERIA	*	SELF	PEER	INSTRUCTOR	COMMENT
1. Assembled the appropriate setup.					
2. Personal protective equipment placed according to procedure.					
3. Cleaned and disinfected the partial or denture for repair.					
4. Aligned the fractured denture parts and applied sticky wax over the fracture line on the external surface of the denture.					
5. Examined the denture and blocked out all undercuts on the internal surface that would be exposed to the plaster using a slurry mix or block out wax.					
6. Prepared a plaster mix using a rubber bowl and spatula.					
7. Slowly poured the plaster into the internal surface of the denture so that the plaster covered the fracture line but not the entire denture.					
8. Placed the denture in an upright position and allowed the plaster to set.					
9. Once the plaster had set, gently removed it from the cast.					
10. Removed the sticky wax and pumice.					

Continued

509

11. With an acrylic bur, widened the fracture lines on the denture and placed retentive grooves along the fracture line.					
12. Applied a thin coat of the acrylic monomer to the fracture lines, followed by placing a small amount of the acrylic powder. Alternated the liquid and powder until the fracture line was filled.					
13. Once the material had cured, smoothed and polished the area on the dental lathe.					
14. Cleaned and disinfected the denture before trying it for fit on the patient.					
15. Procedure documented in patient record.					

ADDITIONAL COMMENTS

Total number of points earned _____

Grade _____ Instructor's initials _____

53 Dental Implants

SHORT-ANSWER QUESTIONS

1. List the indications and contraindications for dental implants.

2. Discuss the selection of patients who can receive dental implants.

3. Identify the different types of dental implants.

4. Describe the surgical procedures for implantation.

5. Describe the home care procedures and follow-up visits required after dental implants have been received.

FILL-IN-THE-BLANK STATEMENTS

Select the best term from the list below and complete the following statements.

- circumoral
- endosteal
- implants
- osseointegration
- stent
- subperiosteal
- titanium
- transosteal

1. A type of implant that is inserted through the inferior border of the mandible is a(n) _____ implant.

2. A type of implant that is surgically embedded into the bone is a(n) _____ implant.

3. _____ is the attachment of healthy bone to a dental implant.

4. _____ means surrounding the mouth.

5. A(n) _____ implant is a type of implant with a metal frame placed under the periosteum that lies on top of the mandible.

6. A clear acrylic template placed over the alveolar ridge to assist in locating the proper placement for dental implants is the _____.

7. _____ are artificial teeth attached to anchors that have been surgically embedded into the bone or surrounding structures.

8. _____ is a type of metal used for implants.

Complete each question by circling the best answer.

1. Which dental specialist has training in dental implants?
   a. Oral and maxillofacial surgeon
   b. Periodontist
   c. Prosthodontist
   d. All of the above

2. The success rate for dental implants is _____.
   a. 50%
   b. 70%
   c. 90%
   d. 100%

3. Which of the following is the minimum number of years a dental implant is expected to last?
   a. 5 years
   b. 10 years
   c. 20 years
   d. 30 years

4. Compared with fixed prosthodontics, what is the financial investment for an implant?
   a. Greater than for fixed prosthodontics
   b. Less than for fixed prosthodontics
   c. About the same cost
   d. Insurance will cover the difference

5. What is the time frame in completing an implant procedure?
   a. Approximately 2 to 4 weeks
   b. Approximately 6 to 8 weeks
   c. Approximately 3 to 9 months
   d. Approximately 1 year

6. Which extraoral radiograph will the dentist commonly use to evaluate a patient for implants?
   a. Panoramic radiograph
   b. Cephalometric radiograph
   c. Tomogram
   d. All of the above

7. How is a surgical stent used for implant surgery?
   a. To hold the tissue in place
   b. To guide placement of the implant screw
   c. To maintain the teeth in an upright position
   d. To assist in the healing process

8. What material is the dental implant commonly fabricated from?
   a. Bone graft
   b. Stainless steel
   c. Titanium
   d. Enamel

9. *Osseo* means _____.
   a. implant
   b. tissue
   c. stent
   d. bone

10. What *component of the* endosteal implant attaches to the artificial tooth or teeth?
    a. Abutment post
    b. Cylinder
    c. Stent
    d. a and b

11. A subperiosteal implant would be recommended for what specific area of the mouth?
    a. Maxillary anterior
    b. Mandibular full
    c. Mandibular posterior
    d. Maxillary full

12. Plaque and calculus are easier to remove from implants than from natural teeth because _____.
    a. implants have a rough surface
    b. implants have a natural cleansing cover
    c. implants have a smooth surface
    d. implants have fluoride embedded in the teeth

13. An example of a cleaning accessory used for implants is a _____.
    a. toothbrush
    b. clasp brush
    c. interproximal brush
    d. All of the above

14. What type of environment should be maintained during a surgical implant procedure?
    a. Aseptic
    b. Sterile
    c. Clean
    d. Free from debris

15. What type of assessment will a prospective implant patient undergo?
    a. Medical history evaluation
    b. Dental examination
    c. Psychological evaluation
    d. All of the above

CASE STUDY

Your patient is considering implants. There are two drawbacks associated with this procedure. One is cost, and the other is that it will take longer for the procedure to be completed.

1. Are there any contraindications that should be reviewed with a patient before an implant is placed?

2. Explain why the process of implants takes so long and the importance of not rushing this type of procedure.

3. What role does infection control play in the procedure of implants?

4. What financial assistance options could the patient be informed of regarding implants?

5. Describe the most important home care advice that this patient should receive regarding implants.

INTERACTIVE DENTAL OFFICE PATIENT CASE EXERCISE Ɵvolve
learning system

Access the *Interactive Dental Office* on *Evolve* and click on the patient case file for Gregory Brooks.
- Review Mr. Brooks's record.
- Complete all exercises on Evolve for Mr. Brooks's case.
- Answer the following questions.

1. Are there any other types of fixed prosthodontics in Mr. Brooks's mouth?

2. Which type of implant did Mr. Brooks decide to have?

3. If Mr. Brooks decided not to proceed with the placement of an implant because of cost, what would be the second choice of treatment?

4. What type of home care is recommended for implants?

5. After the implant procedure is completed, what will Mr. Brooks be scheduled for next?

COMPETENCY 53-1: ASSISTING IN ENDOSTEAL IMPLANT SURGERY

Performance Objective
By following a routine procedure that meets stated protocols, the student will demonstrate the proper techniques to be used when assisting during the stages of implant surgery.

Evaluation and Grading Criteria
 3 Student competently met the stated criteria without assistance.
 2 Student required assistance in order to meet the stated criteria.
 1 Student showed uncertainty when performing the stated criteria.
 0 Student was not prepared and needs to repeat the step.
N/A No evaluation of this step.
Instructor shall define grades for each point range earned on completion of each performance-evaluated task.

Performance Standards
The minimum number of satisfactory performances required before final evaluation is _____.

Instructor shall identify by * those steps considered critical. If step is missed or minimum competency is not met, the evaluated procedure fails and must be repeated.

PERFORMANCE CRITERIA	*	SELF	PEER	INSTRUCTOR	COMMENT
1. Gathered the appropriate setup.					
2. Personal protective equipment placed according to procedure.					
3. Assisted in stage I surgery: implant placement.					
4. Maintained patient comfort and followed appropriate infection control measures throughout the procedure.					
5. Assisted in stage II surgery: implant exposure.					
6. Maintained patient comfort and followed appropriate infection control measures throughout the procedure.					
7. Procedure documented in patient record.					
ADDITIONAL COMMENTS					

Total number of points earned _____

Grade _____ Instructor's initials _____

54 Endodontics

SHORT-ANSWER QUESTIONS

1. List the testing procedures performed for an endodontic diagnosis.

2. List the conclusions of the subjective and objective tests used in the endodontic diagnosis.

3. Describe diagnostic conclusions for endodontic therapy.

4. List the various types of endodontic procedures.

5. Discuss the medicaments and dental materials used in endodontics.

6. Give an overview of root canal therapy.

7. Describe surgical endodontics and explain why it is performed.

FILL-IN-THE-BLANK STATEMENTS

Select the best term from the list below and complete the following statements.

abscess
apical curettage
control tooth
debridement
endodontist
gutta-percha
hemisection
indirect pulp cap
nonvital
palpation

percussion
perforation
periradicular
pulp cap
pulpitis
pulpotomy
retrograde restoration
reversible pulpitis
root amputation
root canal therapy

1. A(n) _____ is the surgical removal of infectious material surrounding the apex of a root.

2. A(n) _____ is a healthy tooth used as a standard to compare questionable teeth of similar size and structure during pulp vitality testing.

3. A(n) _____ is a localized area of pus that originates from an infection.

4. _____ is an examination technique that involves tapping on the incisal or occlusal surface of a tooth to determine vitality.

5. _____ is a plastic type of filling material used in root canal therapy.

6. The surgical separation of a multirooted tooth through the furcation area is a(n) _____.

7. A(n) _____ is the placement of calcium hydroxide over a partially exposed pulp.

8. _____ means not living.

9. _____ is completed to remove or clean out the pulpal canal.

10. _____ is an examination technique of the soft tissues in which the examiner's hand or fingertips are used.

11. A(n) _____ is the removal of one or more roots without removal of the crown of the tooth.

12. _____ is the procedure of removing dental pulp and filling the canal with material.

13. A(n) _____ is the application of calcium hydroxide to a cavity preparation that has an exposed or a nearly exposed dental pulp.

14. To break through and extend beyond the apex of the root is _____.

15. Nerves, blood vessels, and tissue that surround the root of a tooth are called _____.

16. A(n) _____ is the removal of a vital pulp from the coronal portion of a tooth.

17. _____ is inflammation of the dental pulp.

18. A small restoration placed at the apex of a root is _____.

19. A dentist who specializes in the prevention, diagnosis, and treatment of the dental pulp and periradicular tissues is a(n) _____.

20. _____ occurs when there is a form of pulpal inflammation but the pulp may be salvageable.

MULTIPLE-CHOICE QUESTIONS

Complete each question by circling the best answer.

1. Periradicular tissues are _____.
   a. pulp tissues
   b. tissues that surround the root of a tooth
   c. tissues that surround the crown of a tooth
   d. buccal mucosa

2. What specialist is qualified to perform root canal therapy?
   a. Prosthodontist
   b. Implantologist
   c. Endodontist
   d. Periodontist

3. What urgent situation can result if bacteria reach the nerves and blood vessels of a tooth?
   a. Abscess
   b. Decay
   c. Tumor
   d. Calculus

518

4. Is pain a subjective or objective component of a diagnosis?
   a. Subjective
   b. Objective
   c. Neither
   d. Both

5. Tooth #5 is being tested for possible root canal therapy. Which tooth would be used as a control tooth?
   a. #6
   b. #9
   c. #12
   d. #15

6. When the dentist taps on a tooth, what diagnostic test is being performed?
   a. Mobility
   b. Heat
   c. Palpation
   d. Percussion

7. What type of radiograph would be exposed through the course of root canal therapy?
   a. Cephalometric
   b. Bitewing
   c. Periapical
   d. Panorex

8. The diagnosis of inflamed pulp tissues is _____.
   a. pulpitis
   b. pulpotomy
   c. pulpectomy
   d. abscess

9. Another term for necrotic is _____.
   a. living
   b. dead
   c. nonvital
   d. b and c

10. The dental material most commonly selected for pulp capping is _____.
    a. amalgam
    b. zinc phosphate
    c. calcium hydroxide
    d. glass ionomer

11. What portion of the pulp would the dentist remove in a pulpotomy?
    a. Coronal portion
    b. Root portion
    c. Complete pulp
    d. Only the infected portion

12. What instrument has tiny projections and is used to remove pulp tissue?
    a. File
    b. Broach
    c. Reamer
    d. Pesso file

13. What type of file is best suited for canal enlargement?
    a. Broach
    b. Reamer
    c. Pesso
    d. Hedstrom

14. A rubber stop is placed on a file to _____.
    a. prevent perforation
    b. maintain the correct measurement of the canal
    c. identify the file
    d. a and b

15. To *obturate* means to _____.
    a. open a pulpal canal
    b. examine a pulpal canal
    c. fill a pulpal canal
    d. surgically remove a pulpal canal

16. The irrigation material most commonly utilized during root canal therapy is _____.
    a. water from the air-water syringe
    b. diluted sodium hypochlorite
    c. concentrated sodium hypochlorite
    d. phosphoric acid

17. The material commonly selected for obturation of a canal is _____.
    a. amalgam
    b. composite
    c. gutta-percha
    d. IRM

18. The type of moisture control recommended by the ADA for root canal therapy is _____.
    a. cotton pellets
    b. cotton rolls
    c. dry angles
    d. dental dam

19. What surface of a posterior tooth would the dentist enter with a rotary bur when opening a canal for root canal therapy?
    a. Occlusal
    b. Facial
    c. Mesial
    d. Incisal

20. _____ is a surgical procedure that involves the removal of the apex of a root.
    a. Hemisection
    b. Apicoectomy
    c. Forceps extraction
    d. Pulpotomy

CASE STUDY

John Allen is scheduled for a diagnosis on tooth #20. This is Mr. Allen's first time to the endodontist, and his subjective comments describe pain when chewing on the affected side and a constant dull pain lasting for approximately a week.

1. How do you think Mr. Allen knew to come to an endodontist for dental treatment?

2. What type of tooth is #20, and how many canals could be affected?

3. What type of diagnostic testing will the dentist perform to determine the type of endodontic treatment required?

4. What tooth would be used as the control tooth during diagnostic evaluation, and why is there a control tooth?

5. It was determined that the tooth would need a pulpectomy. Describe what this procedure entails.

6. What type of pain control would the endodontist use during the procedure to help alleviate unwarranted stress as well as discomfort?

7. How would tooth #20 be completely restored, and what dentist would complete this procedure?

INTERACTIVE DENTAL OFFICE PATIENT CASE EXERCISE   ⊖volve
learning system

Access the *Interactive Dental Office* on *Evolve* and click on the patient case file for Antonio DeAngelis.
- Review Mr. DeAngelis's record.
- Complete all exercises on Evolve for Mr. DeAngelis's case.
- Answer the following questions.

1. Does Mr. DeAngelis have any existing root canals charted?

2. What tooth was used as a control tooth for electric pulp testing?

3. How would tooth #10 be charted after completion of the root canal?

4. What specialist will Mr. DeAngelis be referred to for the porcelain-fused-to-metal crown?

5. Now that the existing work is completed, should Mr. DeAngelis be rescheduled for anything?

COMPETENCY 54-1: ASSISTING IN AN ELECTRIC PULP VITALITY TEST

Performance Objective

By following a routine procedure that meets stated protocols, in states where it is legal, the student will demonstrate the proper procedure for performing an electric pulp vitality test.

Evaluation and Grading Criteria

__3__ Student competently met the stated criteria without assistance.
__2__ Student required assistance in order to meet the stated criteria.
__1__ Student showed uncertainty when performing the stated criteria.
__0__ Student was not prepared and needs to repeat the step.
__N/A__ No evaluation of this step.
Instructor shall define grades for each point range earned on completion of each performance-evaluated task.

Performance Standards

The minimum number of satisfactory performances required before final evaluation is _____.

Instructor shall identify by * those steps considered critical. If step is missed or minimum competency is not met, the evaluated procedure fails and must be repeated.

PERFORMANCE CRITERIA	*	SELF	PEER	INSTRUCTOR	COMMENT
1. Gathered the appropriate setup.					
2. Personal protective equipment placed according to procedure.					
3. Described the procedure to the patient.					
4. Identified the tooth to be tested and the appropriate control tooth.					
5. Isolated the teeth to be tested and dried them thoroughly.					
6. Set the control dial at zero.					
7. Placed a thin layer of toothpaste on the tip of the pulp tester electrode.					
8. Tested the control tooth first; placed the tip of the electrode on the facial surface of the tooth at the cervical third.					
9. Gradually increased the level of current until the patient felt a response; recorded the response on the patient's record.					
10. Repeated the procedure on the suspected tooth, and recorded the response on the patient's record.					
11. Maintained patient comfort, and followed appropriate infection control measures throughout the procedure.					

Continued

12. Procedure documented in patient record.					

ADDITIONAL COMMENTS

Total number of points earned _____

Grade _____ Instructor's initials _____

COMPETENCY 54-2: ASSISTING IN ROOT CANAL THERAPY

Performance Objective

By following a routine procedure that meets stated protocols, the student will demonstrate the proper procedure for making pretreatment preparations and assisting in root canal therapy.

Evaluation and Grading Criteria

3   Student competently met the stated criteria without assistance.
2   Student required assistance in order to meet the stated criteria.
1   Student showed uncertainty when performing the stated criteria.
0   Student was not prepared and needs to repeat the step.
N/A   No evaluation of this step.

Instructor shall define grades for each point range earned on completion of each performance-evaluated task.

Performance Standards

The minimum number of satisfactory performances required before final evaluation is _____.

Instructor shall identify by * those steps considered critical. If step is missed or minimum competency is not met, the evaluated procedure fails and must be repeated.

PERFORMANCE CRITERIA	*	SELF	PEER	INSTRUCTOR	COMMENT
1. Prepared the appropriate setup.					
2. Personal protective equipment placed according to procedure.					
3. Assisted with the administration of a local anesthetic and with placing and disinfecting the dental dam.					
4. Anticipated the dentist's needs.					
5. Maintained moisture control and a clear operating field throughout the procedure.					
6. Exchanged instruments as necessary.					
7. On request, irrigated the canals gently with a solution of sodium hypochlorite and used the HVE tip to remove excess solution.					
8. On request, placed a rubber stop at the desired working length for that canal.					
9. Assisted in preparation of the trial-point radiograph.					
10. Exposed and processed the trial-point radiograph.					
11. At a signal from the endodontist, prepared the endodontic sealer.					
12. Dipped a file or Lentulo spiral into the cement, and transferred it to the endodontist.					

Continued

13. Dipped the tip of the gutta-percha point into the sealer, and transferred it to the endodontist.				
14. Transferred hand instruments and additional gutta-percha points to the endodontist.				
15. Continued the instrument exchange until the procedure was complete and the tooth was sealed with temporary cement.				
16. Exposed and processed a posttreatment radiograph.				
17. Gave the patient posttreatment instructions.				
18. Maintained patient comfort and followed appropriate infection control measures throughout the procedure.				
19. Procedure documented in patient record.				

ADDITIONAL COMMENTS

Total number of points earned _____

Grade _____ Instructor's initials _____

55 Periodontics

SHORT-ANSWER QUESTIONS

1. Describe the role of the dental assistant in a periodontal practice.

2. Explain the procedures necessary for a comprehensive periodontal examination.

3. Describe the instruments used in periodontal therapy.

4. Give the indications for placement of periodontal surgical dressings, and describe the technique for proper placement.

5. Describe systemic conditions that can have a negative influence on periodontal treatment.

6. Describe the purpose of radiographs in periodontal treatment.

7. Describe the indications for and contraindications to use of the ultrasonic scaler.

8. Describe the various types of nonsurgical periodontal therapy.

9. Describe the various types of surgical periodontal therapy.

FILL-IN-THE-BLANK STATEMENTS

Select the best term from the list below and complete the following statements.

- bleeding index
- furcation probe
- gingivectomy
- gingivoplasty
- laser beam
- mobility
- osseous surgery
- ostectomy
- osteoplasty
- periodontal dressing
- periodontal explorer
- periodontal pocket
- periodontics
- periodontist
- periotomes
- ultrasonic scaler

1. The dental specialty that deals with the diagnosis and treatment of diseases of the supporting tissues is _____.

2. A(n) _____ is a dentist with advanced education in the specialty of periodontics.

3. A(n) _____ is a deepening of the gingival sulcus beyond normal, resulting from periodontal disease.

4. A surgical dressing that is applied to the surgical site for protection, similar to a bandage, is a(n) _____.

5. Movement of the tooth in its socket is called _____.

6. The _____ is a method of scoring the amount of bleeding present.

7. A(n) _____ is a type of explorer that is thin, fine, and easily adapted around root surfaces.

8. A(n) _____ is a device used for rapid calculus removal that operates on high-frequency sound waves.

9. _____ is performed to remove defects in bone.

10. A(n) _____ is the surgical removal of diseased gingival tissues.

11. A type of surgery in which gingival tissues are reshaped and contoured is _____.

12. _____ is a type of surgery in which bone is added, contoured, and reshaped.

13. _____ is a type of surgery that involves the removal of bone.

14. A highly concentrated beam of light is a(n) _____.

15. _____ are used to cut periodontal ligaments for atraumatic tooth extraction.

16. A(n) _____ is used to measure horizontal and vertical pocket depth of multirooted teeth in furcation areas.

MULTIPLE-CHOICE QUESTIONS

Complete each question by circling the best answer.

1. How do patients most often seek periodontal care?
   a. Prescription by their general dentist
   b. Referral by their general dentist
   c. Referral by another specialist
   d. Referral by their insurance company

2. What information is included in periodontal charting?
   a. Pocket readings
   b. Furcations
   c. Tooth mobility
   d. All of the above

3. Should teeth have any mobility?
   a. No
   b. Depends on the teeth
   c. A slight amount
   d. Yes

4. What is the depth of a normal sulcus?
   a. 1 to 3 mm
   b. 2 to 4 mm
   c. 3 to 5 mm
   d. 4 to 6 mm

5. What units of measurement are used on the periodontal probe?
   a. Centimeters
   b. Millimeters
   c. Inches
   d. Milligrams

6. What type of radiograph is especially useful in periodontics?
   a. Panoramic
   b. Occlusal
   c. Bitewing
   d. Periapical

7. Which instrument is used to remove calculus from supragingival surfaces?
   a. Spoon excavator
   b. Scaler
   c. Explorer
   d. Curette

8. Which type of instrument is used to remove calculus from subgingival surfaces?
   a. Spoon excavator
   b. Scaler
   c. Explorer
   d. Curette

9. What is the purpose of explorers in periodontal treatment?
   a. To detect pathology
   b. To provide tactile information
   c. To locate calculus
   d. b and c

10. A type of curette with two cutting edges is a _____.
    a. Universal
    b. Kirkland
    c. Gracey
    d. sickle

11. What is the purpose of a periodontal pocket marker?
    a. To carry items to and from the mouth
    b. To mark bleeding points in the gingival tissue
    c. To measure the sulcus
    d. To remove calculus from the sulcus

12. How do ultrasonic scalers work?
    a. Water pressure
    b. Air pressure
    c. Sound waves
    d. Rpm

13. What oral conditions contraindicate the use of an ultrasonic scaler?
    a. Patients with demineralization
    b. Narrow periodontal pockets
    c. Exposed dentin
    d. All of the above

14. Should an ultrasonic scaler be used on a patient with a communicable disease?
    a. Yes
    b. No
    c. It does not matter

15. What is the more common term for a dental prophylaxis?
    a. Prophy
    b. Sealants
    c. Scaling
    d. Treatment

16. Who can perform a dental prophylaxis?
    a. Dentist
    b. Dental assistant
    c. Dental hygienist
    d. a and c

17. _____ is a surgical periodontal treatment.
    a. Scaling
    b. Root planing
    c. Gingivectomy
    d. Gingival curettage

18. What drug is often used for the treatment of periodontitis, juvenile periodontitis, and rapidly destructive periodontitis?
    a. Fluoride
    b. Tetracycline
    c. Ibuprofen
    d. Acetaminophen

CASE STUDY

You will be assisting Dr. Lanier with an incisional periodontal surgery. Dr. Lanier has noted in the patient record that teeth #23 through #26 do not have adequate tissue coverage, and he will need to move the flap of tissue into position to cover more tooth structure.

1. What type of dental specialist would complete this procedure?

2. What is another name for incisional periodontal surgery?

3. In closing the flap, what would the surgeon most commonly use?

4. To protect the surgical site and promote healing, what would you prepare for placement? Where would this be placed?

MULTIMEDIA PROCEDURES RECOMMENDED REVIEW

- Noneugenol Periodontal Dressing
- Removing Periodontal Dressing

INTERACTIVE PATIENT CASE EXERCISE

Access the *Interactive Dental Office* on *Evolve* and click on the patient case file for Mrs. Louisa Van Doren.
- Review Mrs. Van Doren's record.
- Complete all exercises for Mrs. Van Doren's case.
- Answer the following questions.

1. Are there contraindications to the use of an ultrasonic scaler on Mrs. Van Doren?

2. A gingivectomy is scheduled for which area in Mrs. Van Doren's mouth?

3. Will Dr. Bowman need to place a periodontal dressing?

Access the *Interactive Dental Office* on *Evolve* and click on the patient case file for Mrs. Janet Folkner.
- Review Mrs. Folkner's record.
- Complete all exercises for Mrs. Folkner's case.
- Answer the following questions.

4. Are there any special precautions that should be taken before an ultrasonic scaler is used on Mrs. Folkner?

5. What do you notice regarding the level of bone on Mrs. Folkner's radiographs?

6. What type of instruments would be used to remove the subgingival calculus?

COMPETENCY 55-1: ASSISTING WITH A DENTAL PROPHYLAXIS

Performance Objective
By following a routine procedure that meets stated protocols, the student will demonstrate the proper procedure for assisting with a dental prophylaxis.

Evaluation and Grading Criteria
 3 Student competently met the stated criteria without assistance.
 2 Student required assistance in order to meet the stated criteria.
 1 Student showed uncertainty when performing the stated criteria.
 0 Student was not prepared and needs to repeat the step.
 N/A No evaluation of this step.
Instructor shall define grades for each point range earned on completion of each performance-evaluated task.

Performance Standards
The minimum number of satisfactory performances required before final evaluation is _____.

Instructor shall identify by * those steps considered critical. If step is missed or minimum competency is not met, the evaluated procedure fails and must be repeated.

PERFORMANCE CRITERIA	*	SELF	PEER	INSTRUCTOR	COMMENT
1. Personal protective equipment placed according to procedure.					
2. Adjusted the light as necessary and was prepared to dry teeth with air when requested to do so.					
3. Provided retraction of the lips, tongue, and cheeks.					
4. Rinsed and evacuated fluid from the patient's mouth.					
5. Exchanged instruments with the operator.					
6. Passed the dental floss and/or tape.					
7. Reinforced oral hygiene instructions when requested to do so.					
8. Maintained patient comfort and followed appropriate infection control measures throughout the procedure.					
9. Procedure documented in patient record.					

ADDITIONAL COMMENTS

Total number of points earned _____

Grade _____ Instructor's initials _____

COMPETENCY 55-2: ASSISTING WITH GINGIVECTOMY AND GINGIVOPLASTY

Performance Objective

By following a routine procedure that meets stated protocols, the student will demonstrate the proper procedure for assisting with a gingivectomy and gingivoplasty.

Evaluation and Grading Criteria

3	Student competently met the stated criteria without assistance.
2	Student required assistance in order to meet the stated criteria.
1	Student showed uncertainty when performing the stated criteria.
0	Student was not prepared and needs to repeat the step.
N/A	No evaluation of this step.

Instructor shall define grades for each point range earned on completion of each performance-evaluated task.

Performance Standards

The minimum number of satisfactory performances required before final evaluation is _____.

Instructor shall identify by * those steps considered critical. If step is missed or minimum competency is not met, the evaluated procedure fails and must be repeated.

PERFORMANCE CRITERIA	*	SELF	PEER	INSTRUCTOR	COMMENT
1. Set out patient's health history, radiographs, and periodontal chart.					
2. Personal protective equipment placed according to procedure.					
3. Anticipated the operator's needs and was prepared to pass and retrieve surgical instruments.					
4. Had gauze ready to remove tissue from instruments.					
5. Provided oral evacuation and retraction.					
6. Irrigated with sterile saline.					
7. Assisted with suture placement.					
8. Placed, or assisted with placement of, the periodontal dressing.					
9. Provided postoperative instructions.					
10. Maintained patient comfort and followed appropriate infection control measures throughout the procedure.					
11. Procedure documented in patient record.					
ADDITIONAL COMMENTS					

Total number of points earned _____

Grade _____ Instructor's initials _____

COMPETENCY 55-3: PREPARING AND PLACING A NONEUGENOL PERIODONTAL DRESSING

Performance Objective

By following a routine procedure that meets stated protocols, the student will demonstrate the proper procedure for preparing and placing a noneugenol periodontal dressing.

Evaluation and Grading Criteria

 3   Student competently met the stated criteria without assistance.
 2   Student required assistance in order to meet the stated criteria.
 1   Student showed uncertainty when performing the stated criteria.
 0   Student was not prepared and needs to repeat the step.
 N/A   No evaluation of this step.

Instructor shall define grades for each point range earned on completion of each performance-evaluated task.

Performance Standards

The minimum number of satisfactory performances required before final evaluation is _____.

Instructor shall identify by * those steps considered critical. If step is missed or minimum competency is not met, the evaluated procedure fails and must be repeated.

PERFORMANCE CRITERIA	*	SELF	PEER	INSTRUCTOR	COMMENT
1. Personal protective equipment placed according to procedure.					
Mixing					
2. Extruded equal lengths of the two pastes on a paper pad.					
3. Mixed the pastes until a uniform color was obtained (2 to 3 minutes).					
4. Placed the material in the paper cup.					
5. Lubricated gloved fingers with saline solution.					
6. Rolled the paste into strips.					
Placement					
7. Pressed small triangular pieces of dressing into the interproximal spaces.					
8. Adapted one end of the strip around the distal surface of the last tooth in the surgical site.					
9. Gently pressed the remainder of the strip along the incised gingival margin.					
10. Gently pressed the strip into the interproximal areas.					
11. Applied the second strip from the lingual surface.					

Continued

12. Joined the facial and lingual strips.				
13. Applied gentle pressure on the facial and lingual surfaces.				
15. Checked the dressing for overextension and interference.				
16. Removed any excess dressing and adjusted the new margins.				
17. Procedure documented in patient record.				
18. Maintained patient comfort and followed appropriate infection control measures throughout the procedure.				

ADDITIONAL COMMENTS

Total number of points earned _____

Grade _____ Instructor's initials _____

COMPETENCY 55-4: REMOVING A PERIODONTAL DRESSING

Performance Objective

By following a routine procedure that meets stated protocols, the student will demonstrate the proper procedure for removing a periodontal dressing.

Evaluation and Grading Criteria

<u>3</u>   Student competently met the stated criteria without assistance.
<u>2</u>   Student required assistance in order to meet the stated criteria.
<u>1</u>   Student showed uncertainty when performing the stated criteria.
<u>0</u>   Student was not prepared and needs to repeat the step.
<u>N/A</u>   No evaluation of this step.
Instructor shall define grades for each point range earned on completion of each performance-evaluated task.

Performance Standards

The minimum number of satisfactory performances required before final evaluation is _____ .

Instructor shall identify by * those steps considered critical. If step is missed or minimum competency is not met, the evaluated procedure fails and must be repeated.

PERFORMANCE CRITERIA	*	SELF	PEER	INSTRUCTOR	COMMENT
1. Personal protective equipment placed according to procedure.					
2. Gently inserted the spoon excavator under the margin.					
3. Used lateral pressure to gently pry the dressing away from the tissue.					
4. Checked for sutures and removed any present.					
5. Gently used dental floss to remove all fragments of dressing material.					
6. Irrigated the entire area gently with warm saline solution.					
7. Used the HVE tip or saliva ejector to remove fluid from the patient's mouth.					
8. Procedure documented in patient record.					
9. Maintained patient comfort and followed appropriate infection control measures throughout the procedure.					
ADDITIONAL COMMENTS					

Total number of points earned _____

Grade _____ Instructor's initials _____

56 Oral and Maxillofacial Surgery

SHORT-ANSWER QUESTIONS

1. Define the specialty of oral and maxillofacial surgery.

2. Discuss the role of an oral surgery assistant.

3. State the importance of the chain of asepsis for this specialized area of dentistry.

4. List the instruments used for a forceps extraction.

5. Describe the surgical procedures commonly performed in a general practice.

6. Describe the type of postoperative instructions provided to a patient after a surgical procedure.

7. Discuss possible complications from surgery.

FILL-IN-THE-BLANK STATEMENTS

Select the best term from the list below and complete the following statements.

alveoplasty	mallet
bone file	oral and maxillofacial surgeon
chisel	oral and maxillofacial surgery
donning	oral brush biopsy
elevator	outpatient
forceps	retractor
hard tissue impaction	rongeur
hemostat	scalpel
impacted	soft tissue impaction
incisional biopsy	surgical curette

1. The _____ is a surgical instrument used for cutting or severing the tooth and bone structure.

2. _____ is the surgical instrument used to reflect and retract the periodontal ligament and periosteum.

3. A(n) _____ is when a tooth is partially to fully covered by bone and gingival tissue.

4. An instrument used to hold or grasp items is a(n) _____.

5. The _____ is a surgical instrument used to remove tissue and debris from the tooth socket.

6. _____ is the procedure of surgical reduction and reshaping of the alveolar ridge.

7. A surgical instrument used to smooth rough edges of bone structure is the _____.

8. A(n) _____ is when a tooth is partially to fully covered by gingival tissue.

9. _____ cells are obtained from suspicious oral lesion.

10. A surgical instrument used to grasp and remove a tooth from its socket is _____.

11. _____ is the act of placing an item on, such as gloves.

12. A tooth that has not erupted is called _____.

13. A(n) _____ is the removal of a section of a questionable lesion for evaluation.

14. A(n) _____ is a hammer-like instrument used with a chisel to section teeth or bone.

15. A(n) _____ is a surgical knife.

16. A(n) _____ is a dentist who specializes in surgeries of the head and neck region.

17. _____ is the dental specialty that focuses on treatment of the head and neck.

18. A patient who is seen and treated by a doctor and then is sent home for recovery is considered a(n) _____.

19. A(n) _____ is an instrument used to hold back soft tissue.

20. The _____ is a surgical instrument used to cut and trim the alveolar bone.

MULTIPLE-CHOICE QUESTIONS

Complete each question by circling the best answer.

1. What type of surgical procedures would a general dentist most commonly perform?
   a. Single extractions
   b. Removal of impacted teeth
   c. Reconstructive surgery
   d. Biopsy

2. How would a dental assistant further her/his career as a surgical assistant?
   a. Obtain a dental hygiene degree
   b. Obtain a nursing degree
   c. Obtain continuing education in oral and maxillofacial surgery
   d. Obtain a dental degree

3. In what type of setting are oral surgery procedures completed?
   a. Dental office
   b. Outpatient clinic
   c. Hospital
   d. All of the above

4. Most oral and maxillofacial surgeries are considered
   _____.
   a. major surgery
   b. minor surgery
   c. dental procedures
   d. medical procedures

5. The periosteal elevator is used to reflect and retract _____.
   a. gingival tissue
   b. tooth
   c. periosteum
   d. lips

6. Universal forceps are designed to be used for _____.
   a. right side only
   b. left side only
   c. left or right of opposite arch
   d. left or right of same arch

7. What surgical instrument resembles a spoon excavator?
   a. Rongeur
   b. Surgical curette
   c. Elevator
   d. Scalpel

8. What surgical instrument is used to trim and shape bone?
   a. Rongeur
   b. Surgical curette
   c. Elevator
   d. Scalpel

9. If a chisel is placed on the tray setup, what additional surgical instrument must be set out?
   a. Elevator
   b. Scalpel
   c. Mallet
   d. Hemostat

10. What equipment is used to perform a surgical scrub?
    a. Orange stick
    b. Antimicrobial soap
    c. Scrub brush
    d. All of the above

11. The term *donning* means _____.
    a. taking off
    b. putting on
    c. procedure
    d. prior to

12. What procedure is generally completed by the surgeon following the removal of multiple teeth that are adjacent to one another?
    a. Implants
    b. Sutures
    c. Alveoplasty
    d. b or c

13. When a tooth is directly under gingival tissue, it is said to be _____.
    a. ankylosed
    b. soft tissue impacted
    c. exposed
    d. hard tissue impacted

14. _____ is completed when cells are obtained from a surface lesion.
    a. Incisional biopsy
    b. Excisional biopsy
    c. Oral brush biopsy
    d. Surgical biopsy

15. The term *suture* refers to _____.
    a. impaction
    b. stitching
    c. control of bleeding
    d. multiple extractions

16. Which is an absorbable suture material?
    a. Silk
    b. Polyester
    c. Nylon
    d. Catgut

17. What is the approximate time frame for removing nonabsorbable sutures?
    a. 1 to 3 days
    b. 4 to 6 days
    c. 5 to 7 days
    d. 12 to 14 days

18. How long should a pressure pack remain on the surgical site to control bleeding?
    a. 30 minutes
    b. 2 to 3 hours
    c. 12 hours
    d. 24 hours

19. What analgesic may be prescribed for swelling?
    a. Antibiotic
    b. Ibuprofen
    c. Aspirin
    d. Codeine

20. What should a patient use to control swelling?
    a. Gauze pack
    b. Hydrocolloid
    c. Cold pack
    d. Heat pack

CASE STUDY

Katie Samuels has called the surgeon about extreme pain in her lower right jaw. The business assistant pulls her record and reviews that Katie had teeth #17 and #32 surgically extracted 3 days ago. The teeth were impacted, but the surgeon's progress notes indicate that there were no complications, and the patient tolerated the procedure well. Katie is scheduled to return in a week for a follow-up and suture removal.

1. Why would this patient be referred to a specialist to have these teeth extracted?

2. What does the term *impacted* describe about the teeth that were removed?

3. What type of suture material would the surgeon have placed for the patient to have to return for their removal?

4. Give a possible diagnosis for Katie's pain.

5. Give some of the reasons that can cause this diagnosis.

6. What could have possibly caused this problem? If the diagnosis is correct, what should be performed to alleviate the patient's pain?

7. Can the patient wait until her scheduled checkup to be seen? If not, when should she be seen?

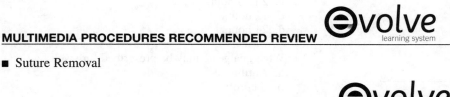

MULTIMEDIA PROCEDURES RECOMMENDED REVIEW

- Suture Removal

INTERACTIVE DENTAL OFFICE PATIENT CASE EXERCISE

Access the *Interactive Dental Office on Evolve,* and click on the patient case file for Mr. Lee Wong.
- Review Mr. Wong's record.
- Complete all exercises on the CD-ROM for Mr. Wong's case.
- Answer the following questions.

1. What does the charting indicate for tooth #30?

2. Could any additional methods of pain control be used to calm Mr. Wong?

3. What type of PPE was worn during the procedure?

4. Were sutures placed after the extraction?

5. How is the medicated dressing placed in the tooth socket for the treatment of alveolitis?

COMPETENCY 56-1: PREPARING A STERILE FIELD FOR INSTRUMENTS AND SUPPLIES

Performance Objective
By following a routine procedure that meets stated protocols, the student will demonstrate the proper procedure for preparing a sterile field for instruments and supplies.

Evaluation and Grading Criteria
<u>3</u>   Student competently met the stated criteria without assistance.
<u>2</u>   Student required assistance in order to meet the stated criteria.
<u>1</u>   Student showed uncertainty when performing the stated criteria.
<u>0</u>   Student was not prepared and needs to repeat the step.
<u>N/A</u> No evaluation of this step.
Instructor shall define grades for each point range earned on completion of each performance-evaluated task.

Performance Standards
The minimum number of satisfactory performances required before final evaluation is _____.

Instructor shall identify by * those steps considered critical. If step is missed or minimum competency is not met, the evaluated procedure fails and must be repeated.

PERFORMANCE CRITERIA	*	SELF	PEER	INSTRUCTOR	COMMENT
1. Washed and dried hands.					
2. Positioned Mayo stand and placed the sterile pack.					
3. Opened the outer wrapping in a direction away from the assistant.					
4. Held outside flaps open and allowed sterile contents to fall on the tray.					
5. Added items to the field.					
ADDITIONAL COMMENTS					

Total number of points earned _____

Grade _____ Instructor's initials _____

COMPETENCY 56-2: PERFORMING A SURGICAL SCRUB

Performance Objective

By following a routine procedure that meets stated protocols, the student will demonstrate the proper procedure for performing a surgical scrub for a sterile surgical procedure.

Evaluation and Grading Criteria

3	Student competently met the stated criteria without assistance.
2	Student required assistance in order to meet the stated criteria.
1	Student showed uncertainty when performing the stated criteria.
0	Student was not prepared and needs to repeat the step.
N/A	No evaluation of this step.

Instructor shall define grades for each point range earned on completion of each performance-evaluated task.

Performance Standards

The minimum number of satisfactory performances required before final evaluation is _____.

Instructor shall identify by * those steps considered critical. If step is missed or minimum competency is not met, the evaluated procedure fails and must be repeated.

PERFORMANCE CRITERIA	*	SELF	PEER	INSTRUCTOR	COMMENT
1. Wet hands and forearms with warm water.					
2. Placed antimicrobial soap on hands.					
3. Scrub each side of each finger, between the fingers, and the back and front of the hand.					
4. Proceed to scrub the arms, keeping the hand higher than the arm at all times.					
5. Wash each side of the arm to three inches above the elbow					
6. Rinse hands and arms by passing them through the water in one direction only, from fingertips to elbow.					
7. Accomplished washing in 7 minutes.					
8. Dried hands using a sterile disposable towel.					
9. Personal protective equipment placed according to procedure.					

ADDITIONAL COMMENTS

Total number of points earned _____

Grade _____ Instructor's initials _____

Chapter **56** **Oral and Maxillofacial Surgery**

COMPETENCY 56-3: PERFORMING STERILE GLOVING

Performance Objective

By following a routine procedure that meets stated protocols, the student will demonstrate the proper procedure for -gloving with the use of a sterile technique.

Evaluation and Grading Criteria

 3 Student competently met the stated criteria without assistance.
 2 Student required assistance in order to meet the stated criteria.
 1 Student showed uncertainty when performing the stated criteria.
 0 Student was not prepared and needs to repeat the step.
 N/A No evaluation of this step.
Instructor shall define grades for each point range earned on completion of each performance-evaluated task.

Performance Standards

The minimum number of satisfactory performances required before final evaluation is _____.

Instructor shall identify by * those steps considered critical. If step is missed or minimum competency is not met, the evaluated procedure fails and must be repeated.

PERFORMANCE CRITERIA	*	SELF	PEER	INSTRUCTOR	COMMENT
1. Opened the glove package before the surgical scrub.					
2. Touched only the inside of the package after the surgical scrub.					
3. Gloved the dominant hand first, touching only the folded cuff.					
4. Placed the other glove on, touching only the sterile portion of the glove with the dominant hand.					
5. Unrolled the cuff from the gloves.					
ADDITIONAL COMMENTS					

Total number of points earned _____

Grade _____ Instructor's initials _____

COMPETENCIES 56-4 TO 56-6: ASSISTING IN SURGICAL EXTRACTION

Performance Objective

By following a routine procedure that meets stated protocols, when provided with information concerning the type of surgery, the tooth, and the anesthetics used, the student will prepare the setup, prepare the patient, and assist in a surgical procedure.

Evaluation and Grading Criteria

__3__   Student competently met the stated criteria without assistance.
__2__   Student required assistance in order to meet the stated criteria.
__1__   Student showed uncertainty when performing the stated criteria.
__0__   Student was not prepared and needs to repeat the step.
__N/A__   No evaluation of this step.
Instructor shall define grades for each point range earned on completion of each performance-evaluated task.

Performance Standards

The minimum number of satisfactory performances required before final evaluation is _____.

Instructor shall identify by * those steps considered critical. If step is missed or minimum competency is not met, the evaluated procedure fails and must be repeated.

PERFORMANCE CRITERIA	*	SELF	PEER	INSTRUCTOR	COMMENT
Preparing the Treatment Room					
1. Prepared the treatment room.					
2. Kept instruments in their sterile wraps until ready for use; if a surgical tray was preset, opened the tray and placed a sterile towel over the instruments.					
3. Placed the appropriate local anesthetic on the tray.					
4. Placed the appropriate forceps on the tray.					
Preparing the Patient					
1. Seated the patient and positioned a sterile patient drape or towel.					
2. Took the patient's vital signs and recorded them in the patient's record.					
3. Adjusted the dental chair to the proper position.					
4. Stayed with the patient until the dentist entered the treatment room.					

Continued

During the Surgical Procedure					
1. Personal protective equipment placed according to procedure.					
2. Maintained the chain of asepsis.					
3. Monitored vital signs.					
4. Aspirated and retracted as needed.					
5. Transferred and received instruments as needed.					
6. Assisted in suture placement as needed.					
7. Maintained a clear operating field with adequate light and irrigation.					
8. Steadied the patient's head and mandible if necessary.					
9. Observed the patient's condition and anticipated the dentist's needs.					
10. Provided post operative instructions.					
11. Maintained patient comfort and followed appropriate infection control measures throughout the procedure.					
12. Procedure documented in patient record.					

ADDITIONAL COMMENTS

Total number of points earned _____

Grade _____ Instructor's initials _____

COMPETENCY 56-7: ASSISTING IN SUTURE PLACEMENT

Performance Objective
By following a routine procedure that meets stated protocols, the student will demonstrate the proper procedure for assisting the surgeon in suture placement.

Evaluation and Grading Criteria
 3 Student competently met the stated criteria without assistance.
 2 Student required assistance in order to meet the stated criteria.
 1 Student showed uncertainty when performing the stated criteria.
 0 Student was not prepared and needs to repeat the step.
 N/A No evaluation of this step.
Instructor shall define grades for each point range earned on completion of each performance-evaluated task.

Performance Standards
The minimum number of satisfactory performances required before final evaluation is _____.

Instructor shall identify by * those steps considered critical. If step is missed or minimum competency is not met, the evaluated procedure fails and must be repeated.

PERFORMANCE CRITERIA	*	SELF	PEER	INSTRUCTOR	COMMENT
1. Personal protective equipment placed according to the procedure.					
2. Removed the suture material from the sterile package.					
3. Clamped the suture needle at the upper third.					
4. Transferred the needle holder to the surgeon.					
5. Retracted during suture placement.					
6. Cut suture where indicated by the surgeon.					
7. Placed suture material on tray.					
8. Recorded the numbers and types of sutures placed in the patient's record.					
ADDITIONAL COMMENTS					

Total number of points earned _____

Grade _____ Instructor's initials _____

COMPETENCY 56-8: PERFORMING SUTURE REMOVAL (EXPANDED FUNCTION)

Performance Objective

By following a routine procedure that meets stated protocols, the student will demonstrate the proper procedure for removing sutures.

Evaluation and Grading Criteria

 3 Student competently met the stated criteria without assistance.
 2 Student required assistance in order to meet the stated criteria.
 1 Student showed uncertainty when performing the stated criteria.
 0 Student was not prepared and needs to repeat the step.
 N/A No evaluation of this step.
Instructor shall define grades for each point range earned on completion of each performance-evaluated task.

Performance Standards

The minimum number of satisfactory performances required before final evaluation is _____.

Instructor shall identify by * those steps considered critical. If step is missed or minimum competency is not met, the evaluated procedure fails and must be repeated.

PERFORMANCE CRITERIA	*	SELF	PEER	INSTRUCTOR	COMMENT
1. Assistant confirmed with surgeon the removal of sutures placed at extraction site.					
2. Instruments were set out correctly.					
3. Personal protective equipment placed according to procedure.					
4. Wiped the area with an antiseptic agent.					
5. Held the suture away from the tissue with cotton pliers.					
6. Cut the suture with suture scissors, ensuring that the scissors were laying flat near the tissue.					
7. Grasped the knot with cotton pliers and removed it, keeping it away from the tissue.					
8. Counted the number of sutures removed and recorded the total in the patient's record.					
9. Maintained patient comfort and followed appropriate infection control measures throughout the procedure.					
10. Procedure documented in patient record.					
ADDITIONAL COMMENTS					

Total number of points earned _____

Grade _____ Instructor's initials _____

555

COMPETENCY 56-9: ASSISTING IN THE TREATMENT OF ALVEOLITIS

Performance Objective

By following a routine procedure that meets stated protocols, the student will assist the surgeon in the treatment of alveolitis.

Evaluation and Grading Criteria

3	Student competently met the stated criteria without assistance.
2	Student required assistance in order to meet the stated criteria.
1	Student showed uncertainty when performing the stated criteria.
0	Student was not prepared and needs to repeat the step.
N/A	No evaluation of this step.

Note: In some states this procedure is legal for the dental assistant to perform.

Instructor shall define grades for each point range earned on completion of each performance-evaluated task.

Performance Standards

The minimum number of satisfactory performances required before final evaluation is _____.

Instructor shall identify by * those steps considered critical. If step is missed or minimum competency is not met, the evaluated procedure fails and must be repeated.

PERFORMANCE CRITERIA	*	PEER	SELF	INSTRUCTOR	COMMENT
1. Gathered the appropriate setup.					
2. Personal protective equipment placed according to procedure.					
3. Assisted the dentist in irrigating the site with saline solution.					
4. Prepared a strip of iodoform gauze in the appropriate length.					
5. Transferred gauze with medication to the site to be packed.					
6. Retrieved prescription pad and pen for surgeon to prescribe analgesics and antibiotics.					
7. Provided postoperative instructions.					
8. Procedure documented in patient record.					
ADDITIONAL COMMENTS					

Total number of points earned _____

Grade _____ Instructor's initials _____

57 Pediatric Dentistry

SHORT-ANSWER QUESTIONS

1. Describe the appearance and setting of a pediatric dental office.

2. List the stages of childhood from birth through adolescence.

3. Discuss the specific behavioral techniques that work as a positive reinforcement in the treatment of children.

4. Describe why children and adults with certain special needs would be seen in a pediatric practice.

5. List the specific areas involved in the diagnosis of and treatment planning for a pediatric patient.

6. Discuss the importance of preventive dentistry in pediatrics.

7. Describe the clinical procedures for treating pediatric patients compared with those used to treat adults.

FILL-IN-THE-BLANK STATEMENTS

Select the best term from the list below and complete the following statements.

athetosis
autonomy
avulsed
cerebral palsy
chronologic age
Down syndrome
extrusion
Frankl scale
intrusion
luxation

mental age
mentally challenged
neural
open bay
papoose board
pediatric dentistry
postnatal
prenatal
pulpotomy
T-band

1. _____ is a neural disorder or loss of motor function caused by brain damage.

2. A child's actual age is the _____.

3. _____ is the process of being independent.

4. A tooth that has been torn away or dislodged by force is said to be _____.

5. _____ is a disorder caused by a chromosomal defect.

6. _____ is a type of involuntary movement of the body, face, arms, and legs.

7. _____ occurs when teeth are displaced from the socket as a result of an injury.

8. When a tooth has been pushed into the socket as a result of injury, it is _____.

9. The _____ is a type of matrix used for primary teeth.

10. _____ means to dislocate.

11. The child's _____ is his or her level of intellectual capacity and development.

12. The _____ is a system designed to evaluate behavior.

13. The specialty of dentistry concerned with the infant through adolescent and the special needs patient is _____.

14. _____ means after birth.

15. _____ is a disorder in which an individual's intelligence is underdeveloped.

16. Another term for referring to the brain, nervous system, and nerve pathways is _____.

17. _____ is a concept of office design used in pediatric dental practices.

18. A(n) _____ is a type of restraining device used to hold hands, arms, and legs still.

19. A(n) _____ is a dental procedure in which the coronal portion of the dental pulp is removed.

20. _____ means before birth.

MULTIPLE-CHOICE QUESTIONS

Complete each question by circling the best answer.

1. At what age would a person most likely be referred to a general dentist from their pediatric dentist?
   a. 12
   b. 14
   c. 17
   d. 25

2. What is unique about the treatment areas of a pediatric practice?
   a. The dental chairs are close together.
   b. More than one dentist can use a treatment area.
   c. Many are designed with the open-bay concept.
   d. There is a chair for a parent.

3. Describe the type of patients seen in a pediatric practice.
   a. Healthy adolescents
   b. Special needs children
   c. Special needs adults
   d. All of the above

4. What are you describing when you say that a child is 10 years old but behaves like a 6-year-old?
   a. Chronologic age
   b. Emotional age
   c. Physical age
   d. Size

5. At what stage of life does a child first want control of, and structure in his or her environment?
   a. 1 to 3 years of age
   b. 3 to 5 years of age
   c. 6 to 9 years of age
   d. 9 to 12 years of age

6. How would Dr. Frankl describe a positive child?
   a. Accepts treatment
   b. Is willing to comply
   c. Follows directions
   d. All of the above

7. Which situation could include the use of a papoose board for the protection of the patient?
   a. Sedation of a 12-year-old
   b. Extraction on a 3-year-old
   c. Placement of sealants on a 10-year-old
   d. Fluoride treatment of a 7-year-old

8. Which of the following have limitations in children who are mentally challenged?
   a. Physical ability
   b. Speech
   c. IQ
   d. b and c

9. Another name for Down syndrome is

   _____.
   a. trisomy 21
   b. mental challenged
   c. cerebral palsy
   d. learning disorder

10. Cerebral palsy is a nonprogressive neural disorder

    caused by _____.
    a. a chromosomal defect
    b. a stroke
    c. brain damage
    d. an overdose

11. At what age should a child first see a dentist for a regular examination?
    a. 2 years
    b. 4 years
    c. 6 years
    d. 8 years

12. If a patient has a high risk of decay, how often should radiographs be taken?
    a. Monthly
    b. Every six months
    c. Once a year
    d. Before each tooth is restored

13. How is fluoride varnish prescribed for children with a high decay rate?
    a. As a direct fluoride application
    b. As prescription fluoride
    c. As a desensitizer
    d. As a liner

14. What procedure is recommended to protect the pits and fissures of posterior teeth?
    a. Pulpotomy
    b. Fluoride rinse
    c. Coronal polishing
    d. Sealants

15. At what phase of orthodontics would a pediatric dentist intercede in getting a patient to stop sucking his or her thumb?
    a. Interceptive
    b. Preventive
    c. Corrective
    d. Elective

16. If you are a competitive swimmer, is it recommended that you wear a mouth guard?
    a. No
    b. Yes

17. What matrices are used on primary teeth?
    a. Metal contoured
    b. T-band
    c. Spot welded
    d. b and c

18. What endodontic procedure would be performed on primary teeth?
    a. Apicoectomy
    b. Pulpectomy
    c. Pulpotomy
    d. Retrograde

19. Would a child be referred to a prosthodontist for the placement of a stainless steel crown?
    a. Yes
    b. No

20. In children, which teeth are most frequently injured?
    a. Mandibular anterior
    b. Mandibular posterior
    c. Maxillary anterior
    d. Maxillary posterior

21. When a tooth is avulsed, it has _____.
    a. been fractured
    b. come out
    c. been pushed back into the socket
    d. become loose

22. How does the dentist stabilize a tooth after an injury?
    a. With a temporary splint
    b. With a thermoplastic resin tray
    c. With wax
    d. With sutures

23. Who in the dental office is legally required to report child abuse?
    a. Dental assistant
    b. Business assistant
    c. Dental hygienist
    d. Dentist

24. What could be a possible sign of child abuse?
    a. Chipped or fractured teeth
    b. Bruises
    c. Scars on the lips or tongue
    d. All of the above

25. What organization should be contacted if someone suspects child abuse?
    a. American Dental Association
    b. Child Protective Services of the Public Health Department
    c. Local hospital
    d. Pediatric Dental Association

CASE STUDY

Ashley is a 12-year-old patient of the practice who is being seen as an emergency patient. Ashley was hit in the face while playing intramural basketball. Her maxillary central incisors were knocked back into the socket.

1. If your schedule is filled for the day, when should Ashley come in for an emergency visit?

2. What type of examination technique should be used to enable the dentist to make a correct diagnosis of the complexity of the damage to the teeth and surrounding area?

3. What is the diagnosis when a person's teeth are knocked inward?

4. Would Ashley's maxillary central incisors be her primary or permanent central incisors?

5. What letter or number would those teeth be called on a charting form?

6. What form of treatment would be provided for Ashley?

Access the *Interactive Dental Office on Evolve* and click on the patient case file for Raul Ortega, Jr.
- Review Raul's record.
- Complete all exercises on the CD-ROM for Raul's case.
- Answer the following questions.

1. What teeth are visible on the maxillary occlusal film taken on Raul?

2. Could the absence of fluoridated water be the reason for Raul's having baby bottle mouth syndrome?

3. What is the normal age range for the eruption of permanent first molars?

4. Would the placement of a stainless steel crown on Raul be considered an expanded function for the dental assistant?

5. Is the cement used for cementation of the stainless steel crown permanent or temporary?

COMPETENCY 57-1: ASSISTING IN PULPOTOMY OF A PRIMARY TOOTH

Performance Objective

By following a routine procedure that meets stated protocols, the student will demonstrate the proper technique when assisting in the pulpotomy of a primary tooth.

Evaluation and Grading Criteria

_3_ Student competently met the stated criteria without assistance.
_2_ Student required assistance in order to meet the stated criteria.
_1_ Student showed uncertainty when performing the stated criteria.
_0_ Student was not prepared and needs to repeat the step.
_N/A_ No evaluation of this step.

Instructor shall define grades for each point range earned on completion of each performance-evaluated task.

Performance Standards

The minimum number of satisfactory performances required before final evaluation is _____.

Instructor shall identify by * those steps considered critical. If step is missed or minimum competency is not met, the evaluated procedure fails and must be repeated.

PERFORMANCE CRITERIA	*	SELF	PEER	INSTRUCTOR	COMMENT
1. Gathered the appropriate setup.					
2. Personal protective equipment placed according to procedure.					
3. Assisted in the administration of the local anesthetic.					
4. Assisted in placement of or placed dental dam.					
5. Assisted in removal of dental caries; used HVE and air-water syringe during removal.					
6. Transferred instruments throughout the procedure.					
7. Prepared formocresol and cotton pellet and transferred when needed.					
8. Mixed ZOE for a base and transferred it to be placed.					
9. Maintained patient comfort and followed appropriate infection control measures throughout the procedure.					
10. Procedure documented in patient record.					

Continued

ADDITIONAL COMMENTS

Total number of points earned _____

Grade _____ Instructor's initials _____

COMPETENCY 57-2: ASSISTING IN PLACEMENT OF A STAINLESS STEEL CROWN

Performance Objective
By following a routine procedure that meets stated protocols, the student will demonstrate the proper technique when assisting in the preparation and placement of a stainless steel crown.

Evaluation and Grading Criteria
  3   Student competently met the stated criteria without assistance.
  2   Student required assistance in order to meet the stated criteria.
  1   Student showed uncertainty when performing the stated criteria.
  0   Student was not prepared and needs to repeat the step.
 N/A   No evaluation of this step.
Instructor shall define grades for each point range earned on completion of each performance-evaluated task.

Performance Standards
The minimum number of satisfactory performances required before final evaluation is _____.

Instructor shall identify by * those steps considered critical. If step is missed or minimum competency is not met, the evaluated procedure fails and must be repeated.

PERFORMANCE CRITERIA	*	SELF	PEER	INSTRUCTOR	COMMENT
1. Gathered the appropriate setup.					
2. Personal protective equipment placed according to procedure.					
3. Assisted in the administration of the local anesthetic.					
4. Assisted in the sizing of the stainless steel crown.					
5. Transferred instruments as requested in the transfer zone.					
6. Assisted in trimming and contouring of the stainless steel crown.					
7. Prepared cement and assisted in the cementation of the stainless steel crown.					
8. Maintained patient comfort and followed appropriate infection control measures throughout the procedure.					
9. Procedure recorded in patient record.					
ADDITIONAL COMMENTS					

Total number of points earned _____

Grade _____ Instructor's initials _____

Coronal Polishing

SHORT-ANSWER QUESTIONS

1. Explain the difference between a prophylaxis and coronal polishing.

2. Explain the indications for and contraindications to coronal polishing.

3. Name and describe the types of extrinsic stains.

4. Name and describe the two categories of intrinsic stains.

5. Describe four types of abrasives used for polishing the teeth.

6. Discuss considerations when esthetic-type restorations are polished.

FILL-IN-THE-BLANK STATEMENTS

Select the best term from the list below and complete the following statements.

calculus
clinical crown
extrinsic stains
fulcrum

intrinsic stains
oral prophylaxis
rubber cup polishing

1. _____ is a hard mineralized deposit attached to the teeth.

2. A(n) _____ is the complete removal of calculus, debris, stain, and plaque from the teeth.

3. The portion of the tooth that is visible in the oral cavity is the _____.

4. Stains that occur within the tooth structure and may not be removed by polishing are _____.

5. Stains that occur on the external surfaces of the teeth and may be removed by polishing are _____.

6. The _____ is a position that provides stability for the operator.

7. _____ is a technique used to remove plaque and stains from the coronal surfaces of teeth.

MULTIPLE-CHOICE QUESTIONS

Complete each question by circling the best answer.

1. What is the purpose of coronal polishing?
   a. To remove calculus
   b. To remove stains and plaque
   c. To prepare teeth for a restoration
   d. To remove inflamed gingiva

2. An oral prophylaxis includes _____.
   a. fluoride treatment
   b. removal of calculus and debris
   c. examination
   d. removal of decay

3. What is the purpose of selective polishing?
   a. To polish only teeth that are visible
   b. To polish the occlusal surfaces of teeth
   c. To polish only teeth with stain
   d. To polish the facial surfaces of teeth

4. Stains that may be removed from the surfaces of the

   teeth are _____.
   a. extrinsic stains
   b. natural stains
   c. intrinsic stains
   d. infected stains

5. Stains that cannot be removed from the surfaces of the

   teeth are _____.
   a. extrinsic stains
   b. natural stains
   c. intrinsic stains
   d. infected stains

6. Which is the most common technique for stain removal?
   a. Using a scaler
   b. Using a toothbrush
   c. Using floss
   d. Rubber cup polishing

7. Which grasp is used to hold the handpiece?
   a. Reverse-palm grasp
   b. Pen grasp
   c. Thumb-to-nose grasp
   d. Palm grasp

8. What is the purpose of a fulcrum?
   a. To provide pressure to the fingers
   b. To provide better retraction
   c. To provide stability to the hand
   d. To provide movement for the arm

9. What precaution should be taken when one is using a bristle brush?
   a. Not to allow the brush to get dry
   b. Not to traumatize the tissue
   c. Not to wear away enamel
   d. Not to use on occlusal surfaces

10. Toward which direction should the polishing stroke be directed?
    a. Toward the incisal
    b. Toward the gingiva
    c. Toward the occlusal
    d. a and c

11. What damage can result from using the prophy angle at high speed?
    a. It can cause frictional heat.
    b. It can remove dentin.
    c. It can cool the tooth.
    d. It can etch enamel.

12. How should the patient's head be positioned for access to the maxillary anterior teeth?
    a. Chin downward
    b. Head turned to the right
    c. Chin upward
    d. Head turned to the left

CASE STUDY

You are a dental assistant in a very busy pediatric office. Your daily schedule usually includes performing coronal polish on 8 to 10 children. You see a variety of conditions in their mouths.

1. Describe what specific procedures you would be responsible for while performing a coronal polish.

2. Is it possible for a pediatric practice not to have a dental hygienist? If so, how?

3. Because you work with children, what contraindications would prevent you from completing a coronal polish on a patient?

4. During the evaluation of a recall patient, you notice calculus located on the lingual surfaces of the lower anteriors. What should you do?

5. Would calculus be removed before the coronal polishing or after?

MULTIMEDIA PROCEDURES RECOMMENDED REVIEW

■ Coronal Polishing

COMPETENCY 58-1: RUBBER CUP CORONAL POLISHING (EXPANDED FUNCTION)

Performance Objective
By following a routine procedure that meets stated protocols, in states where coronal polishing by a dental assistant is legal, the student will demonstrate the proper procedure for a complete mouth coronal polish.

Evaluation and Grading Criteria
3   Student competently met the stated criteria without assistance.
2   Student required assistance in order to meet the stated criteria.
1   Student showed uncertainty when performing the stated criteria.
0   Student was not prepared and needs to repeat the step.
N/A   No evaluation of this step.
Instructor shall define grades for each point range earned on completion of each performance-evaluated task.

Performance Standards
The minimum number of satisfactory performances required before final evaluation is _____.

Instructor shall identify by * those steps considered critical. If step is missed or minimum competency is not met, the evaluated procedure fails and must be repeated.

PERFORMANCE CRITERIA	*	SELF	PEER	INSTRUCTOR	COMMENT
1. Gathered appropriate supplies.					
2. Personal protective equipment placed according to procedure.					
3. Prepared the patient and explained the procedure.					
4. Maintained the correct operator position and posture for each quadrant.					
5. Maintained adequate retraction and an appropriate fulcrum for each quadrant.					
6. Used the rubber polishing cup and abrasive with the proper polishing movements in all quadrants.					
7. Used the bristle brush and abrasive properly in all quadrants.					
8. Controlled the handpiece speed and pressure throughout the procedure while maintaining patient safety and comfort.					
9. Flossed between the patient's teeth.					
10. Rinsed the patient's mouth.					
11. Evaluated the coronal polish; repeated steps as necessary.					

Continued

12. Maintained patient comfort and followed appropriate infection control measures throughout the procedure.					
13. Procedure documented in patient record.					

ADDITIONAL COMMENTS

Total number of points earned _____

Grade _____ Instructor's initials _____

59 Dental Sealants

SHORT-ANSWER QUESTIONS

1. Describe the purpose of dental sealants.

2. Explain the clinical indications for dental sealants.

3. Explain the clinical contraindications to dental sealants.

4. Discuss the differences between filled and unfilled sealant materials.

5. Describe the two types of polymerization.

6. Describe the steps in the application of dental sealants.

7. Describe the safety steps necessary for the patient and the operator during sealant placement.

8. Explain the most important factor in sealant retention.

FILL-IN-THE-BLANK STATEMENTS

Select the best term from the list below and complete the following statements.

acrylate
dental sealant
light-cured
microabrasion
microleakage

polymerization
sealant retention
self-cured
unfilled resin

1. Resin material applied to the pits and fissures of teeth is a(n) _____.

2. _____ is the process of changing a simple chemical into another substance that contains the same elements.

3. A type of material that is polymerized by chemical reactions is _____.

4. A type of material that is polymerized by a curing light is _____.

5. A technique used to open fissures before sealant placement is _____.

6. _____ is a sealant material that does not contain filler particles.

7. _____ is a microscopic leakage at the interface of the tooth structure and the sealant or restoration.

8. _____ is a salt or ester of acrylic acid.

9. The sealant firmly adheres to the tooth surface because of _____.

MULTIPLE-CHOICE QUESTIONS

Complete each question by circling the best answer.

1. The purpose of dental sealants is _____.
   a. to prevent decay from spreading
   b. to prevent decay in pits and fissures of teeth
   c. to promote good oral health
   d. to prevent decay in interproximal spaces

2. Why are pits and fissures susceptible to caries?
   a. Saliva pools in these areas.
   b. Fluoride is less effective in these areas.
   c. These areas are hard to evaluate on a radiograph.
   d. These areas are difficult to clean.
   e. b and d

3. Are sealants the only preventive measure used?
   a. Yes
   b. No

4. What are the ways for sealant materials to harden?
   a. Polymerization
   b. Light-curing
   c. Self-curing
   d. All of the above

5. Why is clear sealant material less desirable?
   a. It is less attractive.
   b. It is more difficult to evaluate.
   c. It does not match tooth color.
   d. It is contraindicated with dental restorations.

6. What is the difference between filled and unfilled sealants with regard to retention rates?
   a. There is no difference.
   b. Filled sealants are much stronger.
   c. Unfilled sealants will last longer.
   d. The filler is weaker.

7. Sealants are placed _____.
   a. in pits and fissures
   b. on cingula
   c. in grooves
   d. on marginal ridges

8. What is the range of shelf life of sealant materials?
   a. 3 to 6 months
   b. 6 to 12 months
   c. 18 to 36 months
   d. Indefinite

9. What patient safety precautions should be considered when one is placing sealants?
   a. Keep the etchant off the soft tissue.
   b. Use only after the patient has been anesthetized.
   c. Have the patient wear eyewear.
   d. a and c

10. What is the main cause of sealant failures?
    a. Polymerization
    b. Moisture contamination
    c. Deep pits and fissures
    d. Occlusion interference

CASE STUDY

Cindy Evans is an 8-year-old patient who is scheduled to have sealants placed on all of her molars. Dr. Allen is running behind and has told you to go ahead with the placement and to call her if you have any questions.

1. What must Dr. Allen complete before you can begin the procedure?

2. How many teeth will receive sealants?

3. Because you are working on your own, what type of moisture control will you use?

4. Describe your plan for preparation and placement of sealants.

5. After placement, Cindy complains of not being able to close her teeth. What is wrong, and how can you fix it?

MULTIMEDIA PROCEDURES RECOMMENDED REVIEW

- Applying Dental Sealants

INTERACTIVE DENTAL OFFICE PATIENT CASE EXERCISE

Access the *Interactive Dental Office on Evolve* and click on the patient case file for Todd Ledbetter.
- Review Todd's record.
- Complete all exercises on the CD-ROM for Todd's case.
- Answer the following questions.

1. Which of Todd's teeth are going to have dental sealants?

2. Why did Dr. Roberts not recommend sealants for Todd's anterior teeth?

3. Identify the materials in the sealant setup.

Access the *Interactive Dental Office on Evolve* and click on the patient case file for Christopher Brooks.
- Review Christopher's record.
- Complete all exercises on the CD-ROM for Christopher's case.
- Answer the following questions.

1. Which of Christopher's teeth are going to have dental sealants?

2. What type of moisture control is used during sealant placement?

3. Before the sealants are placed, how should the teeth be cleaned?

4. What should be done if Christopher accidentally contaminates the conditioned tooth surface with his saliva?

COMPETENCY 59-1: APPLICATION OF DENTAL SEALANTS (EXPANDED FUNCTION)

Performance Objective

By following a routine procedure that meets stated protocols, in states where application of dental sealants by a dental assistant is legal, the student will demonstrate the proper procedure for applying pit-and-fissure sealants.

Evaluation and Grading Criteria

 3 Student competently met the stated criteria without assistance.
 2 Student required assistance in order to meet the stated criteria.
 1 Student showed uncertainty when performing the stated criteria.
 0 Student was not prepared and needs to repeat the step.
N/A No evaluation of this step.
Instructor shall define grades for each point range earned on completion of each performance-evaluated task.

Performance Standards

The minimum number of satisfactory performances required before final evaluation is _____.

Instructor shall identify by * those steps considered critical. If step is missed or minimum competency is not met, the evaluated procedure fails and must be repeated.

PERFORMANCE CRITERIA	*	SELF	PEER	INSTRUCTOR	COMMENT
1. Gathered appropriate supplies.					
2. Personal protective equipment placed according to procedure.					
3. Seated the patient and explained the procedure.					
4. Polished the teeth to be treated.					
5. Used appropriate steps to prevent contamination by moisture or saliva.					
6. Placed the etching agent on the appropriate surfaces for the time specified by the manufacturer.					
7. Rinsed and dried the teeth, and then verified the appearance of the etched surfaces; if the appearance was not satisfactory, etched the surfaces again.					
8. Placed the sealant on the etched surfaces.					
9. Light-cured the material according to the manufacturer's instructions.					
10. Checked the occlusion and made adjustments as necessary.					
11. Wipe the sealant with a cotton applicator to remove the thin, sticky film on the surface. Check occlusion using articulation paper, and adjust if required.					

Continued

12. Asked the dentist to evaluate the result before the patient was dismissed.				
13. Maintained patient comfort and followed appropriate infection control measures throughout the procedure.				
14. Procedure documented in patient record.				

ADDITIONAL COMMENTS

Total number of points earned _____

Grade _____ Instructor's initials _____

Orthodontics

60

SHORT-ANSWER QUESTIONS

1. Describe the environment of an orthodontic practice.

2. Give the three types of malocclusion.

3. Discuss corrective orthodontics and what type of treatment is involved.

4. List the types of diagnostic records used to assess orthodontic problems.

5. Describe the components of the fixed appliance.

6. Describe the use and function of headgear.

7. Describe how you would convey the importance of dietary and good oral hygiene habits in orthodontic treatment.

FILL-IN-THE-BLANK STATEMENTS

Select the best term from the list below and complete the following statements.

- arch wire
- auxiliary
- band
- braces
- bracket
- cephalometric
- cross-bite
- dentofacial
- distoclusion
- fetal molding

- headgear
- ligature tie
- mesioclusion
- open bite
- orthodontics
- overbite
- overjet
- positioner
- retainer
- separator

1. A(n) _____ is a stainless steel ring cemented to molars to hold the arch wire for orthodontics.

2. The common term for fixed orthodontics is _____.

3. A(n) _____ is a small device bonded to teeth to hold the arch wire in place.

581

4. A(n) _____ is used to secure the arch wire within a bracket.

5. An attachment that is located on a bracket or band to hold an arch wire or elastic is a(n) _____.

6. A(n) _____ is a preformed metal wire that provides force when one is guiding teeth in movement for orthodontics.

7. A(n) _____ is a device made from elastic or wire used to wedge molars open before fitting and placement of orthodontic bands.

8. A(n) _____ is a condition that occurs when a tooth is not properly aligned with its opposing tooth.

9. _____ is another term for class III malocclusion.

10. An extraoral radiograph of the bones and tissues of the head is a(n) _____ radiographic image.

11. _____ is another term used for class II malocclusion.

12. An extraoral orthodontic appliance used to control growth and tooth movement is _____.

13. An appliance used for maintaining the positions of teeth and jaws after orthodontic treatment is a(n) _____.

14. The excessive protrusion of the maxillary incisors is diagnosed as _____.

15. A lack of vertical overlap of the maxillary incisors that creates an opening of the anterior teeth is diagnosed as _____.

16. _____ is the specialty of dentistry designed to prevent, intercept, and correct skeletal and dental problems.

17. _____ is a term that describes the structures that include the teeth, jaws, and surrounding facial bones.

18. A(n) _____ is a type of appliance used to retain teeth in their desired position after orthodontic treatment.

19. An increased vertical overlap of the maxillary incisors is a(n) _____.

20. _____ can occur when pressure is applied to the jaw in vitro, causing a distortion.

MULTIPLE-CHOICE QUESTIONS

Complete each question by circling the best answer.

1. Individuals in what age group seek orthodontic care?
   a. Adolescents
   b. Teenagers
   c. Adults
   d. All of the above

2. What could be a genetic cause for malocclusion?
   a. Parent with a small jaw
   b. Ectopic eruption
   c. Fetal molding
   d. Thumb sucking

3. What is the term used for abnormal occlusion?
   a. Distoclusion
   b. Mesioclusion
   c. Malocclusion
   d. Facial occlusion

4. What tooth is used to determine a person's occlusion?
   a. Maxillary central incisor
   b. Mandibular first premolar
   c. Mandibular first molar
   d. Maxillary first molar

582

Chapter **60** Orthodontics

5. If a person's tooth is not properly aligned with its opposing tooth, the malalignment is referred to as

   _____.
   a. overjet
   b. cross-bite
   c. open bite
   d. overbite

6. If a person occludes and you cannot see his or her mandibular anterior teeth, the diagnosis is

   _____.
   a. overjet
   b. cross-bite
   c. open bite
   d. overbite

7. What views will the orthodontist use to evaluate facial symmetry?
   a. Frontal view
   b. Distal view
   c. Profile view
   d. a and c

8. What type of radiograph is most commonly exposed in orthodontics?
   a. Periapical
   b. Cephalometric
   c. Panoramic
   d. Bitewing

9. How many photographs are commonly taken in the diagnostic records appointment?
   a. Two
   b. Four
   c. Five
   d. Six

10. What gypsum material is most commonly used for fabricating orthodontic diagnostic models?
    a. Plaster
    b. Stone
    c. Alginate
    d. Polyether

11. What instrument is part of the setup for seating and cementing a molar band?
    a. Howe pliers
    b. Bite stick
    c. Explorer
    d. Hemostat

12. The orthodontic scaler is used for _____.
    a. removing calculus from around bands and brackets
    b. placing separators
    c. tying in arch wires
    d. removing excess cement or bonding material

13. Another name for #110 pliers is _____.
    a. contouring pliers
    b. Howe pliers
    c. Weingart pliers
    d. band-removing pliers

14. To ease the placement of orthodontic bands, what procedure is completed to open the contact between teeth?
    a. Wearing of a positioner
    b. Placement of a ligature tie
    c. Bonding of a bracket
    d. Placement of a separator

15. When cementing bands, what can be used to prevent cement from getting into the buccal tubes or attachments?
    a. String
    b. Lip balm
    c. Utility wax
    d. b and c

16. How are brackets adhered to a tooth?
    a. Cement
    b. Sealant
    c. Bonding agent
    d. Wax

17. Where are auxiliary attachments found on braces?
    a. Brackets
    b. Arch wire
    c. "Bands"
    d. a and c

18. What shape of arch wire is indicated for correcting malalignment of teeth?
    a. Round wire
    b. Rectangular wire
    c. Braided wire
    d. Twisted wire

19. How would an arch wire be sized for a patient without placing it into the patient's mouth?
    a. Cephalometric radiograph
    b. Study model
    c. Used arch wire
    d. b and c

20. Besides ligature ties, what can be used to hold an arch wire in place?
    a. Cement
    b. Elastomeric ties
    c. Band
    d. Positioner

21. What appliance might the orthodontist use to maintain growth and/or tooth movement?
    a. Space maintainer
    b. Retainer
    c. Headgear
    d. All of the above

22. How could hard foods possibly harm a person's braces?
    a. They can bend a wire.
    b. They can loosen a bracket.
    c. They can pull off a band.
    d. All of the above

23. How can a patient with braces make flossing easier?
    a. Use a floss threader.
    b. Use waxed floss.
    c. Use unwaxed floss.
    d. Have the arch wire positioned toward the incisal or occlusal edge.

24. When braces come off, does that mean treatment is over?
    a. Yes
    b. No

25. An example of a retention appliance is the

    _____.
    a. Hawley retainer
    b. positioner
    c. lingual retainer
    d. All of the above

CASE STUDY

Matt is 14 years old and has completed the diagnostic phase for corrective orthodontics. Through discussion with his parents and the orthodontist, Matt is anxious to get braces to correct crowding in the anterior area and a cross-bite on his left side. He is scheduled today for his first appointment.

1. What diagnostic tools were used to evaluate Matt's case?

2. Discuss the importance of having Matt, his parents, and the orthodontist together when the final decision about having braces is made.

3. What procedure will be completed on Matt today?

4. He should be scheduled for which procedure next time? How long should the appointment last?

5. What is your role in the fitting and cementation of orthodontic bands?

6. After banding, what would be the next procedure to be scheduled?

7. It is common to tell the patient that the length of time he or she will have braces is what?

8. Once the braces come off, what will Matt wear to make sure everything remains aligned?

INTERACTIVE DENTAL OFFICE PATIENT CASE EXERCISE ⊖volve
learning system

Access the *Interactive Dental Office on Evolve* and click on the patient case file for Kevin McClelland.
- Review Kevin's record.
- Complete all exercises on Evolve for Kevin's case.
- Answer the following questions.

1. Looking at Kevin's panoramic, which teeth are banded?

2. What types of ligatures are used for Kevin's orthodontic treatment?

3. The bands have labial hooks. What are these used for?

4. What type of oral hygiene instructions should be provided to Kevin while orthodontic treatment is in progress?

5. Kevin is scheduled to have a sealant placed on tooth #19. Can a sealant be placed while Kevin is receiving orthodontic treatment?

COMPETENCIES 60-1 AND 60-2: PLACING AND REMOVING SEPARATORS (EXPANDED FUNCTION)

Performance Objective

By following a routine procedure that meets stated protocols, the student will demonstrate the proper technique when placing separators.

Evaluation and Grading Criteria

　3　 Student competently met the stated criteria without assistance.
　2　 Student required assistance in order to meet the stated criteria.
　1　 Student showed uncertainty when performing the stated criteria.
　0　 Student was not prepared and needs to repeat the step.
　N/A　 No evaluation of this step.
Instructor shall define grades for each point range earned on completion of each performance-evaluated task.

Performance Standards

The minimum number of satisfactory performances required before final evaluation is ＿＿＿＿＿＿＿.

Instructor shall identify by * those steps considered critical. If step is missed or minimum competency is not met, the evaluated procedure fails and must be repeated.

PERFORMANCE CRITERIA	*	SELF	PEER	INSTRUCTOR	COMMENT
1. Gathered the appropriate setup.					
2. Explained the procedure to the patient.					
3. Personal protective equipment placed according to procedure.					
4. Carried the separator with the appropriate instrument for placement.					
5. Inserted the separator below the proximal contact.					
6. Recorded in the patient record the number of separators used.					
7. Provided postoperative instructions to the patient.					
8. Maintained patient comfort and followed appropriate infection control measures throughout the procedure.					
9. Procedure documented in patient record.					

Continued

Removal of Separators				
1. Used orthodontic scaler to remove eparator				
2. Slid instrument under and continued to remove separator from bracket wings.				
3. Procedure documented in patient record.				
ADDITIONAL COMMENTS				

Total number of points earned _____

Grade _____ Instructor's initials _____

COMPETENCY 60-3: ASSISTING IN THE FITTING AND CEMENTATION OF ORTHODONTIC BANDS (EXPANDED FUNCTION)

Performance Objective

By following a routine procedure that meets stated protocols, the student will prepare the appropriate setup and will assist in the cementation of orthodontic bands.

Evaluation and Grading Criteria

 3 Student competently met the stated criteria without assistance.
 2 Student required assistance in order to meet the stated criteria.
 1 Student showed uncertainty when performing the stated criteria.
 0 Student was not prepared and needs to repeat the step.
 N/A No evaluation of this step.

Instructor shall define grades for each point range earned on completion of each performance-evaluated task.

Performance Standards

The minimum number of satisfactory performances required before final evaluation is _____.

Instructor shall identify by * those steps considered critical. If step is missed or minimum competency is not met, the evaluated procedure fails and must be repeated.

PERFORMANCE CRITERIA	*	SELF	PEER	INSTRUCTOR	COMMENT
1. Gathered the appropriate setup.					
2. Personal protective equipment placed according to procedure.					
3. Placed each preselected orthodontic band on a small square of masking tape with the occlusal surface on the tape.					
4. Wiped any buccal tubes or attachments with the lip balm.					
5. Mixed the cement according to the manufacturer's instructions.					
6. Loaded the bands with cement correctly by flowing cement into the band.					
7. Transferred the band correctly.					
8. For a maxillary band, transferred the band pusher.					
9. For a mandibular band, transferred the band seater.					
10. Repeated the process until all bands were cemented.					

Continued

11. Cleaned the cement spatula and slab.				
12. Used a scaler or explorer to remove excess cement on the enamel surfaces, then rinsed the patient's mouth.				
13. Maintained patient comfort and followed appropriate infection control measures throughout the procedure.				
14. Procedure documented in patient record.				
ADDITIONAL COMMENTS				

Total number of points earned _____

Grade _____ Instructor's initials _____

COMPETENCY 60-4: ASSISTING IN THE DIRECT BONDING OF ORTHODONTIC BRACKETS

Performance Objective
By following a routine procedure that meets stated protocols, the student will prepare the appropriate setup and will assist in the bonding of orthodontic brackets.

Evaluation and Grading Criteria
3	Student competently met the stated criteria without assistance.
2	Student required assistance in order to meet the stated criteria.
1	Student showed uncertainty when performing the stated criteria.
0	Student was not prepared and needs to repeat the step.
N/A	No evaluation of this step.

Instructor shall define grades for each point range earned on completion of each performance-evaluated task.

Performance Standards
The minimum number of satisfactory performances required before final evaluation is _____.

Instructor shall identify by * those steps considered critical. If step is missed or minimum competency is not met, the evaluated procedure fails and must be repeated.

PERFORMANCE CRITERIA	*	SELF	PEER	INSTRUCTOR	COMMENT
1. Gathered the appropriate setup.					
2. Personal protective equipment placed according to procedure.					
3. If stain or plaque was present, prepared tooth surfaces using a rubber cup and a pumice slurry.					
4. Isolated the teeth.					
5. Assisted throughout the etching of the teeth.					
6. Applied a small quantity of bonding material on the back of the bracket.					
7. Used bracket placement tweezers to transfer the brackets to the orthodontist.					
8. Transferred an orthodontic scaler for final placement and removal of excess bonding material.					
9. Maintained patient comfort and followed appropriate infection control measures throughout the procedure.					
10. Procedure documented in patient record.					
ADDITIONAL COMMENTS					

Total number of points earned _____

Grade _____ Instructor's initials _____

COMPETENCIES 60-5 TO 60-7: PLACING AND REMOVING ARCH WIRES AND TIES (EXPANDED FUNCTION)

Performance Objective

By following a routine procedure that meets stated protocols, the student will demonstrate the proper technique for placing and removing ligature wires and elastomeric ties.

Evaluation and Grading Criteria

<u>3</u>   Student competently met the stated criteria without assistance.
<u>2</u>   Student required assistance in order to meet the stated criteria.
<u>1</u>   Student showed uncertainty when performing the stated criteria.
<u>0</u>   Student was not prepared and needs to repeat the step.
<u>N/A</u> No evaluation of this step.
Instructor shall define grades for each point range earned on completion of each performance-evaluated task.

Performance Standards

The minimum number of satisfactory performances required before final evaluation is _____.

Instructor shall identify by * those steps considered critical. If step is missed or minimum competency is not met, the evaluated procedure fails and must be repeated.

PERFORMANCE CRITERIA	*	SELF	PEER	INSTRUCTOR	COMMENT
Placing the Arch Wires					
1. Gathered the appropriate setup.					
2. Personal protective equipment placed according to procedure.					
3. Wire premeasured before placed in the mouth					
4. If additional bends are needed, transferred appropriate plier to orthodontist					
5. Centered arch wire					
6. Distal ends of wire placed in buccal tube with correct length.					
Placing the Ligature Wires					
7. Placed the ligature wire around the bracket and used the ligature director to push the wire against the tie wing.					
8. Used the hemostat to twist the wire snugly against the bracket; repeated the procedure until all brackets were ligated.					
9. Used a ligature cutter to cut the excess wire, leaving a 4- to 5-mm pigtail.					
10. Tucked the pigtails under the arch wire using the correct instruments.					
11. Wire was not protruding to injure the patient.					

Continued

Removing the Ligature Wire					
1. Held the ligature cutter properly and used the beaks of the pliers to cut the wire at the easiest access.					
2. Carefully unwrapped the ligature and removed it.					
3. Did not twist or pull as the ligatures were cut and removed.					
4. Continued cutting and removing until all brackets were untied.					
5. Maintained patient comfort and followed appropriate infection control measures throughout the procedure.					
Placing the Elastomeric Tie					
1. Gathered the appropriate setup.					
2. Used a hemostat and placed the beaks of the pliers on a tie, then locked the pliers.					
3. Placed the tie on the gingival portion of one tie wing and slipped the tie around the edges of the bracket.					
4. Released the pliers.					
Removing the Elastomeric Tie					
1. Used the orthodontic scaler held in a pen grasp, and supported the teeth and tissue with the other hand.					
2. Placed the scaler tie between the bracket and tie wings and pulled the tie at the gingival position with a rolling motion.					
3. Removed the tie in an occlusal direction.					
4. Maintained patient comfort and followed appropriate infection control measures throughout the procedure.					
5. Procedure documented in patient record.					

ADDITIONAL COMMENTS

Total number of points earned _____

Grade _____ Instructor's initials _____

61 Communication in the Dental Office

SHORT-ANSWER QUESTIONS

1. Describe the type of relationship the patient and dental team should have.

2. Discuss oral communications, and identify the differences between verbal and nonverbal communications.

3. Describe professional phone courtesy.

4. Describe and compare the handling of different types of phone calls.

5. Describe external and internal marketing.

6. Discuss the types of stress that exist in a dental practice.

7. Discuss what the "team" concept can do to improve communication.

FILL-IN-THE-BLANK STATEMENTS

Select the best term from the list below and complete the following statements.

copier
fax machine
letterhead
marketing

nonverbal communication
salutation
verbal communication
word processing software

1. The part of the letter that contains the introductory greeting is the _____.

2. _____ is the type of communication by which we use words to express ourselves.

3. _____ a computer program used to create most business documents.

4. A _____ is a business machine that can make duplicates from an original.

5. The business machine that is attached to a phone line and can send written or typed materials is the _____.

6. _____ is the type of communication that uses body language for expression.

7. The _____ is the part of a letter that contains the name and address of the person sending the letter.

8. _____ is a way of advertising or recruiting people to your business.

MULTIPLE-CHOICE QUESTIONS

Complete each question by circling the best answer.

1. What type of communication describes our body language?
   a. Verbal
   b. Written
   c. Nonverbal
   d. Speech

2. What percent of verbal communication is never heard?
   a. 50%
   b. 75%
   c. 90%
   d. 100%

3. What nonverbal behavior could describe tension and uneasiness?
   a. Restrained gait
   b. Grasping the chair arms
   c. Rapid shallow breathing
   d. All of the above

4. Select a more professional term for "pulling" a tooth.
   a. Luxate
   b. Take
   c. Extract
   d. Tug

5. How is a patient psychologically influenced by attitudes of others?
   a. From subjective fears
   b. From negative fears
   c. From objective fears
   d. a and c

6. How are objective fears attained?
   a. By hearing others express their experiences
   b. By learning fears from past experiences
   c. By dreaming up fears
   d. By reading about fears

7. What are some of the best ways to calm an irate patient?
   a. Listen.
   b. Maintain eye contact.
   c. Nod your head when the patient is talking.
   d. All of the above

8. The most important piece of equipment used in a dental office for public relations is the _____.
   a. professional letter
   b. fax machine
   c. telephone
   d. newsletter

9. At what ring should the telephone be answered?
   a. First
   b. Second
   c. Third
   d. Does not matter

10. When the dental office is closed, how should telephone messages be obtained?
    a. Answering service
    b. Answering machine
    c. Email
    d. a and b

11. What piece of equipment allows you to send and receive typed documents?
    a. Phone
    b. Fax machine
    c. Photocopier
    d. Pager

12. Which component is included in the salutation of a letter?
    a. Date
    b. Inside address
    c. Greeting
    d. Closing

13. Besides the patient, who would the business assistant correspond with?
    a. Other dental professionals
    b. Physicians
    c. Dental insurance companies
    d. All of the above

14. Which dental professional would not be involved in the marketing of a practice?
    a. Dentist
    b. Business assistant
    c. Dental laboratory technician
    d. Dental assistant

15. What percentage of revenue should a dental practice invest in marketing?
    a. 1% to 2% of gross revenue
    b. 3% to 5% of gross revenue
    c. 8% to 10% of gross revenue
    d. 15% to 20% of gross revenue

16. An example of an external marketing activity is _____.
    a. preparing and distributing a newsletter for current patients
    b. attending a health fair
    c. sending flowers
    d. All of the above

17. What is the key to a successful work environment?
    a. High salaries
    b. Teamwork
    c. Good benefits
    d. Job flexibility

18. What would not be a stress factor for working in a dental office?
    a. Job flexibility
    b. Overbooking of patients
    c. Performance of multiple tasks
    d. Little opportunity for job advancement

19. Americans spend more time with their _____ than anyone else.
    a. family
    b. friends
    c. coworkers
    d. patients

20. What is a valuable communication tool for a dental practice?
    a. Business letter
    b. Practice newsletter
    c. Personal phone call
    d. Health fair

ACTIVITY

Create a professional letter using the following directions:

1. Use the dental practice heading.

2. Write about the introduction of a new dentist to the practice, how it will affect scheduling, and any changes in staff that will occur.

3. Send the letter to all patients of the practice.

COMPETENCY 61-1: ANSWERING THE PHONE

Performance Objective
By following a routine procedure that meets stated protocols, the student will demonstrate the proper technique when answering the phone in a place of business.

Evaluation and Grading Criteria
 3   Student competently met the stated criteria without assistance.
 2   Student required assistance in order to meet the stated criteria.
 1   Student showed uncertainty when performing the stated criteria.
 0   Student was not prepared and needs to repeat the step.
 N/A No evaluation of this step.
Instructor shall define grades for each point range earned on completion of each performance-evaluated task.

Performance Standards
The minimum number of satisfactory performances required before final evaluation is _____.

Instructor shall identify by * those steps considered critical. If step is missed or minimum competency is not met, the evaluated procedure fails and must be repeated.

PERFORMANCE CRITERIA	*	SELF	PEER	INSTRUCTOR	COMMENT
1. Answered the phone on the first ring.					
2. Spoke directly into the receiver.					
3. Identified the office and self.					
4. Acknowledged the caller by name.					
5. Followed through on the caller's specific inquiry.					
6. Took a message if appropriate.					
7. Completed the call in a professional manner.					
8. Replaced the receiver after the caller hung up.					
ADDITIONAL COMMENTS					

Total number of points earned _____

Grade _____ Instructor's initials _____

COMPETENCY 61-2: COMPOSING A BUSINESS LETTER

Performance Objective

By following a routine procedure that meets stated protocols, the student will demonstrate the proper technique when composing and typing a professional letter.

Evaluation and Grading Criteria

  3 Student competently met the stated criteria without assistance.
  2 Student required assistance in order to meet the stated criteria.
  1 Student showed uncertainty when performing the stated criteria.
  0 Student was not prepared and needs to repeat the step.
 N/A No evaluation of this step.
Instructor shall define grades for each point range earned on completion of each performance-evaluated task.

Performance Standards

The minimum number of satisfactory performances required before final evaluation is _____.

Instructor shall identify by * those steps considered critical. If step is missed or minimum competency is not met, the evaluated procedure fails and must be repeated.

PERFORMANCE CRITERIA	*	SELF	PEER	INSTRUCTOR	COMMENT
1. Prepared the first draft for review.					
2. Checked for correct information, grammar, spelling, and punctuation.					
3. Ensured that the letter had correct margins, font, spacing, and order of text.					
4. Signed name to close the letter.					
ADDITIONAL COMMENTS					

Total number of points earned _____

Grade _____ Instructor's initials _____

62 Business Operating Systems

SHORT-ANSWER QUESTIONS

1. Discuss the role of the office manager and business assistant in the dental office.

2. Define three types of practice records or files commonly used in a dental practice.

3. Describe how each of the following filing systems is used: alphabetic, numeric, cross-reference, chronologic, and subject.

4. Describe the importance of appointment scheduling for maximum productivity.

5. Identify three types of preventive recall systems, and state the benefits of each.

6. Describe the function of computerized practice management systems versus manual bookkeeping systems.

7. Discuss the management of inventory systems.

FILL-IN-THE-BLANK STATEMENTS

Select the best term from the list below and complete the following statements.

active	outguide
buffer time	patient of record
call list	purchase order
chronologic file	rate of use
cross-reference file	reorder tags
daily schedule	requisition
filing	shelf life
inactive	units
lead time	want list
ledger	warranty

1. The _____ is the time estimated to allow for delays when materials are ordered or backordered materials are shipped.

2. A(n) _____ patient is one who has been seen within the past 2 to 3 years.

603

3. A filing system that divides materials into months and days of the month is called a(n) _____.

4. Time reserved on the schedule for emergency patients is the _____.

5. A patient who has not been seen in the office for the past 5 years is considered _____.

6. A(n) _____ is a filing system that uses alphabetic order by name and provides a document number.

7. A(n) _____ is a list of patients who can come in for an appointment on short notice.

8. A printed schedule of the day's procedures that is copied and placed throughout the office for viewing by staff is a(n) _____.

9. _____ is the act of classifying and arranging records to be easily retrieved when needed.

10. A(n) _____ is a type of file or statement that contains the patient's financial records.

11. A(n) _____ is like a bookmark for a filing system.

12. A written statement that outlines the manufacturer's responsibility for replacement and repair of a particular product is a(n) _____.

13. A(n) _____ is a form that authorizes the purchase of supplies from the supplier.

14. A(n) _____ means the person is being seen in the dental practice on a routine schedule.

15. The _____ of something is the time a product may be stored before it begins to deteriorate and is no longer usable.

16. Time increments used in scheduling appointments are _____.

17. A(n) _____ is a list of supplies to be ordered.

18. The _____ is how many or how much of a product is used within a given time.

19. A(n) _____ is a formal request for supplies.

20. _____ are placed when the supply of a certain item is close to being low and the item needs to be replaced.

MULTIPLE-CHOICE QUESTIONS

Complete each question by circling the best answer.

1. Who oversees the financial activities of a dental practice?
   a. Dentist
   b. Clinical assistant
   c. Outside accountant
   d. Business assistant

2. How should a new employee learn about office protocol?
   a. During the interview
   b. From an office procedure manual
   c. From a continuing education course
   d. From the dentist

604

3. What continues to replace manual work in the business office?
   a. Temporary service
   b. Typewriter
   c. Tape recorder
   d. Computer

4. Another term used for a "patient statement" is

   _____.
   a. patient record
   b. ledger
   c. file
   d. document

5. How much free space should be left on each shelf of a filing cabinet?
   a. 2 inches
   b. 4 inches
   c. 6 inches
   d. 1 foot

6. What is used to mark a space where a file has been taken?
   a. Bookmark
   b. Empty file
   c. Ledger
   d. Outguide

7. What is the easiest filing system used?
   a. Chronologic
   b. Alphabetic
   c. Numeric
   d. Color-coded

8. If a patient has not been seen within the past 4 years, what is his or her status as a patient of the practice?
   a. Active
   b. On recall
   c. Backorder
   d. Inactive

9. How many minutes commonly make up 1 unit of time for scheduling?
   a. 5 to 7 minutes
   b. 10 to 15 minutes
   c. 20 to 40 minutes
   d. 60 minutes

10. What elements should be outlined in an appointment book?
    a. Office hours
    b. Buffer times
    c. Meetings
    d. All of the above

11. If a patient does not keep his or her appointment, where should this be recorded?
    a. On the ledger
    b. In the patient record
    c. In the appointment book
    d. b and c

12. What is the most common time frame for scheduling recall appointments?
    a. 3 months
    b. 6 months
    c. 9 months
    d. 1 year

13. If a patient is seen in September, what is his or her recall time for a 6-month appointment?
    a. August
    b. September
    c. February
    d. March

14. What factors must be determined when a product has to be reordered?
    a. Rate of use
    b. Shelf life
    c. Lead time
    d. All of the above

15. How is an item marked for reorder?
    a. Reorder tag
    b. Blue slip
    c. Outguide
    d. Inguide

16. How are supplies ordered?
    a. From a sales representative
    b. By telephone or fax
    c. From a catalog
    d. All of the above

17. What happens when an item is not available from a supply company?
    a. You are referred to another company.
    b. You call other offices to order the product.
    c. It goes on backorder.
    d. You wait until a new shipment is received.

18. What is not considered an expendable item?
    a. Handpiece
    b. Plastic suction tip
    c. Patient napkin
    d. Gloves

19. When a dental unit breaks down, how does this affect a dental practice?
   a. Loss of income
   b. Inconvenience to the dental team
   c. Scheduling conflicts
   d. All of the above

20. A written statement that the dentist receives from the manufacturer that describes the responsibility of equipment replacement and repair is a

   _____.
   a. requisition
   b. warranty
   c. contract
   d. a and c

TOPICS FOR DISCUSSION

As the business assistant in the office, your job is to organize and maintain the operating systems of the dental practice. During your weekly team meeting, the dentist has expressed concern for the decline in patients being scheduled. Because of this decrease, the revenue of the practice has also decreased.

1. Does this issue concern the clinical or business staff of the practice?

2. How could the decrease in revenue affect the staff?

3. Describe how the following could increase the number of daily patients who are active patients of the practice.
   a. Scheduling
   b. Recall
   c. Broken appointments
   d. Quality assurance

4. Describe different methods that may be used to increase the number of new patients in the practice.

DENTRIX EXERCISE

The Dentrix Appointment Book is an electronic scheduler that allows you to manage your patient appointments without paper. Convenient toolbars and exclusive Flip Tabs help you navigate through appointments, search for available time slots, organize appointments and notes, and handle all the common tasks need to run the dental office schedule. Please refer to the Dentrix *User's Guide,* Chapter 7, to review how to complete scheduling.

Exercise: Scheduling Appointments

Please refer to the information on the Evolve website on **Scheduling Appointments** and **Moving Appointments.** Then complete scheduling for the Brooks family. They would all like to schedule appointments in the third week of February. Listed below are the preferences for each family member, along with the procedures that are to be completed on the day of the appointment.

1. Gregory Brooks (prefers afternoon appointment)
   - Complete examination
   - Four bitewing radiographs
   - Prophylaxis

2. Jessica Brooks (prefers morning appointment)
   - MOD composite resin: Tooth #5
   - DO composite resin: Tooth #7

3. Christopher Brooks (prefers to be scheduled with his mother)
   - Periodic oral examination
   - Two bitewing radiographs
   - Prophylaxis
   - Fluoride treatment

63 Financial Management in the Dental Office

SHORT-ANSWER QUESTIONS

1. Describe the functions of computerized practice management systems and manual bookkeeping systems.

2. Describe how to make financial arrangements with a patient.

3. Describe the importance and management of collections in the dental office.

4. Describe check writing.

5. Explain the purpose of business summaries.

6. Identify common payroll withholding taxes, and discuss the financial responsibility of the employer regarding this practice.

7. Discuss the purpose of dental insurance.

8. Identify insurance fraud.

9. Identify the parties involved with dental insurance.

10. Identify the various types of prepaid dental programs.

11. Define managed care.

12. Discuss and define basic dental terminology.

13. Explain dual coverage.

14. Identify dental procedures and coding.

15. Detail claim forms processing.

16. Describe the procedure and purpose of claim forms follow-up.

FILL-IN-THE-BLANK STATEMENTS

Select the best term from the list below and complete the following statements.

accounting	ledger
accounts payable	net income
carrier	petty cash
CDT	posted
check	provider
customary	reasonable
deposit slip	responsible party
expenses	statement
gross income	transaction
invoice	walkout statement

1. Expenses and disbursements paid out from a business are called _____.

2. A(n) _____ is a draft or an order on a bank for payment of a specific amount of money.

3. _____ constitute the overhead that a business requires in order to keep operating.

4. _____ is a system designed to maintain the financial records of a business.

5. A fee that is within the range of the usual fee charged for a service is the _____ fee.

6. A(n) _____ is an itemized list of the funds to be deposited into the bank.

7. A(n) _____ is the insurance company that pays the claims and collects premiums.

8. _____ are procedure codes that are assigned to dental services in the process of dental insurance.

9. _____ is the total of all professional income received.

10. A(n) _____ is an itemized list of goods that specifies the prices and terms of sale.

11. A financial statement that maintains all account transactions of a patient is a(n) _____.

12. _____ is the income minus the expenses taken out.

610

13. _____ is the term used for documenting money transactions within a business.

14. The _____ is the dentist who offers treatment to a patient.

15. The _____ is similar to a receipt in that it shows the account balance.

16. A fee that is considered fair for an extensive or complex treatment is called _____.

17. The person who has agreed to pay for an account is the _____.

18. A small amount of money kept on hand for small daily expenses is _____.

19. The _____ is a summary of all charges, payments, credits, and debits for the month.

20. The _____ is a change in payment or an adjustment made to a financial account.

MULTIPLE-CHOICE QUESTIONS

Complete each question by circling the best answer.

1. What types of bookkeeping systems are used in a dental practice?
   a. Accounts receivable
   b. Accounts payable
   c. Accounts taxable
   d. a and b

2. What form will you use to gather financial information from a patient?
   a. Treatment plan
   b. Consent form
   c. Registration form
   d. Ledger

3. Where should the business assistant discuss financial arrangements with a patient?
   a. Dental treatment area
   b. Dental laboratory
   c. Reception area
   d. Private setting

4. Money that is owed to the practice is considered _____.
   a. accounts payable
   b. revenue
   c. accounts receivable
   d. gross income

5. If a dental office does not have a computerized accounts receivable system, what manual system would be used?
   a. Check register
   b. Posting slip
   c. Pegboard system
   d. Ledger

6. What form is used to transmit a patient's fee for service from the treatment area to the business office?
   a. Receipt
   b. Patient record
   c. Ledger
   d. Charge slip

7. What means of payment can a patient use for his or her account?
   a. Cash
   b. Credit
   c. Insurance
   d. All of the above

8. How often should bank deposits be made?
   a. Daily
   b. Weekly
   c. Monthly
   d. Quarterly

9. When should an office begin collection efforts on a past due account?
   a. After 15 days
   b. After 30 days
   c. After 60 days
   d. After 90 days

10. How would a business follow through on the collection of fees?
    a. Letters
    b. Phone call
    c. Collection agency
    d. All of the above

11. An example of fixed overhead is _____.
    a. dental supplies
    b. continuing education
    c. salaries
    d. business supplies

12. A paycheck is a person's _____.
    a. gross income
    b. net income
    c. reimbursement
    d. accounts receivable

13. Which document will arrive with the shipment of supplies?
    a. Packing slip
    b. Invoice
    c. Statement
    d. All of the above

14. C.O.D. means _____.
    a. cancel order delivered
    b. cost of dental service
    c. cash on delivery
    d. cash order delinquent

15. Where would you record check deposits made on an account?
    a. Daily schedule
    b. Check register
    c. Recall system
    d. Patient registration

16. What term indicates that an account does not have enough money to cover a check?
    a. Insufficient funds
    b. Bounced
    c. Inadequate funds
    d. Delinquent

17. The method of calculating fee-for-service benefits is _____.
    a. UCR
    b. schedule of benefits
    c. fixed fee
    d. All of the above

18. What is the specified amount of money that an insured person must pay before his or her insurance goes into effect?
    a. Overhead
    b. Deductible
    c. Customary fee
    d. Reimbursement fee

19. A child or spouse of an insurance subscriber is considered to be a(n) _____.
    a. uninsured
    b. copayer
    c. dependent
    d. deductible

20. A patient's insurance information is submitted by means of _____.
    a. a fax
    b. registered mail
    c. a claim form
    d. a table of allowances

ACTIVITY

Complete the insurance form on the next page. Use the information listed on the back of the insurance form on the following page.

ADA American Dental Association® Dental Claim Form

HEADER INFORMATION

1. Type of Transaction (Mark all applicable boxes)

☐ Statement of Actual Services   ☐ Request for Predetermination/Preauthorization
☐ EPSDT / Title XIX

2. Predetermination/Preauthorization Number

INSURANCE COMPANY/DENTAL BENEFIT PLAN INFORMATION

3. Company/Plan Name, Address, City, State, Zip Code

OTHER COVERAGE (Mark applicable box and complete items 5-11. If none, leave blank.)

4. Dental? ☐   Medical? ☐   (If both, complete 5-11 for dental only.)

5. Name of Policyholder/Subscriber in #4 (Last, First, Middle Initial, Suffix)

6. Date of Birth (MM/DD/CCYY)   7. Gender ☐ M ☐ F   8. Policyholder/Subscriber ID (SSN or ID#)

9. Plan/Group Number   10. Patient's Relationship to Person named in #5 ☐ Self ☐ Spouse ☐ Dependent ☐ Other

11. Other Insurance Company/Dental Benefit Plan Name, Address, City, State, Zip Code

POLICYHOLDER/SUBSCRIBER INFORMATION (For Insurance Company Named in #3)

12. Policyholder/Subscriber Name (Last, First, Middle Initial, Suffix), Address, City, State, Zip Code

13. Date of Birth (MM/DD/CCYY)   14. Gender ☐ M ☐ F   15. Policyholder/Subscriber ID (SSN or ID#)

16. Plan/Group Number   17. Employer Name

PATIENT INFORMATION

18. Relationship to Policyholder/Subscriber in #12 Above ☐ Self ☐ Spouse ☐ Dependent Child ☐ Other   19. Reserved For Future Use

20. Name (Last, First, Middle Initial, Suffix), Address, City, State, Zip Code

21. Date of Birth (MM/DD/CCYY)   22. Gender ☐ M ☐ F   23. Patient ID/Account # (Assigned by Dentist)

RECORD OF SERVICES PROVIDED

	24. Procedure Date (MM/DD/CCYY)	25. Area of Oral Cavity	26. Tooth System	27. Tooth Number(s) or Letter(s)	28. Tooth Surface	29. Procedure Code	29a. Diag. Pointer	29b. Qty.	30. Description	31. Fee
1										
2										
3										
4										
5										
6										
7										
8										
9										
10										

33. Missing Teeth Information   (Place an "X" on each missing tooth.)

1	2	3	4	5	6	7	8	9	10	11	12	13	14	15	16
32	31	30	29	28	27	26	25	24	23	22	21	20	19	18	17

34. Diagnosis Code List Qualifier ☐   (ICD-9 = B; ICD-10 = AB)

34a. Diagnosis Code(s)   A _____   C _____
(Primary diagnosis in "A")   B _____   D _____

31a. Other Fee(s)

32. Total Fee

35. Remarks

AUTHORIZATIONS

36. I have been informed of the treatment plan and associated fees. I agree to be responsible for all charges for dental services and materials not paid by my dental benefit plan, unless prohibited by law, or the treating dentist or dental practice has a contractual agreement with my plan prohibiting all or a portion of such charges. To the extent permitted by law, I consent to your use and disclosure of my protected health information to carry out payment activities in connection with this claim.

X _____
Patient/Guardian Signature   Date

37. I hereby authorize and direct payment of the dental benefits otherwise payable to me, directly to the below named dentist or dental entity.

X _____
Subscriber Signature   Date

BILLING DENTIST OR DENTAL ENTITY (Leave blank if dentist or dental entity is not submitting claim on behalf of the patient or insured/subscriber.)

48. Name, Address, City, State, Zip Code

49. NPI   50. License Number   51. SSN or TIN

52. Phone Number ( ) -   52a. Additional Provider ID

ANCILLARY CLAIM/TREATMENT INFORMATION

38. Place of Treatment ☐ (e.g. 11=office; 22=O/P Hospital)
(Use "Place of Service Codes for Professional Claims")

39. Enclosures (Y or N) ☐

40. Is Treatment for Orthodontics? ☐ No (Skip 41-42) ☐ Yes (Complete 41-42)

41. Date Appliance Placed (MM/DD/CCYY)

42. Months of Treatment   43. Replacement of Prosthesis ☐ No ☐ Yes (Complete 44)   44. Date of Prior Placement (MM/DD/CCYY)

45. Treatment Resulting from ☐ Occupational illness/injury ☐ Auto accident ☐ Other accident

46. Date of Accident (MM/DD/CCYY)   47. Auto Accident State

TREATING DENTIST AND TREATMENT LOCATION INFORMATION

53. I hereby certify that the procedures as indicated by date are in progress (for procedures that require multiple visits) or have been completed.

X _____
Signed (Treating Dentist)   Date

54. NPI   55. License Number

56. Address, City, State, Zip Code   56a. Provider Specialty Code

57. Phone Number ( ) -   58. Additional Provider ID

To reorder call 800.947.4746
or go online at adacatalog.org

613

Personal Information

Birth Date:	5-22-79
Social Security Number:	402-38-2853
Name:	Jason F. Scott
Address:	8402 Alexander Drive
	Colorado Springs, CO 39720
Home Phone:	486-555-1847
Employer:	U.S. Olympic Association
Work Phone:	486-555-4910
Responsible Party:	Same as above

Dental Insurance Information

Name of Insured:	Jason F. Scott
Insurance Company:	Dental Support
Group Number:	48204
Employee Certificate Number:	40238285-20
Address:	P.O. Box 313
	Denver, CO 13750
Annual Benefits:	1800.00

Treatment to Be Recorded

Date	Tooth and Surface	Treatment	Fee
3/12/11		Periodic Oral Evaluation	75.00
3/12/11		Full Mouth Series	65.00
3/12/11		Oral Prophylaxis	80.00
4/29/11	3 MOD	Amalgam	90.00
4/29/11	4 DO	Amalgam	60.00
5/03/11	10 F	Composite	32.00
5/03/11	11 DI	Composite	64.00
6/10/11	20	Root Canal	700.00
6/20/11	20	PFM Crown	800.00

The Dentrix Ledger component works just like a paper ledger, only it's faster, easier, and more powerful. The main Ledger screen packs a wealth of information in an easy-to-read format, making it possible to find necessary information without toggling among endless screens and menus. The Ledger facilitates entry of payments, claim filing, statement printouts, and much more – all from a single location.

Exercise: Patient Checkout Procedures

Please refer to the information on the Evolve website on **Creating a Pretreatment Estimate, Generating a Payment Agreement, Posting Scheduled Work,** and **Completing a Patient Checkout.** Then complete the following procedures for the Brooks family.

1. Pretreatment Estimate
   - Create a pretreatment estimate for Gregory Brooks.
   - Create a pretreatment estimate for Jessica Brooks.
   - Create a pretreatment estimate for Christopher Brooks.

   a. What is the total estimated charge for each patient?

   b. What is the estimated insurance payment for each patient?

   c. What is the total out-of-pocket payment for the Brooks family?

2. Payment Agreement
   - Complete a Payment Agreement for Gregory Brooks.
   - Print a Truth in Lending Disclosure Statement for Gregory Brooks.
   - Print a Coupon Book for Scheduled Payments.

3. Patient Checkout
   - The Brooks family has completed their treatment.

   a. Post the procedures attached to Gregory Brooks' appointment to show that they have been completed.
   b. Print the Insurance Claim for Gregory Brooks.
   c. Print a Walkout Statement for Gregory Brooks.

64 Marketing Your Skills

1. Determine your career goals, and describe your own personal philosophy.

2. Identify potential career opportunities.

3. Describe the procedures required for a job interview.

4. Discuss factors to consider when negotiating salary.

5. Discuss the elements of an employment agreement.

6. Describe the steps taken to achieve career objectives.

7. Describe the steps that lead to job termination.

FILL-IN-THE-BLANK STATEMENTS

Select the best term from the list below and complete the following statements.

career   **professional**
employment   **resume**
interview   **termination**

1. A(n) _____ is a formal meeting held in person to assess the qualifications of an applicant.

2. When an employee is coming to the end of a contract period, he or she is in _____.

3. A profession or occupation is one's _____.

4. A(n) _____ is the term used to describe a person who conforms to the standards of his or her job.

5. A(n) _____ is a written description of one's professional or work experience and qualifications.

6. An activity or service performed on a routine basis is one's _____.

MULTIPLE-CHOICE QUESTIONS

Complete each question by circling the best answer.

1. What would not be an employment opportunity that a dental assistant may choose?
   a. Teaching
   b. Sales
   c. Dental hygiene
   d. Insurance

2. Where might you find a job position for a dental assistant advertised?
   a. Newspaper
   b. Dental-assisting program
   c. Dental society newsletter
   d. All of the above

3. What is the most common means of communication for your first contact with a potential future employer?
   a. Letter
   b. Phone
   c. Fax
   d. Email

4. A cover letter _____.
   a. gives your educational background
   b. describes your past work experience
   c. covers your resume
   d. introduces you

5. What should not be included in a resume?
   a. Marital status
   b. Race
   c. Religion
   d. All of the above

6. How long should a resume be?
   a. One paragraph
   b. One page
   c. Two pages
   d. It does not matter.

7. The most critical part of an interview is _____.
   a. the closing remarks
   b. the salary discussion
   c. the first 10 minutes
   d. the follow-up

8. Termination without notice or severance pay is considered _____.
   a. summary dismissal
   b. negligence
   c. discrimination
   d. unprofessional

9. What is the most important factor in achieving professional success?
   a. The amount of money you make
   b. Liking the people you work with
   c. Having a positive attitude
   d. Your professional title

10. What time frame is routinely considered provisional employment?
    a. 1 week
    b. 1 month
    c. 3 months
    d. 1 year

ACTIVITIES

1. Prepare a cover letter to be used for seeking employment.

2. Prepare a resume to be used for seeking employment.

3. Prepare a follow-up letter to be used after an interview.

COMPETENCY 64-1: PREPARING A PROFESSIONAL RÉSUMÉ

Performance Objective

By following a routine procedure that meets stated protocols, given a computer, printer, and paper, the student will prepare a one-page resume.

Evaluation and Grading Criteria

 3   Student competently met the stated criteria without assistance.
 2   Student required assistance in order to meet the stated criteria.
 1   Student showed uncertainty when performing the stated criteria.
 0   Student was not prepared and needs to repeat the step.
 N/A No evaluation of this step.

Instructor shall define grades for each point range earned on completion of each performance-evaluated task.

Performance Standards

The minimum number of satisfactory performances required before final evaluation is _____.

Instructor shall identify by * those steps considered critical. If step is missed or minimum competency is not met, the evaluated procedure fails and must be repeated.

PERFORMANCE CRITERIA	*	SELF	PEER	INSTRUCTOR	COMMENT
1. Used common typefaces.					
2. Used a 10-, 12-, or 14-point font size.					
3. Used 1-inch margins on all sides.					
4. Resume was one page in length.					
5. Resume was neat and error free.					
6. Resume was concise and easy to read.					
ADDITIONAL COMMENTS					

Total number of points earned _____

Grade _____ Instructor's initials _____

Types of Teeth

Describe the location and function of the four types of teeth:

1. Incisors   3. Canine
2. Premolars   4. Molars

Surfaces of Teeth

Describe the surface location of the six types of teeth.

1. Facial   3. Occlusal   5. Mesial
2. Lingual   4. Incisal   6. Distal

Tooth Eruption

Describe the age of eruption for the following permanent maxillary and mandibular teeth.

1. Central incisors   5. Lateral incisors
2. Canines   6. First premolars
3. Second premolars   7. First molars
4. Second molars   8. Third molars

Bones of the Skull

Describe the location of the following cranial bones:

1. Frontal   3. Parietal   5. Occipital
2. Temporal   4. Sphenoid   6. Ethmoid

Bones of the Face

Describe the location of the following facial bones:

1. Zygomatic   4. Maxillary   7. Palatine
2. Nasal   5. Lacrimal   8. Vomer
3. Inferior conchae 6. Mandible

Tissues of the Teeth

Identify the four tissues of the teeth and their makeup.

Types of Teeth

1. Front of mouth/cutting food
2. Corner of mouth/cutting and tearing
3. Back of mouth/grasping and tearing
4. Back of mouth/chewing and grinding

Bones of the Skull

1. Forehead
2. Sides
3. Roof
4. Anterior base
5. Base
6. Orbit and floor

Surfaces of Teeth

1. Toward the lips
2. Toward the tongue
3. Back chewing surface
4. Front chewing surface
5. Interproximal surface closest to midline
6. Interproximal surface away from midline

Bones of the Face

1. Cheeks
2. Nose
3. Interior nose
4. Upper jaw
5. Orbit
6. Lower jaw
7. Hard palate
8. Base of nose

Tooth Eruption

1. 6–8 years
2. 9–12 years
3. 10–13 years
4. 11–13 years
5. 7–9 years
6. 10–11 years
7. 6–17 years
8. 17–21 years

Tissues of the Teeth

1. Enamel—the outer covering of the coronal portion of the tooth
2. Dentin—makes up most of the tooth and is reparative
3. Cementum—the outer layer of the root structure for attachment
4. Pulp—contains the nerves and blood of the tooth

Emergency Situation

How would you respond to a patient with hypoglycemia?

Cardiopulmonary Resuscitation

Describe *C-A-B*

Emergency Drugs

The following drugs can be found in an emergency kit. For what emergency is each drug prepared?

1. Epinephrine
2. Antihistamine
3. Diazepam
4. Nitroglycerin
5. Inhaler
6. Ammonia inhalant

Emergency Preparedness

Describe the roles of each profesional in an emergency situation.

1. Business assistant
2. Chairside assistant
3. Dentist

Emergency Situation

How would you respond to a patient with syncope?

Emergency Situation

How would you respond to a patient with anaphylaxis?

Emergency Situation

1. Administer concentrated sugar under patient's tongue.
2. Ready CPR if needed.
3. Monitor and record vital signs.

Emergency Preparedness

1. Calls emergency services.
2. Retrieves oxygen/drug kit and assesses patient.
3. Remains with patient and determines patient needs.

Cardiopulmonary Resuscitation

C = Compressions - You should push hard and fast on the center of the victim's chest.

A = Airway - You should tilt the victim's head back and lift the chin to open the airway.

B = Breathing - You should give mouth to mouth rescue breathing.

Emergency Situation

1. Place patient in supine position.
2. Prepare ammonia inhalant.
3. Prepare oxygen if needed.
4. Monitor and record vital signs.

Emergency Drugs

1. Acute allergic reaction
2. Allergic response
3. Seizure
4. Chest pain
5. Asthma attack
6. Respiratory stimulant

Emergency Situation

1. Position patient in supine position.
2. Prepare epinephrine for administration.
3. Prepare for CPR if needed.
4. Monitor and record vital signs.

Disinfection Procedures

Describe the following.

1. Define disinfection.

2. Describe the spray-wipe-spray technique.

Sterilization Procedures

Describe the following sterilization methods:

1. Steam sterilization

2. Chemical vapor sterilization

3. Dry-heat sterilization

Hazard Communication

Describe the following parts of a hazard communication program.

1. Written program
2. Chemical inventory
3. MSDS
4. Labeling
5. Training

Disease Transmission

Describe the following methods of disease transmission.

1. Direct
2. Indirect
3. Splash/splatter
4. Airborne
5. Dental unit waterlines

Diseases of Major Concern

Describe the following diseases and their effects.

1. Hepatitis B

2. Human immunodeficiency virus

3. Tuberculosis

Personal Protective Equipment

What are the four components of PPE, and how do they protect the caregiver?

Disinfection Procedures

1. Killing or inhibiting pathogens from growth by the use of a chemical agent
2. Spray—Thoroughly spray the surface. Wipe—Wipe the surface clean. Spray—Spray with disinfectant for recommended time.

Sterilization Procedures

1. Superheated steam under pressure for a recommended time (250° F, 20 minutes, 15–20 PSI)
2. Superheated chemical under pressure for a recommended time (270° F, 20–40 minutes, 20 PSI)
3. Superheat with no moisture or chemical for a recommended time (340° F, 60 minutes)

Hazard Communication

1. Document maintained to identify employees who are exposed to hazardous materials
2. Comprehensive list of chemicals used in the dental office
3. Information by the manufacturer describing the physical and chemical properties of a product
4. All containers labeled with name of product and any hazardous material
5. Training required for (1) new employees, (2) when a new chemical is acquired, and (3) yearly for continuing education

Disease Transmission

1. Contact with infectious lesions
2. Contact with a contaminated object
3. Blood, saliva, and body fluids
4. Microorganisms in sprays, mists, and aerosols
5. Microorganisms in water from dental unit

Diseases of Major Concern

1. Bloodborne virus that affects the liver and is transmitted by body fluids
2. Bloodborne virus that affects the immune system and is transmitted by body fluids
3. Bacterial infection that mostly affects the lungs

Personal Protective Equipment

1. Protective clothing protects the skin and underclothing from exposure.
2. A protective mask prevents the inhalation of infectious organisms.
3. Protective eyewear protects the eye from aerosol and debris.
4. Protective gloves prevent direct contact with contaminated objects.

Processing Radiographs

1. Describe the role of developer in the processing of exposed radiographs.

2. Describe the role of fixer in the processing of exposed radiographs.

Technique Errors

Describe how the following errors occur:

1. Elongation
2. Overlapping
3. Underexposure
4. Cone cutting
5. Foreshortening
6. Herringbone pattern
7. Double exposure
8. Bent film

Types of Extraoral Films

Define the use for the following extraoral films:

1. Panoramic
2. Cephalometric
3. Tomogram

Radiation Protection

1. Define three types of radiation protection methods for the patient.

2. Define two types of radiation protection methods for the operator.

Concept of Paralleling Technique

Describe the positioning of the film, tooth, and central ray for the paralleling technique.

Concept of Bisecting Technique

Describe the positioning of the film, tooth, and central ray for the bisecting technique.

Processing Radiographs

1. Developer reacts with silver halide crystals on the film that were affected by radiation. These crystals form the images.

2. Fixer removes any crystals that did not react, hardens the emulsion, and preserves the image.

Radiation Protection

1.
- Proper film-exposure technique
- Use of film-holding instruments
- Lead apron and thyroid collar

2.
- Personnel monitoring
- Equipment monitoring

Technique Errors

1. Not enough vertical angulation
2. Central ray not directed through interproximal space
3. Settings too low
4. X-ray beam did not expose entire film
5. Too much vertical angulation
6. Film reversed
7. Film exposed twice
8. Film bent in mouth

Concept of Paralleling Technique

- The film is parallel to the long axis of the tooth.
- The x-ray beam is directed to the right angle of the film and the long axis of the tooth.

Types of Extraoral Films

1. Provides a view of the entire maxilla and mandible
2. Provides a lateral view of the skull
3. Provides a view of sections of the temporomandibular joint (TMJ)

Concept of Bisecting Technique

- The film is angled to the long axis of the tooth.
- The space between the film and tooth is bisected.
- The x-ray beam is directed perpendicular to the bisecting line.

Endodontic Instruments

Identify the use for the following instruments:

1. Broach
2. File
3. Rubber stopper
4. Endodontic explorer
5. Spreader
6. Plugger

Oral Surgery Instruments

Identify the use for the following instruments:

1. Elevator
2. Forceps
3. Surgical curette
4. Rongeur
5. Bone file
6. Scalpel
7. Hemostat
8. Needle holder

Orthodontic Instruments

Identify the use for the following instruments:

1. Ligature director
2. Band plugger
3. Bite stick
4. Bird beak pliers
5. Distal end cutter
6. Pin and ligature cutter
7. Band remover
8. Howe pliers

Hand Cutting Instruments

Define the use for the following instruments:

1. Excavator
2. Hatchet
3. Hoe
4. Chisel
5. Gingival margin trimmer

Restorative Instruments

Define the use for the following instruments:

1. Amalgam carrier
2. Amalgam condenser
3. Burnisher
4. Discoid-cleoid carver
5. Hollenback carver
6. Composite instrument

Handpiece and Rotary Instruments

Define the use for the following instruments:

1. High-speed handpiece
2. Low-speed handpiece
3. Straight attachment
4. Contra-angle attachment
5. Friction-grip bur
6. Latch-type bur

Endodontic Instruments

1. To remove most of pulp tissue
2. To smooth and enlarge the canal
3. Small piece of rubber to measure the length of the file
4. Long and straight explorer to locate canal openings
5. Pointed end to assist in filling the canal
6. Flat end to assist in filling the canal

Oral Surgery Instruments

1. To reflect and retract the periosteum from the bone
2. To remove the tooth from the socket
3. To clean and remove diseased tissue from the socket
4. To trim alveolar bone
5. To smooth the surface of the bone
6. Surgical knife
7. To grasp and hold items
8. To hold the surgical needle firmly during suturing

Orthodontic Instruments

1. To guide and tuck ligature ties under the archwire
2. To aid in seating molar bands
3. To aid in seating molar bands
4. To form and bend the archwire
5. To cut and hold the end of the archwire
6. To cut ligature wire
7. To remove bands
8. Versatile pliers used to bend wires

Hand Cutting Instruments

1. To remove decay and debris from the tooth
2. To smooth the walls and floors of a prepared tooth
3. To smooth the floors of a prepared tooth
4. To smooth the enamel margin, and form sharp lines, point angles, and retention grooves
5. To place bevels along the gingival margin

Restorative Instruments

1. To carry amalgam to the prepared tooth
2. To pack amalgam into the tooth
3. To smooth amalgam
4. To carve the occlusal anatomy of amalgam
5. To carve the interproximal anatomy of amalgam
6. To place composite material into the prepared tooth

Handpiece and Rotary Instruments

1. Runs at 450,000 rpm to remove decay and large amount of tooth structure
2. Runs at 25,000 rpm to finish, contour, and polish
3. Fits on low-speed handpiece, and holds long-shank lab burs
4. Fits on low-speed handpiece, and holds latch-type burs, prophy cups, and brushes
5. Available in assorted shapes and fits on high-speed handpiece
6. Available in assorted shapes and fits on contra-angle of low-speed handpiece

Preventive Materials

Describe the following preventive materials and their use:

1. Systemic fluoride

2. Topical fluoride

3. Sealants

Impression Materials

Describe the following impression materials and their use:

1. Hydrocolloids

2. Reversible hydrocolloids

3. Elastomeric

Laboratory Procedures

Describe the following procedures completed in the dental laboratory:

1. Diagnostic cast

2. Custom tray

3. Temporary crown

4. Vacuum-formed tray

Amalgam

Describe the makeup of amalgam.

Composite Resin

Describe the makeup of composite resin.

Cements

Identify the use for the following cements:

1. Glass ionomer

2. Zinc phosphate

3. Zinc-oxide eugenol

4. Polycarboxylate

5. Intermediate restorative material

Preventive Materials

1. Mineral found in water, food, and supplements to prevent decay

2. Mineral found in toothpaste, mouthrinses, concentrated gel, and foam to prevent decay

3. Liquid resin applied and cured in the pits and fissures of teeth to prevent decay

Impression Materials

1. Referred to as alginate; used to obtain preliminary impressions for diagnostic purposes

2. Type of impression material with the ability to change its physical state

3. Referred to as a final impression; these materials get the most accurate impression

Laboratory Procedures

1. To diagnose, to fabricate an appliance, and for records

2. Type of tray that is fabricated specifically for a patient's mouth

3. Temporary coverage of a tooth or teeth made from acrylic or prefabricated material

4. Light-gauge plastic material that is form-fitted over a cast and then trimmed to fit over a patient arch

Amalgam

- Silver (to strengthen)
- Tin (to strengthen, and for workability)
- Copper (to strengthen, and for low corrosive properties)
- Mercury (to provide easy application and adaptability to tooth structure)

Composite Resin

- Resin matrix (also known as BIS-GMA, a material used to make synthetic resins)
- Inorganic fillers (quartz, glass, silica)
- Coupling agent (to strengthen and chemically bond the filler to the resin matrix)

Cements

1. Permanent cementation, restorations, liners, and bonding

2. Permanent cementation and insulating base

3. Permanent cementation, temporary cementation, and insulating base

4. Permanent cementation and insulating base

5. Temporary restorative material

Preventive Procedures

Define the following procedures:

3. Coronal polishing
4. Fluoride treatment

1. Flossing
2. Toothbrushing

Oral Surgery

Define the following procedures:

1. Forceps extraction
2. Impaction
3. Alveoloplasty
4. Suture
5. Biopsy

Restorative Classifications

Define the following cavity classifications:

1. Class I restorations
2. Class II restorations
3. Class III restorations
4. Class IV restorations
5. Class V restorations
6. Class VI restorations

Endodontics

Define the following procedures:

1. Indirect pulp capping
2. Direct pulp capping
3. Pulpotomy
4. Pulpectomy
5. Apicoectomy

Prosthodontics

Define the following procedures:

1. Inlay
2. Onlay
3. Veneer
4. Crown
5. Fixed bridge
6. Partial denture
7. Full denture

Periodontics

Define the following procedures:

1. Scaling
2. Root planing
3. Gingival curettage
4. Gingivectomy
5. Gingivoplasty
6. Osteoplasty

Oral Surgery

1. Removal of a fully erupted tooth
2. Removal of a tooth partially or totally covered by tissue and bone
3. Surgical contour of the bone and soft tissue after an extraction
4. Application of a material to control bleeding and promote healing
5. Surgical removal of tissue for analysis

Endodontics

1. Application of calcium hydroxide when the dental pulp is not exposed
2. Application of calcium hydroxide when the dental pulp has a slight exposure
3. Partial removal of the dental pulp
4. Complete removal of the dental pulp
5. Surgical removal of the apical portion of the root

Periodontics

1. Removal of calculus from a tooth surface
2. Removal of calculus and necrotic cementum
3. Removal of necrotic tissue from the gingival wall of the periodontal pocket
4. Surgical removal of diseased gingiva
5. Surgical reshaping of the gingival tissues
6. Surgical reshaping of bone

Preventive Procedures

1. To remove plaque from interproximal tooth surfaces
2. To remove plaque from tooth surfaces
3. To remove plaque and stains from teeth after calculus is removed
4. To apply topical fluoride to clean teeth

Restorative Classifications

1. Pit-and-fissure cavities
2. Posterior interproximal cavities
3. Anterior interproximal cavities
4. Anterior interproximal cavities involving the incisal edge
5. Smooth-surface cavities
6. Cavities or abrasions involving the incisal edge or occlusal cusp

Prosthodontics

1. Fixed restoration involving a portion of the occlusal and interproximal surface
2. Fixed restoration involving most of the occlusal and interproximal surface
3. Thin-shelled, tooth-colored restoration for facial surfaces
4. Fixed restoration covering all of the anatomic crown of a tooth
5. Fixed restoration replacing one or more teeth in the same arch
6. Removable prosthesis replacing one or more teeth in the same arch
7. Removable prosthesis replacing all teeth in the same arch

Orthodontics

Describe the Following Procedure for Fixed Appliances:

1. Placement of separators

2. Cementation of molar bands

3. Bonding of brackets

4. Insertion of arch wire

Tooth Whitening

Name and describe the categories of stains

1. Endogenous

2. Exogenous

3. Extrinsic

4. Intrinsic

Contraindications to Sealants

List six contraindications to the placement of dental sealants.

Stages of Tooth Development

Name the 5 stages of tooth development

Muscles of Mastication

Name the 4 muscles of mastication

Angles Classification of Malocclusion

Define the following Classifications:

Class I

Class II Division I

Class II Division II

Class III

Orthodontics

1. **Placement of Separators**—Separators are made from steel, brass or Elastomeric material. Separators are placed one week prior to the banding appointment to slightly separate the first molar from its adjacent teeth.
2. **Cementation of Molar Bands**—Bands are fitted and cemented to first molars. Bands aids in anchoring the arch wire for each arch, and can also have buttons, tubes and cleats for auxiliary products.
3. **Bonding of Brackets**—Brackets can be made of either stainless steel or ceramic and are bonded to the facial surface of the anterior and premolar teeth. The bracket holds and stabilized the arch wire horizontally around the arch.
4. **Insertion of Arch Wire**—The arch wire is placed in the slots of each bracket and then held into position by a ligature or Elastomeric tie. The force of the arch wire guides the teeth in movement.

Tooth Whitening

1. **Endogenous**—Stains that originate within the tooth from developmental and systemic disturbances
2. **Exogenous**—Stains that are caused by environmental agents
3. **Extrinsic**—Stains that are on the exterior of the tooth and can be removed. Examples of causes include food, drink, and tobacco.
4. **Intrinsic**—Stains that are caused by an environmental source but cannot be removed. An example would be stains from dental amalgam.

Contraindications to Sealants

1. Lack of deep pits and fissures.
2. Obvious dental caries
3. Any proximal surface decay
4. Insufficiently erupted teeth
5. Primary tooth that is expected to be lost soon
6. Poor patient cooperation of the patient in the dental chair

Stages of Tooth Development

1. Induction
2. Proliferation
3. Differentiation
4. Morphogenesis
5. Maturation

Muscles of Mastication

1. Temporal
2. Masseter
3. Internal (medial) pterygoid
4. External (lateral) pterygoid

Angles Classification of Malocclusion

Class I—Mesialbuccal cusp of maxillary 1st occluded with mesialbuccal grove of mandibular 1st molar. Anterior crowding or spacing present.

Class II Division I—Mesialbuccal cusp of maxillary 1st molar occludes mesial to the mesialbuccal grove of mandibular 1st molar. Maxillary anteriors protrude facially with deep overbite. Retrognathic profile.

Class II Division II—Mesialbuccal cusp of maxillary 1st molar occludes mesial to the mesialbuccal grove of mandibular 1st molar. Maxillary central incisors are either upright or retruded and laterals are tipped labially. Mesiognathic profile.

Class III—Mesialbuccal cusp of maxillary 1st molar occludes distal to mesialbuccal grove of mandibular 1st molar. Mandibular incisor in complete cross bite. Prognathic profile.